D1552034

The Neuroscience of Clinical Psychiatry

The Pathophysiology of Behavior and Mental Illness

The Neuroscience of Clinical Psychiatry

The Pathophysiology of Behavior and Mental Illness

Second Edition

Edmund S. Higgins, MD
Clinical Associate Professor of Psychiatry and Family Medicine
Medical University of South Carolina
Charleston, South Carolina

Mark S. George, MD
Distinguished Professor of Psychiatry, Radiology, and Neurosciences
Director, MUSC Center for Advanced Imaging Research
Medical University of South Carolina
Charleston, South Carolina

Illustrations by Edmund S. Higgins, MD

. Wolters Kluwer | Lippincott Williams & Wilkins
Health
Philadelphia · Baltimore · New York · London
Buenos Aires · Hong Kong · Sydney · Tokyo

Acquisitions Editor: Julie Goolsby
Product Manager: Tom Gibbons
Vendor Manager: Alicia Jackson
Senior Manufacturing Manager: Benjamin Rivera
Marketing Manager: Alexander Burns
Design Coordinator: Teresa Mallon
Production Service: Integra Software Services, Pvt. Ltd.

Second Edition © 2013 by LIPPINCOTT WILLIAMS & WILKINS, a WOLTERS KLUWER business
Two Commerce Square
2001 Market Street
Philadelphia, PA 19103 USA
LWW.com

© 2007 by Lippincott Williams & Wilkins, a Wolters Kluwer business.

Printed in USA

Library of Congress Cataloging-in-Publication Data

Higgins, Edmund S.
  Neuroscience of clinical psychiatry: the pathophysiology of behavior and mental illness/Edmund S. Higgins, MD, clinical associate professor of family medicine and psychiatry, Medical University of South Carolina, Charleston, South Carolina, Mark S. George, MD, distinguished professor of psychiatry, radiology, and neurosciences, director, MUSC Center for Advanced Imaging Research, Medical University of South Carolina, Charleston, South Carolina; illustrations by Edmund S. Higgins, MD.—Second edition.
     pages cm
  Includes bibliographical references and index.
  ISBN 978-1-4511-0154-6 (hardback)
  1. Mental illness—Pathophysiology. 2. Psychiatry. I. George, Mark S. (Mark Stork), 1958- II. Title.
  RC483.H54 2013
  616.89—dc23
                                                                        2012043162

Care has been taken to confirm the accuracy of the information presented and to describe generally accepted practices. However, the authors, editors, and publisher are not responsible for errors or omissions or for any consequences from application of the information in this book and make no warranty, expressed or implied, with respect to the currency, completeness, or accuracy of the contents of the publication. Application of the information in a particular situation remains the professional responsibility of the practitioner.

The authors, editors, and publisher have exerted every effort to ensure that drug selection and dosage set forth in this text are in accordance with current recommendations and practice at the time of publication. However, in view of ongoing research, changes in government regulations, and the constant flow of information relating to drug therapy and drug reactions, the reader is urged to check the package insert for each drug for any change in indications and dosage and for added warnings and precautions. This is particularly important when the recommended agent is a new or infrequently employed drug.

Some drugs and medical devices presented in the publication have Food and Drug Administration (FDA) clearance for limited use in restricted research settings. It is the responsibility of the health care provider to ascertain the FDA status of each drug or device planned for use in their clinical practice.

To purchase additional copies of this book, call our customer service department at (800) 638-3030 or fax orders to (301) 223-2320. International customers should call (301) 223-2300.

Visit Lippincott Williams & Wilkins on the Internet: at LWW.com. Lippincott Williams & Wilkins customer service representatives are available from 8:30 am to 6 pm, EST.

10 9 8 7 6 5

To my eldest son Fess, for his assistance with the artwork on Tuesday mornings at local coffee shops while waiting for school to open.

—ESH

To Eloise, my dance partner for 27 years now, who has acetylated large portions of my DNA through wonderful shared life experiences.

—MSG

Preface

Neuroscience is the basic science of psychiatry. Neuroscience describes the brain mechanisms that

- gather information from the external and internal world,
- analyze the information, and
- execute the best response.

Psychiatric disorders are the result of problems with these mechanisms.

The increased accessibility to the workings of the brain in the last 25 years has resulted in an explosion of information about neuroscience. Different lines of research such as brain imaging and animal studies along with more traditional postmortem analysis, medication effects, and genetic studies have transformed the way we conceptualize normal and abnormal behavior.

Bits and pieces of the neuroscience literature have filtered up to the practicing clinician, but a comprehensive understanding of the field is almost inaccessible to all but the most dedicated self-educators. The jargon is foreign and difficult to navigate. The standard textbooks are thick with contributions from multiple authors and almost impossible to read cover to cover. The relevance to the practice of psychiatry can sometimes be hard to appreciate.

We hope this book will provide a way for residents and practicing clinicians to gain a thorough appreciation for the mechanisms within the brain that are stimulating (or failing to stimulate) their patients. We also hope that the reader will have more accurate answers for the patient who asks, "What's causing my problem?" Likewise, we hope the reader will be better prepared for the increasingly difficult neuroscience questions that appear on board certification tests.

If we've learned anything from our studies of the brain, it is that LEARNING IS WORK! The brain increases its metabolism when conducting academic assignments. The process of focusing one's attention, understanding the concepts, and storing the new information requires energy. There is no passive learning.

Consequently, when learning is interesting and relevant it requires less energy. We have made every effort to make this material appealing and easy to consume. Pictures, drawings, and graphs have been liberally incorporated to allow the reader to learn the concepts quickly and efficiently. Every effort has been made to keep the material short and concise, but not too simple. Finally, we think information that is relevant to the reader is easier to retain, so we have tried to keep bringing the focus back to the practice of psychiatry.

We intend our book to be for three populations. First, it is for those in training: psychiatrists, psychologists, counselors, and allied physicians. Second, it is for psychiatric residents seeking to review the topics in preparation for their board examinations. And last, it is for the practicing clinician who was trained before the revolution in neuroscience and who would like to become more up-to-date and familiar with the field.

We hope that the reader will have a thorough—soup to nuts—understanding of the important topics in neuroscience and will henceforth be able to read and comprehend the future research in this field.

Edmund S. Higgins, MD
Mark S. George, MD

Acknowledgments

The authors wish to thank the following people for their assistance with this manuscript: Sherri A. Brown for her assistance with the artwork; Pamela J. Wright-Etter, MD, and Robert J. Malcolm Jr, MD, who reviewed individual chapters; and Laura G. Hancock, DO, and L. William Mulbry, MD, residents, who reviewed the entire book. We also wish to thank all those readers who pointed out the typos in the first edition.

Figures 3.5, 3.6, 3.7 and 22.1 and the dolphin in the sleep chapter were drawn by Fess Higgins.

About the Authors

Edmund S. Higgins, MD

Mark S. George, MD

Edmund S. Higgins, MD, is a clinical associate professor of psychiatry and family medicine at the Medical University of South Carolina (MUSC). He received his medical degree from Case Western Reserve University School of Medicine. He completed residencies in family practice and psychiatry at MUSC. He provides psychiatric services at several jails and prisons in South Carolina and has a private psychiatric practice. He has written one other book with Mark George: *Brain Stimulation Therapies for Clinicians*. He lives on Sullivan's Island, South Carolina.

Mark S. George, MD, is a distinguished professor of psychiatry, radiology, and neuroscience as well as director of the Brain Stimulation Laboratory, Psychiatry, at the Medical University of South Carolina, Charleston. He received his medical degree and completed dual residencies at MUSC in both neurology and psychiatry and is board certified in both areas. After a fellowship in London and 4 years at NIMH, he returned to Charleston where he has conducted pioneering work with functional imaging of the brain, transcranial magnetic stimulation, and vagus nerve stimulation. He is the editor in chief of the journal *Brain Stimulation*, is on several editorial review boards, has published over 400 scientific articles or book chapters, has 2 patents, and has written or edited 5 books. He too resides on Sullivan's Island, South Carolina.

Contents

SECTION IV **Disorders**

The Neuroscience Model

CHAPTER 1

Historical Perspective and Neuroscience Methods

One of the most remarkable paradigm shifts that has occurred during our lives has been the recognition that most of our behavior is inherited: eccentric, compassionate, outgoing, irritable, and so on. Traits such as these travel in families from generation to generation. The same is true with many forms of mental illness. With schizophrenia, if one family member has the illness, the likelihood that a relative will also develop the disease increases as the percentage of shared DNA increases (Figure 1.1).

The domestication of animals provides another example of the genetic control of behavior. Charles Darwin, without any knowledge of genes, believed the temperament of domestic animals was inherited. Dmitry Belyaev, a Russian geneticist, validated this with his famous farm-fox experiment in Siberia.

Belyaev domesticated wild foxes simply by selecting and breeding the tamest animals. He started with 130 wild foxes and administered a little test of tameness. Animals were approached by humans. Those that were most tolerant were mated to each other and the process was repeated with the offspring. Within 20 years, the foxes were domesticated. Within 40 years, they were literally house pets. Furthermore, the domesticated foxes produced less corticosteroids (the stress hormones) and higher levels of serotonin than did control foxes.

But what role does the environment play in the development of our personalities? Bouchard and others have eloquently addressed this question by looking at personality characteristics in monozygotic (identical) and dizygotic (fraternal) twins—reared together and reared apart. Using personality tests to assess five major personality traits, they found more correlations for monozygotic twins compared with dizygotic twins

regardless of whether they were raised together or apart (Table 1.1). In other words, the monozygotic twins reared apart shared more personality characteristics than did the dizygotic twins reared in the same household. Bouchard's conclusion was that these personality traits are strongly influenced by inheritance and only modesty affected by environment. (The lay press unfortunately summarized this research as "Parents Don't Matter.")

The mean correlations are surprisingly similar to the lifetime risk of developing schizophrenia for identical (monozygotic) and fraternal (dizygotic) twins as shown in Figure 1.1.

Figure 1.2 shows a remarkable example of identical twins separated when 5 days old and raised in different households—one in Brooklyn and the other in New Jersey. They did not meet again until they were 31 years old. Both are firemen, bachelors, with mustaches, and metal frame glasses. Not only do they have the same mannerisms, but they laugh at the same jokes and enjoy the same hobbies. Yet, they were exposed to entirely different environmental influences throughout their lives. Our individuality—who we are, how we socialize, what we like, even our religious beliefs—is influenced more by the brain we are born with than by the experiences we have along the way.

An alternative perspective on the twin studies, however, makes us cautious about ignoring the role of environment on behavior. For example, even though there is about a 50% concurrence between monozygotic twins for schizophrenia (Figure 1.1) or extraversion (Table 1.1), the other 50% do not have the same condition—**yet they share the same DNA**. This is also true for bipolar disorder, alcoholism, and panic disorder. About half the monozygotic twins have the same illnesses while the other half do not.

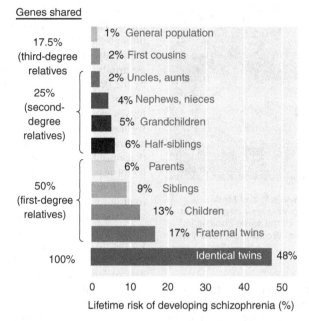

Genes shared

17.5%
(third-degree
relatives

25%
(second-
degree
relatives)

50%
(first-degree
relatives)

100%

1% General population
2% First cousins
2% Uncles, aunts
4% Nephews, nieces
5% Grandchildren
6% Half-siblings
6% Parents
9% Siblings
13% Children
17% Fraternal twins
Identical twins 48%

0   10   20   30   40   50
Lifetime risk of developing schizophrenia (%)

FIGURE 1.1 ● As the shared genetic profile with someone having schizophrenia increases, the risk of developing schizophrenia also increases. (Adapted from Gottesman II. *Schizophrenia Genesis*. New York, NY: WH Freeman; 1991.)

Clearly, our brains are more programmed by our genes than we previously believed, but that does not explain everything. Experiences during our lives can affect the outcome, particularly trauma, and especially when the trauma occurs early in life. The challenge for us in trying to understand the brain and complex behaviors is to conceptualize and begin to unravel the brain mechanisms that are predetermined by genetics but can change in response to the environment.

BRIEF HISTORY OF NEUROSCIENCE

The brain has not always been of interest to humankind. Most ancient cultures did not consider the brain to be an important organ. Both the Bible and Talmud fail to mention diseases related to the central nervous system (CNS). Egyptians carefully embalmed the liver and the heart but had no use for the brain; they actually scooped it out and threw it away. (If there really is an Egyptian afterlife—

TABLE 1.1

The Correlations for Five Personality Traits in Monozygotic Twins Reared Apart and Together, and Dizygotic Twins Reared Apart and Together

Personality Trait	Monozygotic, Apart	Monozygotic, Together	Dizygotic, Apart	Dizygotic, Together
Extraversion	0.41	0.54	0	0.19
Neuroticism	0.49	0.48	0.44	0.19
Conscientiousness	0.54	0.54	0.07	0.29
Agreeableness	0.24	0.39	0.09	0.11
Openness	0.57	0.43	0.09	0.11
Mean	**0.45**	**0.48**	**0.17**	**0.18**

FIGURE 1.2 ● Gerald Levy (*left*) and Mark Newman are identical twins who were separated at birth, yet have made many of the same choices in life. (From The Image Works, Woodstock, New York.)

those poor pharaohs are spending eternity without a brain.) So how did humans go from ignoring the brain to seeing it as the most complex organ in the universe?

Thomas Willis—after whom the Circle of Willis at the base of the brain was named—was the first neurologist. In the 17th century, he moved us into what one author has called the *Neurocentric Age*. Before Willis—and actually for a considerable time after him—physicians based their understandings of illness on the writings of the great physicians from antiquity. Willis took the unusual approach of describing a patient's behavior, then examining the brain after death and making correlations.

He was the first to coin terms such as *lobe, hemisphere*, and *corpus striatum*—terms that we still use. Comparing the human CNS anatomy with that of animals and conducting postmortem dissection of interesting cases, he made surprisingly accurate conclusions about higher brain functions versus lower brain functions. For example, he deduced that human functions such as memory were likely to reside in the "outmost banks" (gray matter) of the cerebral hemispheres because these areas were smaller in animals and damaged in individuals with severe head injuries who had lost memory. He believed that the brainstem likely controlled basic functions such as breathing and heart rate. However, he also thought that the white matter was the seat of imagination. He was not entirely on target, but he started the process of matching structures with behaviors.

At the start of the 18th century, it was still not clear how nerves transmitted information. *Luigi Galvani*, an Italian physician (memorialized by the term *galvanic skin response*), demonstrated through extensive experimentation that a frog

muscle would twitch when stimulated with electricity. This established that the substance flowing through the nerves was not air, fluid, or spirits, but electricity. Galvani proposed that the brain secretes electricity, which is then distributed to the muscles by the nerves. He also believed that the electricity did not leak into the surrounding tissue because the nerves were covered with a fatty insulation, which we now know is myelin. Not all his beliefs were accurate, but he made the big leap to recognizing that muscle movement in mammals is stimulated by intrinsic electrical activity.

Before the 1860s the brain was seen as a single multipurpose organ, much the way we currently view the liver or pancreas. The French physician *Paul Broca* with his famous case in 1861 confirmed for the first time that certain functions were localized to specific regions of the brain (Figure 1.3). The patient exhibited a loss of articulate speech. All he could express was one syllable: "tan." His utterances could convey great emotional tone, but the syllable never changed. However, he retained oral dexterity, and he could hear and comprehend. After his death, an autopsy revealed a lesion of his left frontal lobe—what is now called *Broca's aphasia*. The fact that almost all similar cases were on the left hemisphere and that similar right hemispheric lesions did not affect speech also led Broca to identify left/right dominance for some functions.

David Ferrier of Scotland and *Eduard Hitzig* of Germany independently identified the specialized cortical areas controlling motor function. Using the techniques of stimulation and ablation in

Central sulcus

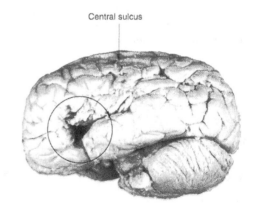

FIGURE 1.3 ● The preserved brain of the patient who helped Broca convince physicians that some functions—in this case the ability to speak—were localized in the cerebrum. (Adapted from Bear MF, Connors BW, Paradiso MA, eds. *Neuroscience: Exploring the Brain*. 3rd ed. Baltimore, MD: Lippincott Williams & Wilkins; 2007.)

experimental animals, they localized and mapped out what we now call the motor cortex. This new understanding of the brain provided the first examples of useful neurosurgical treatment given on the basis of the patient's motor symptoms. There is a case reported from 1879 of a teenage girl with seizures of the right face and arm who had a left meningioma accurately diagnosed and removed. With the development of antiseptic techniques and effective anesthesia, surgeons could successfully localize and remove some tumors using Ferrier's map of the motor cortex.

It is noteworthy that both men speculated about higher brain functions and the lobes in front of the motor cortex—the prefrontal cortex. Ferrier noted problems with attention in monkeys with damaged frontal lobes. Experimenting with dogs, Hitzig came to believe that the frontal cortex played an important role in abstract thought.

The discovery of individual neurons was a major step in the development of neuroscience. In order to be able to see nerve cells, it was necessary to be able to fix the brain (which can have the consistency of gelatin) and to cut thin slices; in addition, microscopes of sufficient power were needed. An Italian physician, *Camillo Golgi*, discovered a selective silver stain that allowed researchers to visualize the individual nerve cells in what was otherwise a uniform blob of color. For the first time, researchers could see sharp black images of the nerve cells and identify specific parts such as the cell body and the dendritic branches (Figure 1.4). Termed the *Golgi stain*, this technique is still used today.

Santiago Ramón y Cajal, a Spanish physician, used Golgi's stain, a Zeiss light microscope, and 25 years of patient observation to become perhaps the first modern neuroscientist. He proposed that individual nerve cells are the singular unit of the brain—a new concept at that time, which has since been called the *neuron doctrine*. By tracing neurons from sensory organs such as the eye back to the cortex and from the motor cortex to the muscles, he concluded that the dendrites are receptive, the cell body is executive, and the axon transmits the information over a long distance.

Ramón y Cajal went on to show that nerve impulses flow only in one direction—what he called his *law of dynamic polarization*. Figure 1.5 is one of his drawings, with little arrows showing the direction of the impulses between two communicating neurons. Additionally, Ramón y Cajal observed and meticulously drew the embryonic development of neurons. He was the first to document the growth of an axon that ultimately branches with dendrites and collateral axons. In 1894, Ramón y Cajal stated in a lecture to the Royal Society of London, "the ability of neurons to grow in an adult and their power to create

FIGURE 1.4 ● Pyramidal nerve cells after incubation with Golgi's silver stain. Only about 1% of the neurons absorb the stain, which allows for the identification of individual cells in what would otherwise be a very crowded slice. (Adapted from Bear MF, Connors BW, Paradiso MA, eds. *Neuroscience: Exploring the Brain*. 3rd ed. Baltimore, MD: Lippincott Williams & Wilkins; 2007.)

FIGURE 1.5 ● Drawing of neurons by Ramón y Cajal showing the unidirectional nature of impulses in the communication between neurons A and B. (From Ramón y Cajal S. *Recollections on My Life. Transactions of the American Philosophical Society*. Vol. 8, Part 2. Philadelphia, PA: The American Philosophical Society; 1937.)

new connections can explain learning." This is often cited as the origin of the synaptic theory of memory. Both Golgi and Ramón y Cajal received the Nobel Prize for Physiology and Medicine in 1906.

Charles Sherrington, an English neurophysiologist, did extensive studies of animal nerves. Focusing mostly on the spinal and peripheral nerves, he advanced the understanding of sensory dermatomes and reflexes. He is best known for giving us the term *synapse*—although he never actually saw one. Sherrington theorized that a physical junction existed between nerves to pass along an impulse. The synapse would not be seen until the development of the electron microscope in the 1950s.

Another English neurophysiologist (who shared the 1932 Nobel Prize with Sherrington), *Edgar Adrian*, is best known for recognizing the "all-or-nothing" properties of the action potentials. With regard to behavior and the brain, his major discoveries dealt with habituation and the sensory cortex. Adrian found that a stimulus to a nerve cell is followed by a burst of action potentials coursing down the axon. However, the quantity of action potentials decreases over time even if the stimulus remains unchanged. This may explain at the level of the neuron the basis for a well-known treatment for anxiety: exposure therapy.

In the beginning of the 20th century, it was not known how neurons communicate with each other or how a neuron can make a muscle contract. Some believed the communication was electrical—as though a spark jumped from one neuron to another. Others believed that a chemical process transmitted the signal. No one had evidence establishing one system or another. *Henry Dale* and *Otto Loewi*, an Englishman and a German, shared the Nobel Prize in 1936 for their work in establishing the chemical transmission of nerve impulses. Dale was working with the autonomic nervous system and found that an epinephrine-like compound had activating effects on the sympathetic nervous system, and that acetylcholine could activate the parasympathetic nervous system as well as skeletal muscles. Unfortunately, Dale was unable to show that epinephrine (or really norepinephrine) and acetylcholine were excreted by the neurons to elicit these effects.

It was Otto Loewi who in 1921 performed the elegant little experiment that proved the neurochemical transmission of nerve impulses. Legend has it that Loewi dreamed the experiment and, upon awaking early in the morning, rushed down to the laboratory and performed it. The experiment is depicted in Figure 1.6. Loewi's clever

FIGURE 1.6 ● Otto Loewi's famous experiment establishing that a chemical from the vagus nerve of one heart can induce bradycardia in a second unstimulated heart.

experiment showed that stimulating the vagus nerve slowed down the beating of the frog heart bathed in Ringer's solution. He then transferred some of that solution to another isolated frog heart and, without electrical stimulation, its rhythm also slowed down—as though its vagus nerve had been stimulated. He concluded that a chemical was excreted from the synapses of the first heart when the vagal nerve was stimulated. This chemical then flowed into the container holding the second heart and induced bradycardia.

In 1939, *Hodgkin* and *Huxley* published the first intracellular recording of an action potential (Figure 1.7). Before this time, no one had directly measured the electrical charge in an axon as an

FIGURE 1.7 ● First published intracellular recording of an action potential. (From Hodgkin AL, Huxley AF. Action potentials recorded from inside a nerve fibre. *Nature*. 1939;144:710-711.)

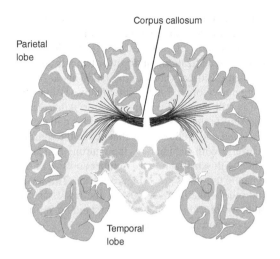

Parietal
lobe

Corpus callosum

Temporal
lobe

FIGURE 1.8 ● The corpus callosum contains millions of axons crossing between the two hemispheres. Sperry established that surgical resection of this structure interrupts the passage of information from one hemisphere to another.

action potential passed. Hodgkin and Huxley were able to accomplish this by inserting microelectrodes into the giant axons of squids.

By the 1940s, neurosurgeons were transecting the corpus callosum for a few patients with intractable seizures (Figure 1.8). The procedure prevented the spread of electrical activity across the corpus callosum into the opposite hemisphere and often provided significant relief for the patient. Remarkably, the patient's personality and intellectual functioning appeared unaffected by the drastic procedure. *Robert Sperry*, with careful experimentation, established that the left and right hemispheres no longer share information after this procedure. Furthermore, he was able to prove that the hemispheres have different functions. The left hemisphere is more involved with linear reasoning, language, and routine. The right hemisphere controls language intonation, spatial orientation, and processing novel situations.

Sperry won the 1981 Noble Prize in Medicine for his work with "split-brain" research. He shared the prize with *David Hubel* and *Torsten Wiesel* (see Chapter 6 for more on Hubel and Wiesel).

The CNS contains small quantities of proteins that some people call "brain fertilizer." It is an apt description, as these molecules facilitate the growth of nerve cells. *Rita Levi-Montalcini* and her colleagues accidentally discovered the first of this class of proteins, now called nerve growth factors (NGFs) or trophic factors. They observed sensory nerve cells exploding with growth when cultured next to a mouse sarcoma. Recognizing the significance of their discovery, they painstakingly isolated the protein that they called as *nerve growth factor*. Figure 1.9 shows the profound impact NGF has on the growth of sensory neurons. Since this landmark discovery, many other growth factors have been isolated. Some of these growth factors, or the absence of these growth factors, appear to play important roles in how the brain develops and changes with experience. They are thus key targets in trying to understand many psychiatric diseases.

Without a doubt, proving that the adult brain can change in response to experience (plasticity) has

A   B

FIGURE 1.9 ● The sensory nerves in (**A**) show robust growth when exposed to nerve growth factor. (From Levi-Montalcini R. The nerve growth factor. *Ann NY Acad Sci.* 1964;118:149-170.)

been the most exciting discovery in neuroscience. While many individuals have been involved in this research, no single individual has done more than *Eric Kandel.* Kandel was able to prove what Cajal could only speculate about—that learning changes the cells of the brain, and even the chemical composition of those cells. Kandel worked with the simple sea snail *Aplysia* because it can remember and has only about 20,000 neurons in its entire CNS (compared with 100 billion in humans). Kandel taught the snail a few simple tasks—habituation (gradually ignoring an innocuous stimuli) and sensitization (remembering an aversive stimuli) (Figure 1.10A).

For *Aplysia*, the gill with its siphon is a sensitive and important organ—one that it quickly withdraws

with any sign of danger. Habituation is induced by sequentially touching the siphon with a soft brush. With repetition, the snail learns to ignore the gentle stimuli. Sensitization, on the other hand, is elicited with an electrical shock to the tail. This is something not to forget. Indeed, after many sessions the gill is still retracted with great vigor. After teaching *Aplysia* these skills, Kandel and his colleagues dissected and analyzed the changes in the sensory neurons. With habituation, the neurons regressed while with sensitization the number and size of the synaptic terminals grew (Figure 1.10B). This study and others like it are serving as the basic science building blocks for better understanding normal behavior and mental illness.

FIGURE 1.10 ● **A.** Animals learn to ignore a benign stimulus but continue to react to noxious stimuli. **B.** Cellular changes occurred in *Aplysia* with habituation and sensitization. (Adapted from Kandel ER. *In Search of Memory. The Emergence of a New Science of Mind.* New York, NY: W. W. Norton & Co.; 2006.)

MODERN RESEARCH

Imaging

Researchers such as Willis and Broca were forced to wait for a patient to die before they could examine the brain. These scientists were studying patients with damaged brains using what some have called the *lesion method*. Although this remains an important tool for the modern neuroscientist (now there are large "brain banks" preserving brains of patients with similar illnesses), the noninvasive analysis of the CNS has transformed the way we study behavior and mental disorders.

Early attempts to image the brain were unhelpful, painful, and even dangerous. An ordinary x-ray provides little information because the brain is soft tissue and not radiopaque. Searching for the displacement of calcified structures could provide indirect evidence of a mass. Pneumoencephalography, in which cerebrospinal fluid is removed and replaced with air to enhance visualization of the CNS, is an example of the painful and dangerous extremes that were foisted on patients in earlier times.

The development of noninvasive imaging techniques (Table 1.2) has led to another small revolution in neuroscience. Although the functional studies (positron emission tomography, single photon emission computerized tomography [SPECT], and functional magnetic resonance imaging) remain largely limited to research, the noninvasive structural analyses (computed tomography and magnetic resonance imaging [MRI]) have transformed the practice of neurology. Diffusion tensor imaging, a technique using MRI scans to measure the movement of water in tissue, creates images of white matter tracts.

A word of caution regarding brain imaging studies and psychiatric disorders. Throughout this book, we mention numerous studies examining brain volume or brain function for various psychiatric disorders. However, Ioannidis recently reviewed brain volume studies and found that the reported number of positive studies far exceeded what would be expected based on the power estimates of the studies. He believes the studies that do *not* find a significant difference between control subjects and patients are seldom published. The Ioannidis review reminds us that, in spite of the wonderful images of the brain shown in these studies, these studies may be misleading.

TABLE 1.2

A Brief History of Imaging Methods Used to Analyze the Central Nervous System

Date	Initials	Name	Method	Specifics
1918	X-ray	Pneumoencephalography	Replacing CSF with air	Painful and dangerous
1927	X-ray	Cerebral angiography	Injecting contrast into circulation	Visualizes the cerebral vasculature
1970s	CT	Computed tomography	Ionizing radiation	Changed the way we practice medicine
	PET	Positron emission tomography	Decay of positron-emitting radionuclides	Measures the activity of the brain by analyzing blood flow
	SPECT	Single photon emission computed tomography	Single photon emission	More widely available than PET; lower resolution
1980s	MRI	Magnetic resonance imaging	Magnetic changes induced in molecules	No radiation; noninvasive; high resolution
	fMRI	Functional magnetic resonance imaging	Measures changes in blood oxygen used by brain regions	Has allowed extensive explorations of brain localization of function
1990s	DTI	Diffusion tensor imaging	Assesses the direction of movement of water in tissue	Allows visualization of white matter tracts

CSF, cerebrospinal fluid.

POINT OF INTEREST

The figure shows a method of using imaging studies frequently found in the literature. That is, one functional study is subtracted from another and the result is superimposed on a structural image. In this case, the subject is performing a finger opposition task with his right fingers while in a SPECT scanner (A). The white arrow shows the activation of the left motor cortex. B. A SPECT scan in the controlled state (not moving) is also produced. C. The control image is subtracted from the task image. D. The results are superimposed on an MRI of the same location, and drawings of the human homunculus along the motor cortex are added for further understanding.

(A) Finger opposition task   (B) Control   (C) Task minus control   (D) Superimposed on MRI

Functional imaging subtraction study superimposed on a structural image.

Nonhuman Animal Studies

Nonhuman animal studies provide another technique for understanding the marvels of the brain. The nonhuman animal brain is accessible in ways that are beyond the ethics of human research. Although they might have paws and whiskers, our human brains have much in common with those of nonhumans. The protein-coding regions of the mouse and human genomes are 85% identical. Nature is conservative and many of the molecular and cellular mechanisms that underlie the behavior are preserved from one species to the next. However, animals do not possess a similarly developed human cerebral cortex, nor can we ever be sure they actually have the psychiatric symptoms being studied. Besides the well-known microelectrode stimulation or ablation studies, there are several modern techniques that can be used on nonhuman brains that are worth reviewing.

Markers of Gene Activation

Two words of advice we would like to give to any student interested in neuroscience: *gene expression*. The DNA that gets turned on (or turned off) is called "gene expression" and this then controls the growth and activity of the brain. Understanding which genes are responsible is the key to understanding the brain and behavior. Researchers can now measure mRNA or proteins that result from gene expression. Cyclic adenosine monophosphate responsive element binding (CREB) protein and proteins in the Fos family are two transcription factors that are frequently used as markers of gene expression. Identifying CREB or FOS in a postmortem brain slice helps pinpoint the areas in the brain that were active in the animal during the experimental manipulation.

Knockout Mice

Animals (typically mice) can be engineered so that certain genes are turned off. Animals with silenced genes are called *knockout mice*. They are raised (if possible) and observed for changes in behavior compared with control mice—often called "wild" mice. Knockout mice have been used to understand obesity, substance abuse, and anxiety. While these studies represent a valuable research tool, one has to be cautious about generalizing from the results. The downstream effects of silencing the gene during development can never be fully appreciated.

Transgenic Mice

Transgenic mice are genetically engineered creatures. DNA from one organism is introduced into the DNA of a mouse egg, which is then fertilized. The adult mouse incorporates the foreign DNA into its genome. For example, DNA from jellyfish

Microarray
chip

Spot containing copies
of single-stranded DNA

Single-
stranded
DNA

FIGURE 1.11 ● The microarray chip contains multiple copies of many different genes so that a broad spectrum of gene activity can be analyzed quickly in a scanner. (Adapted from Friend SH, Stoughton RB. The magic of microarrays. *Sci Am*. 2002;286:44-53.)

encoding for fluorescent proteins has been inserted into the mouse genome. Brain slices from these mice "light up" when viewed under fluorescent microscopes. Likewise, the ability to insert disease-causing DNA into mice and then observe the damage it causes to the brain has revolutionized neurology.

Viral-Mediated Gene Transfer
Viruses can be used as a vehicle to insert a section of DNA into the brain of living animals at specific locations. When the DNA is incorporated into the host DNA, new genes are expressed with possible alterations in behavior. For example, a virus was used to implant the DNA for the vasopressin receptor in the ventral pallidum of promiscuous voles. Responding voles were transformed into monogamous, family-oriented, church-going, and card-carrying conservatives (see Chapter 14 for details).

DNA Microarrays—Also Called Gene Chips
DNA microarrays enable researchers to compare the mRNA (and therefore gene activity) found in a tissue sample with the DNA of known identity. The microarray is a chip no bigger than a postage stamp with thousands of different DNA molecules, multiplied, segregated, and attached in separate tiny locations (Figure 1.11).

The mRNA from the tissue being studied is transcribed to DNA, labeled with fluorescent markers, and dropped onto the microarray chip. The single-stranded DNA from the tissue sample will bind with similar single-stranded DNA on the microarray. The chip is then read in a scanner that calculates the amount of binding between the tissue DNA and the chip DNA in each discrete spot, giving an estimate of that specific gene activity in the tissue. As an example, this procedure was done with small samples from the prefrontal cortex of schizophrenic and control postmortem brain. The schizophrenic brains showed reduced expression of myelination-related genes, suggesting a disruption in the myelin as part of the pathogenesis of schizophrenia (see Chapter 23).

The Controlled Trial
It is discouraging to realize that the brain is so resistant to change. It is more discouraging to read about eccentric clinicians, parents, teachers, and other meddlers expounding the effectiveness of their unproven interventions to reduce symptoms or improve behavior. Sugar and hyperactivity are "known" to have a cause and effect relationship that has unfortunately failed to materialize in controlled trials.

We tend to conceptualize the pathogenesis of psychiatric disorders as the absence of what we are replacing with our treatment (neurotransmitters, a superego, the corrective emotional experience, etc.). It is important to prove that these interventions are actually working. Perhaps, the greatest research tool in health care has been the controlled clinical trial. With this technique we can determine with some confidence how effective interventions might be, which then gives us some insight into the working of the brain.

QUESTIONS

Part 1: Match the names in the right column with the events in the left column

1. Started the Neurocentric Age

2. The brain has intrinsic electric activity

3. Localization of function

4. The motor cortex

5. Silver stain

6. Individual nerve cells are the singular unit of the CNS

7. Coined the term *synapse*

8. "All-or-nothing"

9. Neurochemical transmission of nerve impulses

10. First action potential

11. Chemical guidance of regenerating nerves

12. Nerve growth factors

A. Edgar Adrian

B. Paul Broca

C. Santiago Ramón y Cajal

D. David Ferrier

E. Luigi Galvani

F. Camillo Golgi

G. Hodgkin and Huxley

H. Otto Loewi

I. Rita Levi-Montalcini

J. Charles Sherrington

K. Robert Sperry

L. Thomas Willis

Part 2: Match the columns

13. Implanted micropipette

14. Activation of DNA

15. Missing receptors

16. Single-stranded DNA

17. Implanting specific traits

M. DNA microarray

N. Gene expression

O. Knockout mice

P. Microdialysis

Q. Viral-mediated gene transfer

See Answers section at the end of the book.

CHAPTER 2

Neuroanatomy

CEREBRAL CORTEX

There are many large textbooks with extensive writings and illustrations providing all the known specifics about the anatomy of the nervous system. If you are looking for that sort of detail, then you are reading the wrong book. We—on the other hand—have tried to limit our discussion of neuroanatomy to those structures frequently identified in the scientific articles that are relevant to the clinician treating mental illness. First, we feel compelled to review a bit about the developing brain. You can best understand how the brain anatomy is organized by remembering how it formed itself in the first place.

Development

The fertilized egg quickly divides and differentiates into an embryo with three cell lines: the endoderm, mesoderm, and ectoderm. A portion of the ectoderm folds and forms the neural tube that becomes the rudimentary nervous system. The most anterior cells of the nervous system spend the ensuing weeks proliferating, migrating, and developing into the different regions of the brain.

The process of differentiating is almost unbelievable. How one undeveloped cell decides it should be a neuron while a similar one becomes an astrocyte is simply amazing. The evidence suggests that chemical signals between cells turn the DNA on and off, which then controls the destiny, but orchestrating all this is almost beyond comprehension.

The migration of cells to their appropriate location in the brain is another remarkable aspect of the developing brain. Neuroblasts (undeveloped neural cells) multiply in an area called the ventricular zone. Then they shinny up radial cells (specialized glial cells) that form a kind of scaffolding to build the cerebral cortex (Figure 2.1). As the neuroblasts reach the surface of the brain, they differentiate into the various mature neurons and astrocytes that make up the gray matter.

Other neuroblasts migrate tangentially from the bottom of the ventricles. These neuroblasts typically develop into the inhibitory interneurons. They start in a different location and must come up and around before they intermingle with the other neuroblasts climbing the radial cells. It boggles the mind that all these cells find their correct location and make the right connections while we can barely find what we are looking for in Walmart.

A residual portion of the ventricular zone remains in the adult brain and allows limited neurogenesis to continue beyond the fetal stage (Figure 8.3)—more on this topic in Chapter 8.

The migrating and differentiating neuroblasts slowly form into the six layers of the cerebral

DISORDER	MENTAL RETARDATION

The migration of neurons to their specific location is a critical and venerable period of brain development. Fetal alcohol syndrome may in part be a result of aberrant migration due to the toxic effects of ethanol. Radiation is another insult that deters the traveling neuron. Studies of pregnant Japanese women who were in proximity to the epicenter when the atomic bombs were dropped found that 80% of the children who developed severe mental retardation were exposed to radiation between 8 and 16 weeks after conception—the time of peak migration.

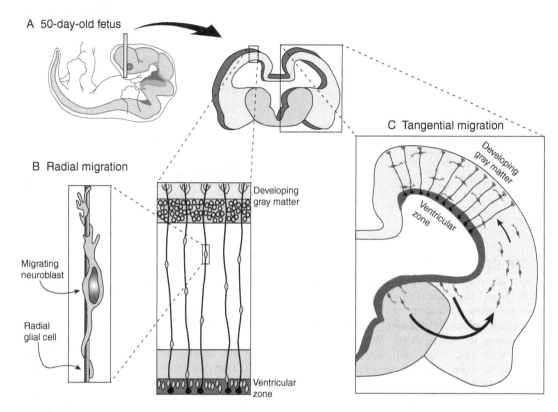

A 50-day-old fetus

B Radial migration

C Tangential migration

Developing gray matter

Developing gray matter

Ventricular zone

Migrating neuroblast

Radial glial cell

Ventricular zone

FIGURE 2.1 ● **A.** Cross section of the brain of a 50-day-old fetus. **B.** Neuroblasts climb up the radial glial cells to the developing gray matter. **C.** Inhibitory neurons develop from neuroblasts that migrate tangentially from lower regions of the brain.

cortex. Figure 2.2 shows how the process proceeds. The inner layers are formed first: layer IV, then layer V, and so on. This means that cells destined for the outer layers must climb past the other neurons before locating their place in the brain.

The cerebral cortex is made up of white matter and gray matter (Figure 2.3). The gray matter is where the nerve cells and synapses reside. This is where the action occurs psychologically—where we think and feel—where depression, schizophrenia, and dementia likely develop. The white matter is primarily myelinated axons transporting impulses between the gray matter and lower brain structures. The white matter makes up the circuits that connect the regions of the brain—connecting cabling.

When we say a "neuron," we are usually thinking of the large pyramidal neurons with their triangular-shaped cell bodies. They make up approximately 75% of the cortical neurons. They have a single apical dendrite pointed toward the pial surface and a number of basilar dendrite branches projecting horizontally. The axons project (and send impulses)

to other cortical regions or the deeper structures of the subcortex.

The pyramidal neurons receive signals from the other brain regions as well as from the local interneurons. The afferent signals from other regions are typically excitatory signals that encourage the neuron to generate its own impulse. The interneurons are typically γ-aminobutyric acid (GABA) neurons, which inhibit the pyramidal neuron and reduce the likelihood it will fire.

Brodmann's Areas
In the early part of the 20th century, many neuro-anatomists were struggling to divide the neocortex into structurally distinct regions. Korbinian Brodmann, a German neurologist, was working in a psychiatric clinic where he was influenced by Alois Alzheimer to pursue a career in neuroscience basic research. After extensive analysis of the human and monkey neocortex, he published in 1909 his classic work *Comparative Localization Studies in the Brain Cortex, Its Fundamentals Represented on the Basis of Its Cellular Architecture.*

FIGURE 2.2 ● The six layers of the cerebral cortex develop in reverse order as the neuroblasts migrate up from the ventricular zone. (Adapted from Bear MF, Connors BW, Paradiso MA, eds. *Neuroscience: Exploring the Brain.* 3rd ed. Baltimore, MD: Lippincott Williams & Wilkins; 2007.)

He had divided the neocortex into 52 regions based on the size, number, and density of the cells as well as the local connections and long tract projects to and from the subcortical regions (Figure 2.4). Brodmann's scheme is still widely used and often mentioned in the scientific literature.

Prefrontal Cortex

Everybody loves the prefrontal cortex (PFC). It is one of the anatomic structures that distinguishes humans from other mammals. Technically, it is the cortex in front of the motor cortex. Brodmann calculated that the PFC as a percentage of the total cortex is 3.5% in the cat, 7% in the dog, 8.5% in the lemur, 11.5% in the macaque, 17% in the chimpanzee, and 29% in humans (Figure 16.10). Dysfunction in the PFC is implicated as a possible source of pathology in many psychiatric disorders—depression, schizophrenia, anxiety, and attention-deficit/hyperactivity disorder (ADHD), as well as disorders of anger and violence.

There are four regions of the PFC that are frequently mentioned in the scientific literature (Figure 2.5): dorsolateral PFC, anterior cingulate gyrus, ventromedial PFC, and orbital PFC. Unfortunately, there is no consensus on the wording of these regions. Different terms are often combined to describe an area of interest, for example, ventrolateral and medial orbital. The ever-expanding jargon of the scientific writers is one of the great challenges of understanding neuroscience.

Neurologists, assessing and following up patients with injuries (e.g., Phineas Gage—see Figure 11.4), have identified three different

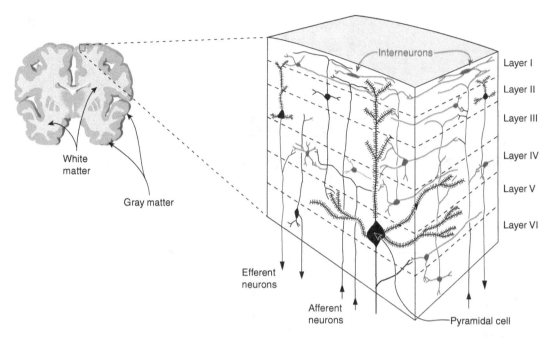

FIGURE 2.3 ● The six layers of the neocortex, from the pial surface above layer 1 to the white matter below layer 6. (Snell RS. *Clinical Neuroanatomy: A Illustrated Review with Questions and Explanations*. 3rd ed. Philadelphia, PA: Lippincott Williams & Wilkins; 2001.)

syndromes associated with frontal lobe damage. The location, core characteristics, and common symptoms are briefly outlined in Table 2.1. The three syndromes roughly correlate with the three regions of the PFC. Although it is appealing to associate a location with specific behavioral pattern, it is not that simple. Most patients have clinical features of more than one of the syndromes because few lesions are confined to one region. Furthermore, recent imaging studies do not always find correlations between the anatomy and the traditional syndromes.

TABLE 2.1

The Three Traditional Frontal Lobe Syndromes and the Associated Regions and Symptoms

Location	Syndrome	Symptoms
Orbital (orbitofrontal)	Disinhibited	Poor impulse control
		Explosive outburst
		Inappropriate behavior
Dorsolateral (dorsal convexity)	Disorganized	Cognitive dysfunction
		Diminished judgment, planning, and insight
		Concrete and inflexible
		Decreased spontaneous behavior
Medial (ventromedial)	Apathetic	Paucity of spontaneous behavior
		Sparse verbal output

FIGURE 2.4 ● The human cerebral cortex as delineated by Brodmann in his 1909 publication. The different regions are defined by the composition of the gray matter. Four examples are shown.

Hippocampus

The hippocampus and the amygdala are the essential structures of what is commonly called the *limbic lobe*—although there is no specific lobe. The hippocampus is a folded structure incorporated within the temporal lobe—dorsal to other important cortical structures of the rhinal sulcus (or primitive smell brain). The hippocampus is made up of two thin sets of neurons that look like facing "C"s—the dentate gyrus and the Ammon's horn. Ammon's horn has four regions of which only CA3 and CA1 are shown in Figure 2.6.

The hippocampus plays an essential role in the development of memories (see Chapter 18) and is one of the few locations in the brain where neurogenesis persists in adults (see Chapter 8). Additionally, the volume of the hippocampus is decreased in various psychiatric disorders (e.g., PTSD, Alzheimer's disease, and major depression), suggesting that this region may play a role in the pathogenesis of these disorders.

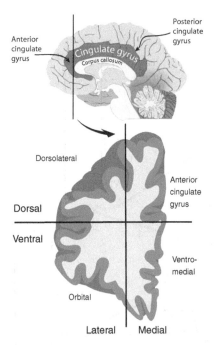

FIGURE 2.5 ● The important regions of the prefrontal cortex frequently mentioned in studies of normal behavior and mental illness. (Adapted from Lewis DA. Structure of the human prefrontal cortex. *Am J Psychiatry.* 2004;161(8):1366.)

Amygdala

The amygdala lies within the temporal lobe just anterior to the hippocampus (Figure 2.7). Using the anatomy and connections, the amygdala can be divided into three regions: the medial group, the central group, and the basolateral group. The basolateral group, which is particularly large in humans, receives input from all the major sensory systems. The central nucleus sends output to the hypothalamus and brain stem regions. Therefore, the amygdala links sensory input from cortical regions with hypothalamic and brain stem effectors. The amygdala is active when people are anxious and/or angry, which will be discussed further in subsequent chapters. Likewise, when the organ is removed these emotions are impaired.

Hypothalamus

If there is a tiny person that sits inside our head, watching the "control panel" from our body and making decisions about internal settings, they are sitting at the hypothalamus. This small cluster of nuclei makes up less than 1% of the brain mass yet has powerful effects on the body's homeostasis. The hypothalamus controls

TREATMENT PREFRONTAL LOBOTOMY

The infamous prefrontal lobotomy was developed in Portugal in 1935 by the neurologist Egas Moniz. He coined the term *psychosurgery* and later even won the Nobel Prize for Medicine for his work. Oops! The procedure was intended to sever the afferent and efferent fibers of the prefrontal lobe and produce a calming effect in patients with severe psychiatric disease.

Walter Freeman popularized and simplified the procedure in the United States. He developed a minimally invasive technique, shown in the figure, called the *transorbital lobotomy*. An instrument resembling an ice pick was inserted under the eyelid through the orbital roof and blindly swept left and right. It is hard to believe what Freeman reported in 1950—that out of 711 lobotomies 45% yielded good results, 33% produced fair results, and 19% left the patient unimproved or worse.

Although initially received with enthusiasm, in part due to the unavailability of other effective treatments, the development of unacceptable personality changes (unresponsiveness, decreased attention span, disinhibition, etc.) led to a decline in the procedure. Ultimately, the development of effective pharmacologic treatments brought an end to the biggest mistake in the history of psychiatry.

Transorbital frontal lobotomy. (Adapted from Bear MF, Connors BW, Paradiso MA, eds. *Neuroscience: Exploring the Brain*. 3rd ed. Baltimore, MD: Lippincott Williams & Wilkins; 2007.)

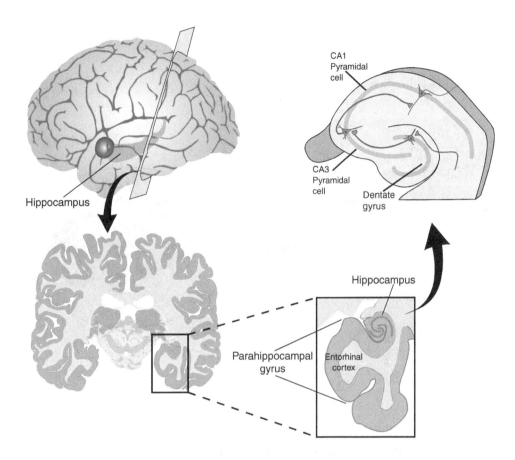

FIGURE 2.6 ● Different views of the hippocampus. (Adapted from Bear MF, Connors BW, Paradiso MA, eds. *Neuroscience: Exploring the Brain*. 3rd ed. Baltimore, MD: Lippincott Williams & Wilkins; 2007 and Kandel ER, Schwartz JH, Jessell TM, eds. *Principles of Neural Science*. 4th ed. New York, NY: McGraw-Hill; 2000.)

such basic functions as eating, drinking, sleeping, and temperature regulation, to name a few. A small lesion in the hypothalamus has devastating effects on the body's basic functions. The suprachiasmatic nucleus is an example of a small cluster of cells within the hypothalamus that has a profound impact on sleep/wake cycles (see Figure 15.8).

DISORDER **LIMBIC LOBE**

The limbic lobe concept is a term that occasionally appears in psychiatric literature, but not the one that we will use. It was originally introduced in 1878 by Broca, who noted that the cingulate gyrus, hippocampus, and their connecting bridges formed a circle on the medial side of the hemispheres. He called the structure *le grand lobe limbique*. Paul MacLean in the mid-1950s popularized the concept by linking the structure to emotional functions. Historically, this was a big step in associating emotions with neuroanatomy and has had a large impact on biologic psychiatry.

Exactly what constitutes the limbic system has never been well defined nor is it clear that the structures involved (amygdala, hippocampus, and cingulate gyrus) have unique connections that process emotions. The problem originates from the attempt to impose emotional functions on to a number of closely related structures, rather than trying to find which structures are responsible for particular emotions. We prefer to identify the neuroanatomy involved with a specific emotion instead of using the more ambiguous limbic system concept.

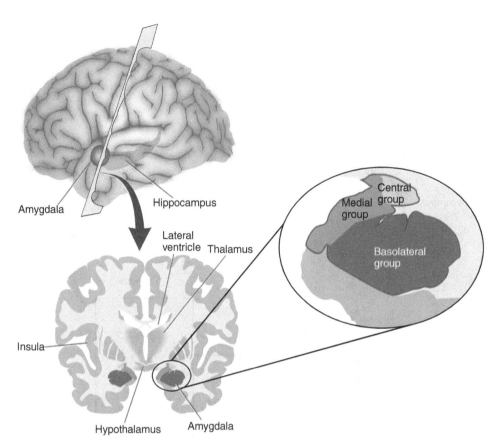

FIGURE 2.7 ● The location and groups (often called *nuclei*) of the amygdala.

The hypothalamus sits in a commanding position within the central nervous system (CNS), between the cortex and brain stem (Figure 2.8). It receives input from four sources: the higher cortex, the brain stem, internal chemoreceptors, and hormonal feedback. The cortex relays filtered cognitive and emotional information about the external environment. The sensory neurons in the body send signals about the internal milieu up through the brain stem. The hypothalamus has its own chemoreceptors that measure glucose, osmolarity, temperature, and so on in the blood. Finally, the hypothalamus receives feedback from the steroid hormones and neuropeptides.

The hypothalamus lies on either side of the third ventricle and is divided into three zones. The lateral zone controls arousal and motivated behavior. The medial zone is more involved with homeostasis and reproduction. The periventricular zone is of most interest to us. It includes the suprachiasmatic nucleus, cells that control the autonomic nervous system (ANS), and the neurosecretory neurons that extend into the pituitary (see Chapter 6).

AUTONOMIC NERVOUS SYSTEM

The ANS can be thought of as the brain's conduit to the vital organs of the body (Figure 2.9). There are two branches. First is the sympathetic division, which originates in the posterolateral region of the periventricular zone of the hypothalamus. The other branch is the parasympathetic division, which originates in the anterior cells of the same zone in the hypothalamus. The sympathetic and parasympathetic divisions appear to operate in parallel but with opposite effects and use different neurotransmitters.

The sympathetic division, in a simplified sense, controls the fight–flight response and plays a prominent role in the physical symptoms of anxiety, for example, racing heart. These neurons send out their axons from the thoracic and lumbar regions to preganglionic neurons, which primarily

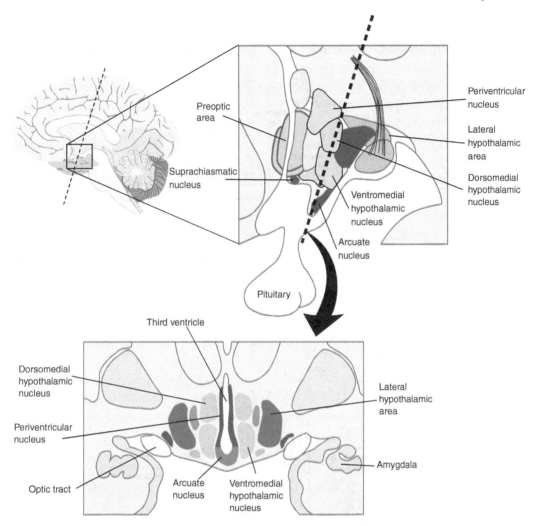

FIGURE 2.8 ● The hypothalamus lies on either side of the third ventricle in close proximity to the pituitary gland. The hypothalamus can be subdivided into multiple nuclei, many of which are not shown. (Adapted from Kandel ER, Schwartz JH, Jessell TM, eds. *Principles of Neural Science*. 4th ed. New York, NY: McGraw-Hill; 2000.)

reside in the sympathetic chain on either side of the spinal cord. The postganglionic sympathetic neurons innervate the smooth muscles of the vital organs as well as the walls of blood vessels. The preganglionic neurons are cholinergic, whereas the postganglionic neurons use norepinephrine. The postganglionic norepinephrine receptors likely explain why β-blockers can be used to quell the physical symptoms of anxiety.

The parasympathetic neurons mediate functions that the body performs in times of calm, for example, digest food. These neurons emerge from the brain stem and sacral region of the spinal cord. The axons travel longer distances and innervate ganglia typically located at the end organ. Unlike the sympathetic neurons, the parasympathetic neurons are exclusively cholinergic.

For the psychiatrist, the ANS occasionally complicates the treatment of mental disorders—particularly when using the tricyclic antidepressants. Side effects such as dry mouth, tachycardia, and constipation can be seen as an imbalance between the sympathetic and parasympathetic divisions. These symptoms are not so much the result of sympathetic stimulation as they are the result of parasympathetic blockade. The likely culprit is blockade of the muscarinic receptor in the cholinergic neurons of the parasympathetic division.

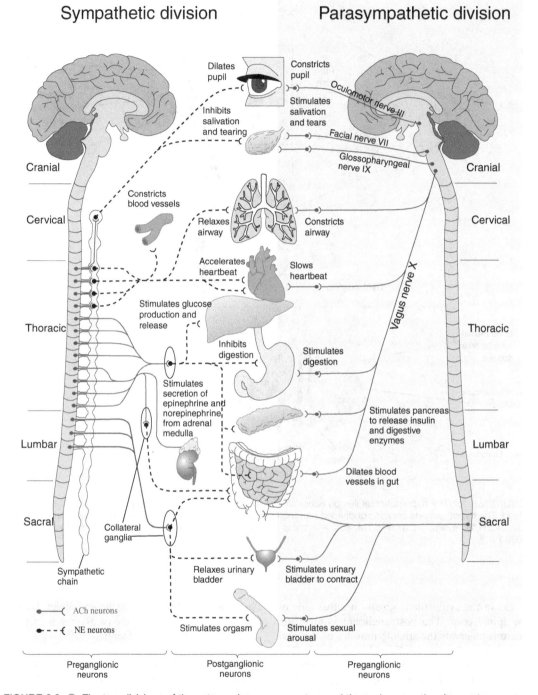

Sympathetic division

Parasympathetic division

Dilates pupil

Constricts pupil

Oculomotor nerve III

Inhibits salivation and tearing

Stimulates salivation and tears

Facial nerve VII

Glossopharyngeal nerve IX

Cranial

Cranial

Constricts blood vessels

Relaxes airway

Constricts airway

Cervical

Cervical

Accelerates heartbeat

Slows heartbeat

Stimulates glucose production and release

Vagus nerve X

Thoracic

Thoracic

Inhibits digestion

Stimulates digestion

Stimulates secretion of epinephrine and norepinephrine from adrenal medulla

Stimulates pancreas to release insulin and digestive enzymes

Lumbar

Lumbar

Dilates blood vessels in gut

Sacral

Collateral ganglia

Sacral

Sympathetic chain

Relaxes urinary bladder

Stimulates urinary bladder to contract

● ───(ACh neurons

●- - -(NE neurons

Stimulates orgasm

Stimulates sexual arousal

Preganglionic neurons

Postganglionic neurons

Preganglionic neurons

FIGURE 2.9 ● The two divisions of the autonomic nervous system and the end organs they innervate. (Adapted from Bear MF, Connors BW, Paradiso MA, eds. *Neuroscience: Exploring the Brain*. 3rd ed. Baltimore, MD: Lippincott Williams & Wilkins; 2007.)

VAGUS NERVE STIMULATION

The ANS is actually a two-way street. That is, signals originating from the internal organs proceed up to the brain. Remarkably 80% of the signals traveling through the vagus nerve are afferent—from the organs toward the CNS. This is why vagus nerve stimulation can reduce seizure activity and improve mood.

CEREBELLUM

The cerebellum sits on top of the brain stem, at the back of the skull, below the cerebral cortex. Once considered the "lesser brain" and only involved with the coordination of movement, more recent functional imaging studies have shown that the cerebellum "lights up" in a wide variety of behaviors. Not only it is active in sensation, cognition, memory, and impulse control but it has also been implicated to be playing a role in the pathophysiology of autism, ADHD, and schizophrenia.

Fossil records document that the cerebellum has grown throughout human evolution and actually contains more neurons than any other part of the brain. Yet, its function is not clearly understood. Of particular interest, if the cerebellum is totally removed, especially in young persons, with time the person can regain almost normal function.

It appears that the cerebellum is a supportive structure for the cerebral cortex. Some have speculated that it grew throughout evolution to provide extra computational support for an overburdened cortex. This reasoning proposes that the cerebellum is not responsible for any one particular task, but rather functions as an auxiliary structure for the entire cerebral cortex—not just movement.

In the future, we anticipate increased reports of the important role of the cerebellum in mental illness.

BLOOD–BRAIN BARRIER

The brain needs to be bathed in a pristine extracellular environment. If the brain is exposed to the fluctuations in hormones, amino acids, or ions that occur in the rest of the body, unexpected neuronal activity could result. The brain uses the *blood–brain barrier* (BBB) to live in a more muted environment buffered from the hysterical fluctuations of the body.

Historically, it was thought that the barrier was produced by the astrocytes that hold the capillaries with their foot processes. Later, it became clear that it is the *tight junctions* between the endothelial cells of the capillaries that prevent many substances from leaking into the CNS (Figure 2.10). There are a few areas of the brain that have gaps in the BBB. The pituitary gland and some parts of the hypothalamus are two examples of these BBB gap regions. This is appropriate because these areas need to receive unfiltered feedback regarding the status of the endocrine system by way of the circulating blood.

The BBB is not an impenetrable wall, as the brain needs constant supplies to perform its functions. Lipid-soluble substances can readily diffuse through the lipophilic cell walls. Conversely, water-soluble substances are deflected by the endothelial cell wall. Yet, the brain needs some water-soluble substances, such as glucose, and indeed there are active transport mechanisms within the endothelial cell wall to bring these essential substances into the brain.

The endothelial cells also actively transport offensive substances out of the brain's extracellular environment. The P-glycoprotein is such a transporter. Found in the gut as well as the brain, this

BREACHING THE BBB

Approximately 98% of small molecules and nearly all large molecules do not cross the BBB. Overcoming this obstacle is of utmost importance if new therapeutic agents are to reach their target. Several options are being explored— some are more reasonable than others.

1. Implants—medications impregnated in biodegradable wafers are placed in the brain. 2. Administering high-frequency ultrasound to disrupt the BBB and increase penetration of the drug into the brain. 3. Intranasal delivery. 4. Trojan horse—attach the medication to a molecule that binds with a transcytosis receptor. The medication then sneaks into the brain by endocytosis. 5. If all else fails, direct injection into the brain—always a favorite.

A

B

FIGURE 2.10 ● **A.** The tight junctions formed by the brain endothelial cells along with the astrocytes make up the blood–brain barrier. **B.** Transport mechanisms facilitate or impede the movement of substances between the brain and blood stream. ((**A**) Adapted from Goldstein GW, Betz AL. The blood-brain barrier. *Sci Am*. 1986;255(3):74-83.)

protein actively removes a wide variety of drugs and deposits them in the capillary lumen. For example, the newer antihistamines are excluded from the CNS by this protein so they can work their magic on allergens in the body but not sedate the brain.

Some psychiatrists speculate that a very active P-glycoprotein transporter contributes to treatment resistance by diminishing the cerebral concentration of medications. For example, olanzapine and risperidone are substrates for P-glycoprotein.

QUESTIONS

1. Brodmann's areas are differentiated by the
   a. Cortical morphology.
   b. Cellular architecture.
   c. Afferent connections.
   d. Predominant neurotransmitter.

2. The orbitofrontal aspect of the PFC describes the area
   a. Above the corpus callosum.
   b. Posterior to the amygdala.
   c. At the base of the PFC.
   d. Anterior to the cingulate gyrus.

3. Lesions of the medial (also ventromedial) PFC are associated with
   a. Paucity of spontaneous behavior—apathetic.
   b. Disorganized cognitive function.
   c. Concrete thinking.
   d. Poor impulse control.

4. All of the following are true about the hippocampus except that it
   a. Is smaller in some psychiatric disorders.
   b. Is involved with memory.
   c. Is disrupted by frontal lobotomy.
   d. Contains undifferentiated stem cells.

5. The "command center" of the brain is the
   a. Hippocampus.
   b. Amygdala.
   c. ANS.
   d. Hypothalamus.

6. All of the following are true about the sympathetic nervous system except that it
   a. Stimulates digestion.
   b. Is associated with anxiety.
   c. Stimulates secretions from the adrenal medulla.
   d. Relaxes the airways.

7. The cerebellum
   a. Solely functions to support movement.
   b. Has been implicated with autism.
   c. Is similar to the motor cortex.
   d. Is relatively small in humans.

8. The BBB can be crossed by all of the following except
   a. Lipid-soluble molecules.
   b. Active transport across the cell wall.
   c. Breaches in the tight junctions.
   d. Most medications.

See Answers section at the end of the book.

CHAPTER 3

Circuits and Cells

THE NEURONAL CELL

The human brain is the most complex organ known to exist in the universe. Its weight is just 3% of the body, but it consumes 17% of the body's energy. The workhorse of the brain is the neuron. It is estimated that we have 100 billion neurons with 100 trillion connections. When we think of a neuron, we are typically thinking of a pyramidal neuron in the cerebral cortex. These neurons have a diamond-shaped cell body and usually reside in layers III or V of the gray matter (Figure 3.1).

Let us start with a brief review of cell biology. The cell body of the neuron is full of the usual assortment of organelles, although not in the same proportions as seen in non-neural cells. Structures such as the *endoplasmic reticulum* (ER) and *mitochondria* are found more frequently in neurons than in other brain cells, presumably because of the increased need for protein synthesis and energy production. The instructions for the functioning of the cell are contained in the DNA, which resides in the nucleus. The instructions are read when the DNA is *transcribed* into messenger ribonucleic acid (mRNA), which is *translated* into proteins in the cytoplasm (Figure 3.2). As mentioned in Chapter 1, this process is often called *gene expression—* two of our favorite words.

The *ribosome* is the organelle in which mRNA is translated into proteins (Figure 3.3). The ribosomes are usually attached to the rough ER, but can also be floating freely in the cytoplasm. The proteins, once they are refined, are used by the cell for structural (e.g., receptors), functional (e.g., enzymes), or communication (e.g., neuropeptides) purposes, to name a few.

The *Golgi apparatus*, which looks like ER without the ribosomes, is where much of the "posttranslation" refinement, sorting, and storage of proteins occurs. This structure enables proteins to be appropriately transported to distant sites within the cell.

The *mitochondria* are the remarkably abundant energy generators of the neuron. The brain requires considerable energy, even at rest, just to maintain an electrical gradient poised to respond at a moment's notice. The mitochondria convert adenosine diphosphate into adenosine triphosphate (ATP) and it is ATP that the cell uses to perform its functions.

The *dendrites* are the part of the neuron that sprout off the cell body and look like tree branches. They are often called the *ears* of the neuron, because they receive input from other neurons and relay the signal to the cell body. Most dendrites have "little knobs" along their stalks that are called *dendritic spines*. Each spine is the postsynaptic receptor for an incoming signal from another neuron (Figure 3.4).

The morphology (structure and density) of the dendritic spines has been a source of considerable interest since Ramón y Cajal first identified them over 100 years ago. Spines can change in shape, volume, and number with remarkable speed and frequency. This plasticity is one of the great discoveries of modern neuroscience. We mention spines throughout this book as their morphology changes in a number of conditions, including substance abuse, mental retardation, schizophrenia, and learning (see Point of Interest).

The *axon* is perhaps the most unique structure of the neuron. Starting at the *axon hillock* and running anywhere from a few micrometers to the entire length of the spinal cord, the axon can transmit a signal quickly without degradation to other

FIGURE 3.1 ● **A.** Cross section of the right prefrontal cortex (PFC). **B.** The six layers of neurons in the gray matter of the PFC. **C.** A stereotypical pyramidal neuron found in layer III of the cerebral cortex. ER, endoplasmic reticulum. (Adapted from Bear MF, Connors BW, Paradiso MA, eds. *Neuroscience: Exploring the Brain.* 3rd ed. Baltimore, MD: Lippincott Williams & Wilkins; 2007.)

neurons or end organs. For this reason, the axon is often conceptualized as the telephone wire of the brain. Because the axon is devoid of ribosomes and incapable of protein synthesis, a process called *axoplasmic transport* enables the neuron to send material down the microtubules to the distal ends of the cell.

The terminal end of the axon forms the synapse (Figure 3.5). This is where one neuron talks to another—if the dendrites are the ears, the synapse is the mouth. Here the electrical signal streaming down the axon is converted into a chemical signal, so the impulse can pass from one cell to another. The neurotransmitters that form the basis of the chemical signal are stored in vesicles. When released, they diffuse across the synaptic cleft to receptors on the postsynaptic dendrite (more on this later in the chapter).

FIGURE 3.2 ● Messenger ribonucleic acid (mRNA) carries the genetic instructions from the nucleus to the cytoplasm where translation into proteins occurs. (Adapted from Bear MF, Connors BW, Paradiso MA, eds. *Neuroscience: Exploring the Brain*. 3rd ed. Baltimore, MD: Lippincott Williams & Wilkins; 2007.)

ELECTRICAL SIGNALING

All living cells maintain a negative internal electronic charge relative to the fluid outside of the cell—roughly –60 mV in a neuron. Nerve cells use the depolarization (rapid change in the electrical charge) to communicate with other nerves or end organs. There are two basic steps in this process. The neuron first receives signals through the dendrites, which are called *postsynaptic potentials*. Second, the cell sums the incoming impulses and

POINT OF INTEREST

Enhanced branching and spine formation have been found consistently in rats raised in enriched environments when compared with rats raised in standard wire cages. The neurons in the figure below are from rats raised in different environments. Note the increased branching (also called *arborization*) of the neuron from the rat raised in the enriched environment. Abundant dendritic branching with multiple connections seems to be a microscopic sign of a healthy active brain.

From Kolb B, Forgie M, Gibb R, et al. Age, experience and the changing brain. *Neurosci Biobehav Rev*. 1998;22(2):143-159.

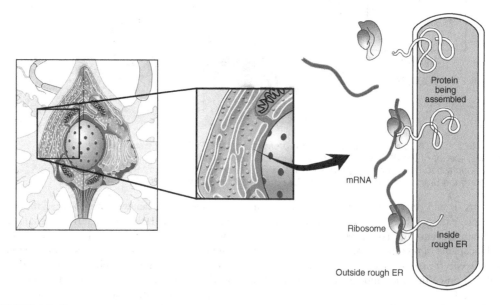

FIGURE 3.3 ● Messenger ribonucleic acid (mRNA) binds to a ribosome, initiating protein synthesis. Proteins synthesized on the rough endoplasmic reticulum (ER) as shown are eventually inserted into the membrane. Proteins synthesized on free ribosomes (not shown) are utilized in the cytosol. (Adapted from Bear MF, Connors BW, Paradiso MA, eds. *Neuroscience: Exploring the Brain*. 3rd ed. Baltimore, MD: Lippincott Williams & Wilkins; 2007.)

FIGURE 3.4 ● Spines are the "little knobs" on the dendrites. They are on the receiving side of the electrochemical signal from other neurons—also called the postsynaptic membrane.

FIGURE 3.5 ● A synapse as seen with an electron microscope (**A**) and in a schematic drawing (**B**). Note the high concentration of vesicles filled with neurotransmitter and mitochondria to power the rapid processing. (Adapted from Bear MF, Connors BW, Paradiso MA, eds. *Neuroscience: Exploring the Brain*. 3rd ed. Baltimore, MD: Lippincott Williams & Wilkins; 2007.)

if they are high enough then it sends an impulse down the axon, which is called an *action potential.*

Postsynaptic Potentials

A single pyramidal cell will receive input from 1 to 100,000 neurons through the postsynaptic synapses (spines) on the dendrites and cell body. When the neurotransmitters bind with the receptor at the postsynaptic synapse, ions flow into the neuron and change the electrical potential making it more positive or more negative—or what is called depolarization and hyperpolarization.

This proceeds in two ways:

Depolarize (excitatory) with an influx of positive ions such as Na⁺.

Hyperpolarize (inhibitory) with an influx of negative ions such as Cl⁻.

These are appropriately called *excitatory postsynaptic potentials* (*EPSPs*) and *inhibitory postsynaptic potentials* (*IPSPs*) (Figures 3.6 and 3.7). The EPSP and IPSP are, respectively, the

accelerator and brake for the brain. An EPSP is more likely to generate an action potential; an IPSP inhibits the generation of an action potential. The goal for a healthy brain is to maintain the correct balance—if there is too much excitation, one can have a seizure; if there is too much inhibition, the brain is sluggish, even comatose. Actually, most of us want our brains to be activated during the day and inhibited at night—something our hunter–gatherer brains are not always wired to accommodate.

The Action Potential

The decision to fire an action potential is made at the axon hillock. Moment to moment, the sum of all the incoming EPSPs and IPSPs at the axon hillock determines whether the neuron sends an impulse down the axon. If the potential has depolarized to the threshold, then an action potential is generated. Figure 3.8 shows how the neuron requires enough depolarization (excitation) but not too much hyperpolarization (inhibition) to generate an action potential.

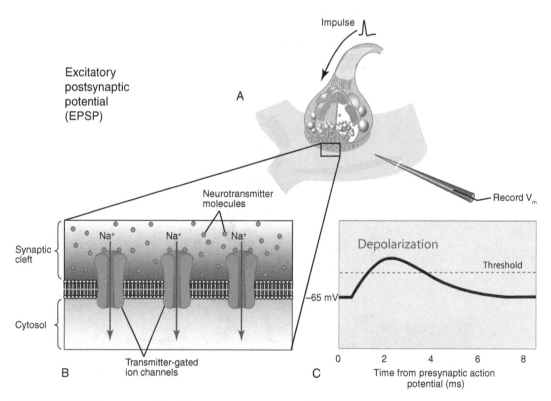

FIGURE 3.6 ● Neurotransmission from an *excitatory* neuron (**A**) promotes the entry of *positively* charged sodium ions into the dendrite (**B**). The resulting depolarization generates an EPSP (**C**). (Adapted from Bear MF, Connors BW, Paradiso MA, eds. *Neuroscience: Exploring the Brain.* 3rd ed. Baltimore, MD: Lippincott Williams & Wilkins; 2007.)

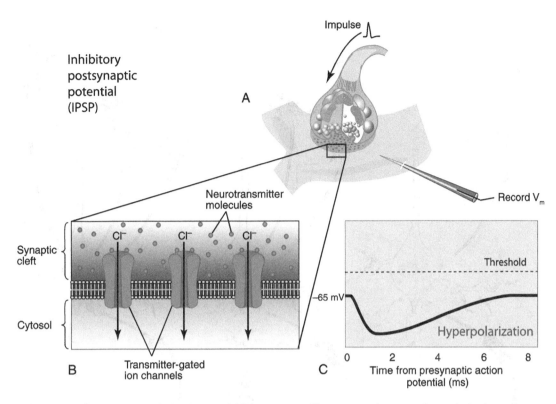

FIGURE 3.7 ● Neurotransmission from an *inhibitory* neuron (**A**) promotes the entry of *negatively* charged chloride ions into the dendrite (**B**). The resulting hyperpolarization generates an IPSP (**C**). (Adapted from Bear MF, Connors BW, Paradiso MA, eds. *Neuroscience: Exploring the Brain*. 3rd ed. Baltimore, MD: Lippincott Williams & Wilkins; 2007.)

Once the threshold (–40 mV) has been reached at the axon hillock, the neuron "pulls the trigger" and shoots an action potential down the axon. Because of the unique design of the *voltage-gated sodium channels*, the action potential maintains its integrity as it proceeds along the axon—there is no diminution in the signal. This occurs because the voltage-gated sodium channels facilitate a rapid influx of positive ions. Like other ion channels, the voltage-gated sodium channel is a protein embedded in the lipid member of the cell. The "gated" nature of the channel allows a large and rapid influx of the ions once the threshold has been

crossed. The voltage-gated channel is like a trap waiting to be sprung. When the switch is tripped, the ions pour into the axon.

Electrochemical Signaling

As Otto Loewi demonstrated in 1921, the communication within the nervous system is *both* electrical and chemical. Figure 3.9 shows a representation of the arrival of the action potential at the synaptic terminal, the release of the neurotransmitters, and the generation of an excitatory or inhibitor postsynaptic potential in the dendrite of the neighboring neuron. This example is of a

TREATMENT **CALM DOWN**

We often treat patients who have too much cerebral activity. Anxiety, attention-deficit/hyperactivity disorder (ADHD), insomnia, and mania are four conditions in which the brain is going too fast. Such patients have too much excitation and not enough inhibition. It

is encouraging that more research is being directed toward treatments that increase inhibitory potentials (e.g., γ-aminobutyric acid). The challenge is to selectively inhibit the annoying trait without slowing down the whole brain: calmer but not stupid.

FIGURE 3.8 ● A signal from one excitatory neuron (**A**) increases the EPSP but is not sufficient to reach the threshold. Two excitatory impulses reaching the neuron at the same time (**B**) generate an EPSP that reaches the threshold at the axon hillock and an action potential is fired. However, with an inhibitory input from a third neuron (**C**), the membrane potential again fails to reach the threshold.

dopamine neuron that is an excitatory neuron, but the same principles apply to all the neurons and neurotransmitters.

The arrival of the action potential at the terminal depolarizes the membrane, which opens the *voltage-gated calcium channels*. The voltage-gated calcium channels are similar to the voltage-gated sodium channels except that they are permeable to Ca^{2+}. Consequently, there is a large and rapid influx of Ca^{2+}, which is required for *exocytosis* and the release of the neurotransmitter.

NON-NEURONAL CELLS

The glial cells that make up the rest of the cells in the central nervous system (CNS) actually outnumber the neurons by 9:1. Traditionally seen as supportive cells with no roll in communication, recent research has shown that glial cells

Electro

1. The action potential arrives at the presynaptic terminal.

2. Depolarization causes voltage-gated calcium channels to open and results in a large influx of Ca^{2+}.

3. Exocytosis: Ca^{2+} causes the vesicles to fuse with the membrane and release the neurotransmitter.

4. Excitatory postsynaptic potentials (EPSP) spread out over the dendrite.

Chemical

A. Precursor molecules and enzymes are transported down the axon from the cell body along the microtubules.

B. Enzymes in the synaptic terminal convert the precursor molecules into active neurotransmitter.

C. The neurotransmitter is stored in the vesicles until released by the influx of Ca^{2+}.

D. The released neurotransmitter binds with the receptors on the post synaptic terminal and generates an EPSP.

E. Reuptake of the neurotransmitter limits the duration of the signal and allows the cell to recycle the neurotransmitter.

Enzymes convert tyrosine to dopamine

Ca^{2+}

Ca^{2+}

Ca^{2+}

EPSP

EPSP

FIGURE 3.9 ● This is an example of the electrochemical signaling from a dopamine neuron. If this were an inhibitory neuron, γ-aminobutyric acid or glycine, for example, the postsynaptic potential would be an inhibitory postsynaptic potential (IPSP) and not an excitatory postsynaptic potential (EPSP).

modulate the synaptic activity. There are three kinds of glial cells: astrocyte, oligodendrocyte, and microglia. The microglia are similar to macrophages found in the peripheral tissue. They respond to injury with a dramatic increase in their numbers and remove cellular debris from the damaged area. (For more information on microglia, refer Chapter 9.)

The oligodendrocyte is considered the CNS equivalent of the Schwann cell in the peripheral nervous system (Figure 3.10; see also Figure 20.12). Schwann cells are the cells that wrap myelin around the axons of the neurons and by acting as an electrical insulator they greatly increase the speed of the transmission of the

action potential. This process of myelinization is not complete at birth and proceeds rapidly in the first years of life, which has a dramatic effect on behavior. In children, this process results in improved motor skills as they mature. Complete myelinization of the prefrontal cortex (PFC) is delayed until the second and even third decade of life. Hence why we worry about our teens—the bodies of adults without the brakes of matured frontal lobes.

Alternatively, demyelinating disorders such as multiple sclerosis and Guillain-Barré have devastating effects on patients. Clearly, a neuron without its myelin is not as effective. Regarding mental illness, recent research suggests that some failure

Oligodendroglial cells

Myelin sheath

Mitochondrion

Node of Ranvier

FIGURE 3.10 ● Oligodendroglial cells wrap a myelin sheath around the axon, providing electrical insulation. This can improve the speed of the transmission of an action potential up to 15 times. (Adapted from Bear MF, Connors BW, Paradiso MA, eds. *Neuroscience: Exploring the Brain*. 3rd ed. Baltimore, MD: Lippincott Williams & Wilkins; 2007.)

in myelinization may play a role in schizophrenia (see Chapter 23).

The astrocyte is the star-shaped cell that fills the spaces between the neurons (Figure 3.11). We have already seen that the astrocyte plays a role in maintaining the blood–brain barrier, but other functions include regulating the chemistry of the extracellular fluid, providing structural support, and bringing nutrients to the neurons. Even more interesting is the role the astrocyte plays in modulating the electrical activity at the synapse. Research has shown that astrocytes encircle the synapse and have receptors that respond to the neurotransmitters released by the neuron. The astrocyte may in turn release its own neurotransmitter, which enhances the transmission of the signal. This may facilitate learning and memory. Additionally, there is evidence that the presence of astrocytes or their proteins increases the number of synapses a neuron will form. Clearly, the glial cells are more involved in the communication within the brain than previously thought.

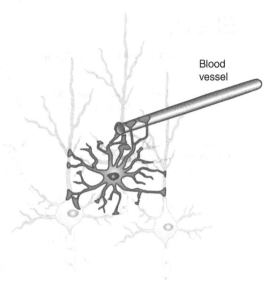

Blood vessel

FIGURE 3.11 ● The astrocyte not only supports the neurons and blood vessels but also has some role in modulating the transmission of information.

CIRCUITS

The capacity to communicate quickly over long distances (relative to the size of a cell) is the most unique feature of the nerve cell. Sending a signal, receiving feedback, and adjusting further responses is the essence of communication—cellular or social. The white matter tracts—bundles of axons just underneath the gray matter—connect the nerve cells with other regions of the cortex, subcortical nuclei, and end organs such as muscles and glands (Figure 3.12).

DISORDER **EPILEPSY**

Increasing evidence is pointing to the astrocyte as playing an instigating role in epilepsy—a problem historically assigned to dysfunctional neurons. Analysis of specimens after surgical resection for epilepsy often shows prominent gliosis. Glutamate released from astrocytes can trigger experimental models of seizures. Finally, several effective antiepileptic drugs (valproate, gabapentin, and phenytoin) potently reduce astrocytic Ca^{2+} signaling—an event believed to precede seizure activity. If aberrant astrocytes are the nidus for seizures, then new treatments might be developed that can calm the astrocytes without dulling the neurons.

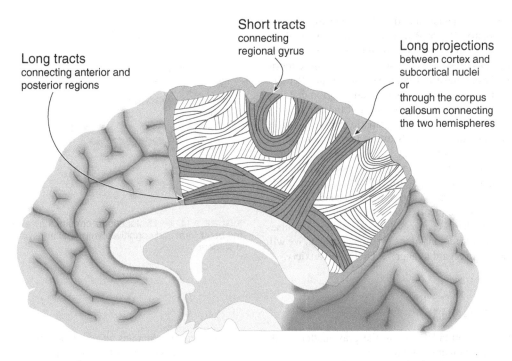

Short tracts
connecting
regional gyrus

Long tracts
connecting anterior and
posterior regions

Long projections
between cortex and
subcortical nuclei
or
through the corpus
callosum connecting
the two hemispheres

FIGURE 3.12 ● Beneath the gray matter are white matter tracts that allow communication between widely separated regions of the brain or between the brain and end organs. (Adapted from Rosenzweig MR, Breedlove SM, Watson NV. *Biological Psychology*. 4th ed. Sunderland, MA: Sinauer; 2005.)

A new imaging technique, called diffusion tensor imaging (DTI), has been developed to assess the quality of the white matter tracks. Using a magnetic resonance imaging scanner, the technique involves following the movement of water (diffusion) in the brain. In most tissues, the water molecules move in every direction. In the white matter tracts, the water molecules tend to move along the length of the axons. Thus, with some Herculean number crunching on the computer, images showing remarkable detail of the white matter tracks can be produced (Figure 3.13). Although still a research tool, DTI is being used to identify white matter abnormalities in patients with psychiatric disorders (see Chapter 23).

The networks formed to coordinate a task are called circuits. We can imagine that catching a Frisbee requires such a circuit. The visual cortex registers the trajectory of the Frisbee, the frontal cortex acknowledges the emotional importance of making the catch, and the motor cortex signals the legs and arms to get in a position to grasp the spinning disc. The interplay between these and other regions of the brain enables the individual to move into the appropriate location and make the grab. We can imagine that the efficiency and accuracy of such a circuit for different people falls along a spectrum from poor to superior—whether due to genes

or practice. It is the coordination of the circuit—not one particular region—that masters that catch.

Increasing evidence suggests that understanding circuits may help us understand the variants in behavior. The elusive nature of the biological

FIGURE 3.13 ● Visualization of white matter tracks in the brain using diffusion tensor imaging (DTI) technology. (Adapted from Brun A, Park HJ, Knutsson H, et al. *Coloring of DT-MRI Fiber Traces Using Laplacian Eigenmaps*. Available at http://lmi. bwh.harvard.edu/papers/papers/brunEUROCAST03. html. 2003.)

causes of mental disorders has been the bane of psychiatry. While Broca could pinpoint the damaged region to explain his aphasic patients, conspicuous lesions corresponding to psychiatric conditions have not been easy to locate. Perhaps this is because it is not one specific region that is at fault, but rather the dysfunction of the circuit.

Figure 3.14 shows a schematic representation of a hypothetical circuit between the PFC, temporal cortex, and subcortical regions. Imaging studies suggest that dysfunction of emotional circuits may explain some psychiatric disorders—particularly depression, anxiety, and substance abuse. One common example involves the PFC. Insufficient activity from the PFC allows the expression of impulses from lower regions of the brain—a problem we will address in regard to anger, ADHD, and anxiety.

FIGURE 3.14 ● Dysfunctional circuits may explain the behavioral and cognitive symptoms in psychiatric disorders.

QUESTIONS

1. The pyramidal cells in the gray matter reside predominantly in which layers?
   a. I and III.
   b. II and IV.
   c. III and V.
   d. IV and VI.

2. Protein synthesis requires all of the following except
   a. Rough ER.
   b. Gene expression.
   c. Transcription and translation.
   d. mRNA.

3. Enhanced arborization of the dendrites is found with
   a. Mental retardation.
   b. Stimulating environments.
   c. Usual laboratory environments.
   d. Schizophrenia.

4. An IPSP
   a. Results from the influx of sodium ions.
   b. Depolarizes the cell.
   c. Can induce seizures.
   d. Hyperpolarizes the cell.

5. The neuron generates an action potential based on the postsynaptic potential at the
   a. Axon hillock.
   b. Synapse.
   c. Nucleus.
   d. Node of Ranvier.

6. Exocytosis of the neurotransmitters at the synapse requires opening of the
   a. Voltage-gated sodium channels.
   b. Voltage-gated calcium channels.
   c. Excitatory postsynaptic channels.
   d. Inhibitory postsynaptic channels.

7. The cell responsible for myelin in the CNS is
   a. Astrocyte.
   b. Microglia.
   c. Schwann cell.
   d. Oligodendrocyte.

8. Modulates electrochemical activity at the synapse:
   a. Astrocyte.
   b. Microglia.
   c. Schwann cell.
   d. Oligodendrocyte.

See Answers section at the end of the book.

CHAPTER 4

Neurotransmitters

A "neurotransmitter" is technically defined by meeting the following three criteria:

1. The substance must be stored in the presynaptic neuron.
2. It must be released with depolarization of the presynaptic neuron induced by the influx of Ca^{2+}.
3. The substance must bind with a specific receptor on the postsynaptic neuron.

Neurotransmitters differ from hormones by their close physical proximity of the release to the receptor—although this turns out to be less straightforward than one might imagine, as we will see in Chapter 6.

The classic neurotransmitters—the ones we frequently discuss—are small molecules designed for the ease of use. For neurotransmitters, the body needs a substrate that can be produced quickly, with ease, and be recycled—much like the daily newspaper. Figure 4.1 shows some representative neurotransmitters compared with a neuropeptide

substance P. The common neurotransmitters such as γ-aminobutyric acid (GABA) and norepinephrine (NE) are small and these are constructed with elements that are easy for the body to find. This facilitates the rapid creation and release of the signals that are the essential feature of neural communication.

An extensive review of all known neurotransmitters is beyond the scope of this book. We will focus on the relevant molecules in the following three basic categories:

1. The classic neurotransmitters.
2. Neuropeptides.
3. Unconventional neurotransmitters.

CLASSIC NEUROTRANSMITTERS

Amino Acids

Glutamate

This is the major workhorse of the brain, with glutamate neurons making up more than half of the *excitatory* neurons. Without glutamate the brain does not get started or keep running. Glutamate

FIGURE 4.1 ● A sample of neurotransmitters showing the relative size of the amino acids (**A**), two of the amines (**B**), and a neuropeptide (**C**). (Adapted from Bear MF, Connors BW, Paradiso MA, eds. *Neuroscience: Exploring the Brain*. 3rd ed. Baltimore, MD: Lippincott Williams & Wilkins; 2007.)

DISORDERS

Glutamate neurons are believed to be involved in the formation and storage of memories. Changes in the receptors—termed *synaptic plasticity*—are well documented and seem to be involved in the physical manifestation of learning. Too much glutamate, as occurs with a stroke, is toxic to the nerve cells. Not only is the cell deprived of oxygen but also the glutamate that is released from the dying cell results in further damage. Efforts are underway to find an agent that will block the toxic effects of glutamate during ischemic events to limit the secondary damage. More recently, glutamate has been implicated as a possible culprit in the pathophysiology of schizophrenia. Postmortem studies and therapeutic trials suggest that glutamatergic dysregulation may be present in patients with schizophrenia.

and another excitatory transmitter *aspartate* are nonessential amino acids that do not cross the blood–brain barrier—an important barrier as otherwise our diet could alter our neural activity. Consequently, glutamate must be synthesized in the brain from glucose and other precursors. Glial cells assist in the reuptake, degradation, and resupply of glutamate for neurons.

γ-Aminobutyric Acid and Glycine

GABA is the major inhibitory transmitter in the brain and is used by approximately 25% of the cortical neurons. Glycine is the other, but less common, inhibitory amino acid. GABA puts the brakes on the brain: not enough GABA and one can have seizures. The GABA neurons are primarily the interneurons in the gray matter. They provide local constraint over too much cortical circuitry. Figure 3.7 shows an example of a GABA neuron

POINT OF INTEREST

Of the classic neurotransmitters, the mono-amines are the ones we typically talk about. Hanging around psychiatrists, one might imagine that the brain is predominately made up of dopamine (DA), serotonin, and NE. Amazingly, these agents are present in minor amounts in the brain. The largest number of neurons and the ones that do the heavy lifting in the brain come from the amino acid group, of which glutamate and GABA are the most prominent. The pie chart gives a very rough estimate of the relative proportion of several important neurotransmitters. The neuropeptides (discussed later) would only be a line on this chart.

A: Without inhibitory input

Inhibitory input from
GABA interneuron

B: With inhibitory input

FIGURE 4.2 ● Effects of inhibitory input.
A. Without GABA inhibition (or any other inhibition)
the neuron fires regularly. **B.** With input from a GABA
interneuron (arrows), some action potentials are
inhibited. GABA, γ-aminobutyric acid.

hyperpolarizing the receiving neuron so that it is
less likely to fire an action potential.

Similarly, Figure 4.2 shows how the input
from a GABA interneuron quiets an overactive
neuron. One can see how increasing GABAergic activity can be an effective treatment for
epilepsy. More recently, increasing GABAergic
activity has been used to treat insomnia, pain,
and anxiety and to assist in the management of
mania—all situations where too much central
nervous system (CNS) activity is a component
of the disorder.

Monoamines

The monoamines modulate the activity of the
excitatory and inhibitory neurons. Although
small in total number compared with glutamate
or GABA, the monoamine neurons project widely
throughout the brain. They have the capacity to
"fine-tune" and coordinate the response of the
major neurons.

There are two principal classes of monoamines:
catecholamines (DA, NE, and epinephrine) and
indoleamines (serotonin and melatonin). After
being released, monoamines are degraded or repro-
cessed by the neuron. (Clinicians often refer to this
as the reuptake pump, but neuroscientists call this
the *transporter*, e.g., the DA transporter.) The class
of enzymes in the terminal that degrades the neurotransmitters is the monoamine oxidases (MAOs).

MAO inhibitors cause an increase in catecholamines (e.g., DA, NE, and serotonin), by limiting
the degradation process, with well-known benefits
for depression and anxiety.

Unfortunately, some food products and medications enhance the release of NE. When the
MAOs are inhibited, an excessive amount of NE
is released. This can result in dangerous elevations
in blood pressure, which has resulted in stroke and
even death in some cases.

Catecholamines

The catecholamines begin as the essential amino
acid tyrosine (Figure 4.3), which must be introduced in the diet. L-DOPA (Figure 4.3A) is
the molecule made famous in the Oliver Sacks

FIGURE 4.3 ● The synthesis of catecholamines
from tyrosine. Dopamine (**B**) cannot cross the blood–
brain barrier although some L-DOPA can sneak
through. By giving patients DOPA decarboxylase
inhibitors, such as carbidopa, along with L-DOPA,
the half-life of L-DOPA is extended and more
crosses into the brain. Furthermore, carbidopa does
not cross the blood–brain barrier, so L-DOPA can
be converted into dopamine in the brain and the
Parkinson's patient moves with greater ease.

story *Awakenings* and remains the gold standard treatment for Parkinson's disease. The structures of DA, NE, and epinephrine are remarkably similar, yet have different functions in the brain.

Dopamine

The DA neurons constitute only about half a million of the cells in the brain—a tiny percentage out of the 100 billion total cells (Figure 4.4). Three nuclei contain the cell bodies that project the three primary branches of the DA network. The *substantia nigra* located in the ventral midbrain has primary projections to the caudate and putamen (collectively called the *striatum*). This pathway is called the *nigrostriatal system* or *mesostriatal system*. As part of the basal ganglia, this pathway is integral to voluntary movement. Parkinson's disease is the result of a loss of DA neurons in the substantia nigra. The extrapyramidal side effects due to antipsychotic medications can induce parkinsonian symptoms by blockade of these neurons.

The cells of the *ventral tegmental area*, also in the ventral midbrain, project to the nucleus accumbens, prefrontal cortex, amygdala, and hippocampus. These innervations, called the *mesolimbocortical DA system*, are particularly dense in primates. Some writers subdivide these branches into the *mesolimbic* (nucleus accumbens, amygdala, and hippocampus) and *mesocortical*

DISORDERS

The branches to the nucleus accumbens are involved with reward and substance abuse. The branches to the prefrontal cortex are involved with attention and cognition and seem to be impaired in patients with attention-deficit/hyperactivity disorder (ADHD). Some speculate that problems with the mesolimbic system cause the positive symptoms of schizophrenia, whereas negative symptoms are caused by impairment in the mesocortical system.

(prefrontal cortex) systems, which seems artificial as they originate from the same cell bodies.

The short tracts in the *arcuate nucleus* of the hypothalamus—called the *tuberoinfundibular DA system*—release the DA into the portal veins of the pituitary gland. The synthesis and release of prolactin in the anterior pituitary is inhibited by dopamine. Any interruption between the DA and the prolactin-producing cells will lead to hyperprolactinemia. Hence, antipsychotic medications that block the DA receptor can cause an increase in prolactin, although it appears to be less with the newer antipsychotic agents for unclear reasons.

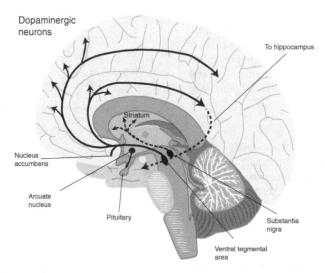

FIGURE 4.4 ● The three major pathways of the dopaminergic system. The substantia nigra forms the nigrostriatal pathways to the caudate and putamen. The ventral tegmental area projects to the nucleus accumbens and cortex. The arcuate nucleus of the hypothalamus projects to the tuberoinfundibular area of the hypothalamus.

Noradrenergic neurons

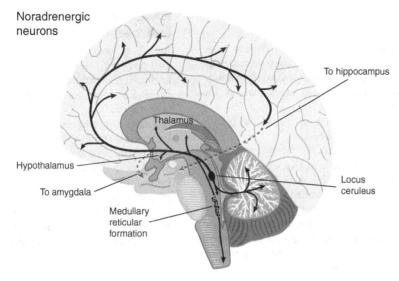

To hippocampus

Thalamus

Hypothalamus

To amygdala

Locus ceruleus

Medullary reticular formation

FIGURE 4.5 ● The noradrenergic system. With projections to almost every area of the brain and spinal cord, the NE system plays an important role in alertness and anxiety. NE, norepinephrine.

Norepinephrine is called *noradrenaline* in the UK and hence neurons that produce noradrenaline are called noradrenergic neurons. These neurons contain an additional enzyme in their terminal buds that converts DA to NE. Approximately 50% of the NE neurons have their cell bodies located in the locus coeruleus—small nuclei, one on each side of the brain stem. In total, there are only about 24,000 neurons in both nuclei. The remainder of the NE neurons as found in loose clusters in the medullary reticular formation (Figure 4.5).

The noradrenergic neurons project to virtually every area of the brain and spinal cord. Although small in number, they are essential for survival of the organism. For example, knockout mice that are deficient in NE cannot survive. The NE neurons play an important role in alertness. The firing of the locus coeruleus increases along a spectrum from drowsy to alert, with the lowest found when we sleep and the highest when we are hypervigilant. Clearly, the noradrenergic neurons are important in handling danger. In a threatening situation, the locus coeruleus is active as are the sympathetic neurons of the autonomic nervous system (ANS), where the peripheral noradrenergic neurons are found.

NE is cleared from the synaptic cleft by a reuptake transporter that is also capable of taking up DA—most likely due to the structural similarity of these two transmitters (Figure 4.4). This may explain why atomoxetine, an NE reuptake inhibitor, results in an increase in DA (as well as NE) in the prefrontal cortex even though it does not inhibit the DA reuptake pump.

TREATMENT

Inappropriate noradrenergic activity, both centrally and peripherally, plays an important role in anxiety and depression. Not only is a rapid heart rate a symptom of anxiety but also a high resting heart rate after a motor vehicle accident is a predictor of later post-traumatic stress disorder. Reducing the activity of these neurons is one goal of pharmacological treatment.

Recently, the Food and Drug Administration (FDA) approved vagus nerve stimulation (VNS) as a treatment for medication-resistant depression. Incoming signals to the brain from the vagus nerve provide the locus coeruleus with information about the state of the internal organs. In a hypervigilant condition such as chronic anxiety, the information from vagus nerve increases the activity of the locus coeruleus and the NE neurons. VNS may work by regulating the locus coeruleus and the NE system.

Epinephrine

The *epinephrine* (or adrenaline) neurons are few and play a minor role in the CNS. Most of the epinephrine in the body is produced in the adrenal medulla and excreted with sympathetic stimulation. Epinephrine plays a much greater role outside of the brain as a hormone, compared with its role as a CNS neurotransmitter.

Indoleamines
Serotonin (5-Hydroxytryptamine)

No other neurotransmitter is more closely associated with modern neuropsychopharmacology than serotonin. Also called *5-hydroxytryptamine (5-HT)*, serotonin is found in many parts of the body outside of the CNS, such as platelets and mast cells. Only about 1% to 2% of the body's serotonin is located in the brain.

Serotonin is synthesized from tryptophan, another essential amino acid that cannot be synthesized in the body (Figure 4.6). Unlike the catecholamines, levels of serotonin in the brain can be significantly lowered with insufficient dietary tryptophan (grains, meats, and dairy products are good sources of tryptophan). In the pineal gland, there are two additional enzymes that convert serotonin to *melatonin*, the other indoleamine.

The location of the cell bodies and distribution of the serotonin neurons are similar to that of the catecholamines (Figure 4.7). The cell bodies are relatively few in number (approximately 200,000) and reside in the raphe nuclei in the brain stem. As with NE, the serotonin neurons project to virtually all areas of the brain.

Histamine

Histamine is not just for itching anymore. Although histamine is released from mast cells as part of an allergic reaction in the peripheral tissue, in the brain it is involved in arousal and attention. Most of the cell bodies start in the tuberomammillary nucleus of the posterior hypothalamus, with

DISORDERS

As we all know, the serotonin neurons play an important role in depression and anxiety and are also implicated in the sleep–wake cycle. Serotonin, as with the catecholamines, is removed from the synaptic cleft by the reuptake of the transmitter with the serotonin transporter. It is the blockade of this process that is believed to result in the therapeutic effect of the commonly prescribed antidepressants. Although increasing the availability of serotonin in the synaptic cleft has proven therapeutic value for the treatment of depression, it remains unclear if insufficient serotonin is part of the etiology of the disorder.

TREATMENT

As prescribers, we are often struggling with unintended sedation due to blocking of the histamine neurons (antihistamines), for example, tricyclic antidepressants (TCAs), clozapine, and olanzapine. More recently, there has been increased interest in activating the histamine neurons as a treatment for fatigue. Modafinil, the only agent in the class, indirectly activates the histamine neurons and has been used successfully as a treatment for narcolepsy, excessive sleepiness, and ADHD.

FIGURE 4.6 ● Serotonin synthesis.

Serotonergic
neurons

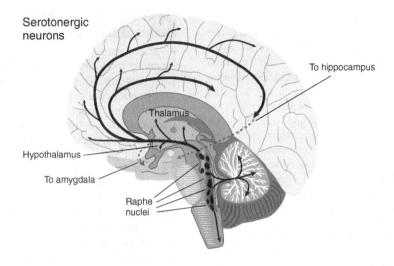

FIGURE 4.7 ● The serotonergic system. The cluster of raphe nuclei along the brainstem has projections to most of the brain and spinal cord. These neurons play an important role in the mood, anxiety, and sleep–wake cycle.

sparse but widespread projections to all regions of the brain and spinal cord. When animals are alert, the histamine neurons are active. Histamine neurons are quiet when animals are sleeping.

Acetylcholine
In the 1920s, acetylcholine (ACh) was the first molecule to be identified as a neurotransmitter (Figure 1.6). ACh is the only small molecule transmitter that is not an amino acid or directly derived from one. ACh is actually not a monoamine but is often grouped with these neurotransmitters due to similar size and distribution.

ACh plays a prominent role in the peripheral ANS and is the neurotransmitter at the neuromuscular junction. Its relative ease of accessibility outside the cranium is one reason it was discovered first. The neurons in the CNS arise from cell bodies in the brain stem and forebrain with prominent projects to the cortex and hippocampus. These latter projections to the hippocampus are involved with learning and memory and are disrupted in Alzheimer's disease.

NEUROPEPTIDES
In the late 1960s and early 1970s, it was established that many peptides initially discovered in the body, for example, gut and heart, are also produced and are active in the brain. This is another example of the parsimonious evolution of neurotransmitters: The same transmitter has different functions in various organs or brain regions depending on its location.

TREATMENT
ACh is also synthesized in interneurons in the CNS. In the striatum, the ACh neurons balance the dopaminergic input from the substantia nigra to coordinate extrapyramidal motor control. Disruption of this balance with DA-blocking antipsychotic agents can result in extrapyramidal side effects. The anticholinergic agents are administered to restore the ACh/DA balance and allow normal movement.

POINT OF INTEREST
Henry Dale, who shared the 1936 Nobel Prize with Otto Loewi, started the convention of identifying neurons by the neurotransmitter they release, for example, "adrenergic" and "cholinergic." This was based on Dale's belief that a neuron can synthesize just one neurotransmitter. We now know that neurons can release different transmitters with opposing functions, for example, the excitatory ACh and inhibitory glycine have been found in the same neuron. Furthermore, small molecule neurotransmitters such as those discussed in the preceding text often inhabit the same neuron with neuropeptides—referred to as *colocalization*.

Neuropeptides such as adrenocorticotropic hormone, luteinizing hormone, somatostatin, and vasopressin (to name a few) have important endocrine functions in the body, such as the regulation of reproduction, growth, water intake, salt metabolism, and temperature control. In the last 30 years, it has been established that these same peptides are synthesized in the nerve cells and have effects on behaviors such as learning, attachment, mood, and anxiety. This has generated tremendous interest in further analysis of the effects of these neuroactive peptides on behavior. Table 4.1 gives examples of neuropeptides from the five classes.

The neuropeptides are small chains of amino acids (Figure 4.1) and are considerably larger than the classic neurotransmitters. Furthermore, the formation, release, and inactivation of the neuropeptides differ from that of the monoamines. Figure 4.8 shows the life of a neuropeptide in relation to a classic neurotransmitter. Peptides must be transcribed from mRNA on the ribosomes of the endoplasmic reticulum. Initially, the peptide is a large *propeptide* precursor, which is cleaved into an active neuropeptide as it is moved from

POINT OF INTEREST

In some cases, the neuropeptides travel relatively long distances from their release to a receptor. This begs the question: Are they transmitters or hormones? Further complicating our understanding of the role of neuropeptides, it has been shown that they do not always evoke an action potential. They can play a gentle role—often called *modulation*—in facilitating or enhancing the effects elicited by the classic neurotransmitters, and they are often stored in the same neuron as 5-HT, NE, or DA. It appears that neuropeptides act as transmitters, hormones, or modulators depending on the tissue, synapse, and frequency of stimulation.

the Golgi apparatus into large dense core vesicles that are stored at the terminal bud of the neuron. Unlike the monoamines, neuropeptides are not recycled by the neuron, but rather are broken down by degradative enzymes (*peptidases*) on the receptor membrane.

UNCONVENTIONAL NEUROTRANSMITTERS

It would be foolish to think that we have discovered all the neurotransmitters—or even all the transmitter classes. For example, two unconventional neurotransmitters (nitric oxide [NO] and the endocannabinoids) are being studied that are expanding our understanding of how the brain communicates and what constitutes being a neurotransmitter.

Gases

Most commonly associated with erectile dysfunction, *NO* is a gas that is formed in glutamate neurons when arginine is converted into citrulline and NO. NO has the ability to diffuse (without obstruction) out of the originating cell, through the extracellular medium and into any neighboring cell that it meets. NO converts guanosine triphosphate (GTP) into cyclic guanosine monophosphate (cGMP), which acts as a second messenger. Cells containing the NO synthase (the enzyme that creates NO) constitute only approximately 1% of neuronal cells in the brain, but reach out so extensively that nearly every cell in the brain may encounter NO. It is hard to imagine this gas as a neurotransmitter in the traditional sense if for no other reason than that it cannot be stored in vesicles awaiting the

TABLE 4.1

The Five Classes of Neuropeptides and Some Examples

Peptide Class	Example
Gut–brain peptides	Substance P
	Cholecystokinin
	Galanin
Pituitary peptides	Adrenocorticotropic hormone
	Luteinizing hormone
	Oxytocin
	Vasopressin
Hypothalamic releasing peptides	Corticotropin-releasing factor
	Gonadotropin-releasing hormone
	Thyrotropin-releasing hormone
	Somatostatin
Opioid peptides	β-Endorphin
	Enkephalins
Other peptides	Angiotensin
	Bradykinin

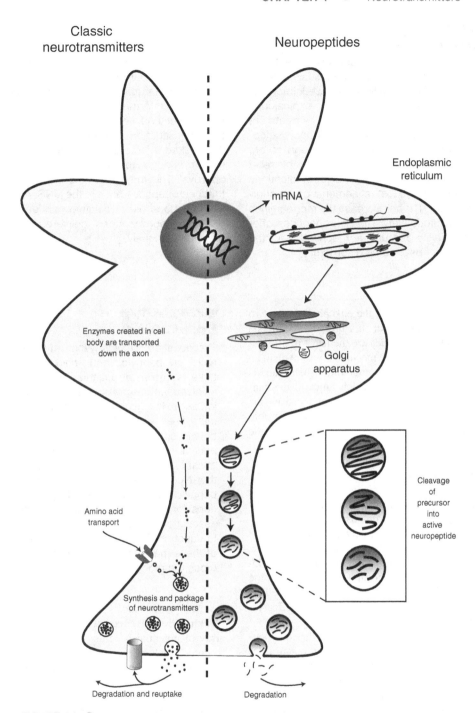

FIGURE 4.8 ● Comparison of classic neurotransmitters and neuropeptides.

appropriate signal to be released. But NO does send a message to the neighboring cells that signals an increase in activity—almost like turning the porch lights on shows our neighbors that we are home.

Endocannabinoids

The journey from recognizing an effect of a substance on behavior to identifying the endogenous substrate and receptor is a common and fascinating story. Reserpine and the monoamines,

TREATMENT

Since the serendipitous discovery in the 1950s that patients treated for tuberculosis with an agent that inhibited MAO showed improvement in mood, there has been an explosion in the manipulation of monoamines as treatment for depression and anxiety: TCAs, selective serotonin reuptake inhibitors, and so on. Although this has resulted in incalculable relief for millions of patients, the newer medications are in many ways just refinements of the original concept. They all increase the monoamines in the synaptic cleft. The neuropeptides offer the possibility of a unique mechanism for the treatment of psychiatric disorders.

Several pharmaceutical companies are investigating neuropeptide systems as novel therapeutic targets for depression, anxiety, and pain. Unfortunately, none have come to the market and some have been withdrawn from investigation. The problem may be that the desired effects are only mild and are not robust enough to justify seeking full FDA approval. This may reflect the modulating role that neuropeptides have in the CNS. Additionally, the blood has circulating peptidases that degrade neuropeptides delivered orally or even intravenously.

as well as morphine and the enkephalins, are two well-known examples of this process. Marijuana and the endocannabinoids are the latest in this history of searching for the mechanisms to explain an effect. The main active compound of marijuana is Δ^9-tetrahydrocannabinol, which binds to the cannabinoid receptor type 1 (CB_1) and causes the well-known euphoria, calm, distorted cognition, and "munchies." Following the discovery of the receptor, there was an active search for the naturally occurring neurotransmitter that activates the receptor. Subsequently, the endogenous cannabinoids, called *endocannabinoids*, were identified.

The CB_1 is widely expressed throughout the brain on presynaptic terminals. The endocannabinoids are retrograde messengers residing in the postsynaptic neuron. When released, they diffuse back across the synaptic space. When coupled with a CB_1 receptor, the endocannabinoids inhibit the release of the presynaptic neurotransmitter. This simple description explains the calming effect of marijuana—it reduces neural activity.

There is considerable interest in the therapeutic effects of pharmacological manipulation of various components of the endocannabinoid signaling pathways. The issue of medical marijuana highlights the potential benefits of activating the CB_1 receptor for pain, nausea, and glaucoma. But this is also not without potential CNS problems,

DISORDERS

The question remains: What effect does NO have on behavior and mental disorders? Little is known about this, but NO may be involved with aggression and sexual behavior, as well as migraine headaches. Knockout mice, bred without NO synthase, are extraordinarily aggressive and sexual, although their behavior is mediated by testosterone and absent in females. These findings suggest that NO may restrain aggressive and sexual behavior. It is worth noting that the medications for erectile dysfunction have not been associated with any adverse effects on mental function. This may be due to the inability of these medications in their current form to cross the blood–brain barrier.

for example, psychosis and depression. Likewise, blocking the CB_1 receptor offers an alternative array of potential benefits. For a short time, CB_1 receptor blockers (antagonists) were available in Europe to treat obesity and smoking cessation but were eventually removed due to psychiatric complications. Medications that enhance or reduce the endocannabinoids will likely continue to be developed as this neurotransmitter has such potential.

QUESTIONS

1. Which is an indoleamine?
   a. DA.
   b. NE.
   c. Melatonin.
   d. Aspartate.

2. Which pathway is believed to result in the negative symptoms of schizophrenia?
   a. Nigrostriatal.
   b. Mesocortical.
   c. Mesolimbic.
   d. Tuberoinfundibular.

3. Which pathway mediates prolactin?
   a. Nigrostriatal.
   b. Mesocortical.
   c. Mesolimbic.
   d. Tuberoinfundibular.

4. The cell bodies of the NE neurons are located in the locus coeruleus and the
   a. Medullary reticular formation.
   b. Raphe nuclei.
   c. Arcuate nucleus.
   d. Tuberomammillary nucleus.

5. Most of the cell bodies for histamine neurons reside in the
   a. Medullary reticular formation.
   b. Raphe nuclei.
   c. Arcuate nucleus.
   d. Tuberomammillary nucleus.

6. Which statement is not true regarding NO?
   a. It is quickly degraded.
   b. It converts GTP into cGMP.
   c. It is stored in dense core vesicles.
   d. It is formed from arginine.

7. All of the following are neuropeptides except
   a. Cannabinoid peptides.
   b. Pituitary peptides.
   c. Opioid peptides.
   d. Hypothalamic releasing peptides.

8. The most common neurotransmitter in the brain is
   a. Serotonin.
   b. DA.
   c. GABA.
   d. Glutamate.

See Answers section at the end of the book.

CHAPTER 5

Receptors and Signaling the Nucleus

INTRODUCTION

In this chapter, we continue a discussion about events at the cellular level and explore what happens at receptors after neurotransmitters make contact.

Electrochemical communication continues at the receptor on the postsynaptic membrane. Without a receptor, the neurotransmitter is like a tree falling in the woods with no one to hear it. The binding of the neurotransmitter with the receptor initiates a series of events that change the postsynaptic cell in some way. Receptors are protein units embedded in the lipid layer of the cell membrane. There are two basic types of receptors activated by neurotransmitters (more on this below), and the response generated depends on what type of receptor is engaged.

Agonists and Antagonists

Most neuropsychiatric medications work their magic by enhancing or limiting the effects of the neurotransmitter at the receptor. Figure 5.1 shows a schematic representation of a receptor, a neurotransmitter, and the opposing effects of contrasting medications. Pharmacologists and neuroscientists use the terms *ligand*, *agonist*, and *antagonists*, but in this book we also use the more self-explanatory terms such as *transmitter*, *drug/medication*, *stimulate*, and *block*.

FAST RECEPTORS: CHEMICAL

There are two basic types of receptors for neurotransmitters. The one we usually think of is shown in Figure 5.1—an ion channel (also called *transmitter-gated ion channel*). A neurotransmitter or medication stimulates the opening of the pore inside the receptor and ions rapidly flow into the cell. Receptors that allow the entry of positive ions such as Na^+ or Ca^{2+} result in an excitatory postsynaptic potential (EPSP). Acetylcholine

(ACh) and glutamate result in such activation and are considered excitatory.

Receptors permeable to negative ions, such as Cl^-, will result in inhibitory postsynaptic potentials. γ-Aminobutyric acid (GABA) and glycine, both considered inhibitory, cause this kind of activation. The essential point regarding these transmitter-gated ion channels is that they are fast. These receptors are magnificent little machines that rapidly allow the entry of large currents with great precision. The ions pour into the cell and the signal from the proceeding neuron, whether excitatory or inhibitory, is quickly propagated along the membrane of the target cell. As we reviewed in Chapter 3, an action potential is only generated if enough EPSPs bring the resting potential of the postsynaptic cell above the threshold at the axon hillock.

Amino Acid Receptors

The amino acid receptors mediate most of the fast transmitter-gated channels in the brain. The two prominent ones are glutamate and GABA, which are reviewed in the subsequent text.

POINT OF INTEREST

The receptors, unlike the transmitter, come in a variety of styles—a relationship that is much like feet and shoes. You only have two feet, but many shoes. Serotonin is one example: there are 14 different receptor subtypes for this one neurotransmitter. Some receptors are categorized as different classes, whereas others are just different subtypes within a class. It is not entirely clear why some differences constitute a new class and others just warrant a new subtype. Most likely a committee decided.

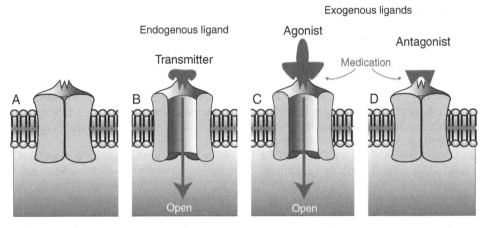

FIGURE 5.1 ● An unbound receptor in closed state (**A**). A natural ligand (neurotransmitter) stimulates the receptor, which then opens to allow entry of ions (**B**). Medication *simulates* the action of the natural ligand and the receptor opens (**C**). An antagonist *blocks* the action of the ligand so the receptor cannot be opened (**D**).

Glutamate

There are three prominent glutamate receptors: *N-methyl-d-aspartate (NMDA)*, α-*amino-3-hydroxy-5-methyl-4-isoxazole propionate (AMPA)*, and *kainate*, each with several subtypes. They are named after the artificial agonist that selectively activates them. For example, NMDA activates the NMDA receptor, but not the AMPA or kainate receptors. NMDA and AMPA constitute the bulk of fast excitatory synaptic transmission in the brain. The role of kainate is not clearly understood.

Both NMDA and AMPA receptors, which often coexist on the same postsynaptic receptor, allow the rapid entry of Na^+ into the cell (and the simultaneous exit of K^+) that generates the depolarization of the postsynaptic cell. NMDA receptors are unique in that they also allow the entry of Ca^{2+} that can act as a second messenger inside the cell. This can have a profound impact on the cell resulting in lasting changes, as will be shown at the end of this chapter when we discuss long-term memory.

The NMDA receptor is further unique in that it requires both the glutamate transmitter and a change in the voltage to open before it will allow the entry of Na^+ and Ca^{2+}. This property is due to the presence of Mg^{2+} ions, which clog the NMDA receptor at resting voltage. Figure 5.2 shows how the AMPA receptor works in conjunction with

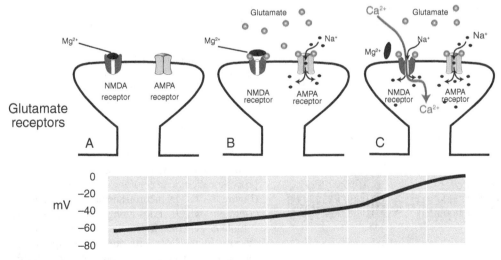

FIGURE 5.2 ● **A.** A postsynaptic glutamate terminal with both receptors closed. **B.** The presence of glutamate transmitters opens the AMPA receptor but not the NMDA receptor. **C.** When the voltage in the postsynaptic neuron gets above –35 mV, the magnesium ion blocking the receptor falls off and Na^+ as well as Ca^{2+} ions pour into the cell. AMPA, α-amino-3-hydroxy-5-methyl-4-isoxazole propionate; NMDA, *N*-methyl-ᴅ-aspartate.

the NMDA receptor to depolarize the cell and bring Ca^{2+} into the cell. This property has a significant impact on the capacity of the neurons to change.

The glutamate receptor is increasingly being explored as a novel target for psychiatric conditions. Preliminary studies have shown that a single IV injection of ketamine (an NMDA antagonist) can rapidly and temporarily reduce depression. With schizophrenia, glutamate has long been suspected as a possible culprit, and Eli Lilly is conducting clinical trials with a medication that reduces glutamate release. Figure 15.3 shows the benefits of a partial NMDA agonist that, in conjunction with exposure therapy, reduces fear.

γ-Aminobutyric Acid

GABA and *glycine* are the primary inhibitory neurons in the brain; inhibition is a process that must be tightly regulated. Too much inhibition causes the brain to slow down—even lose consciousness. Not enough inhibition and the electrical activity can get out of control—evoke a seizure. GABA is the most common inhibitory receptor.

The GABA receptor is made up of five protein subunits, which vary for different subclasses of the receptor. The GABA$_A$ receptor (Figure 5.3) is the focus of much pharmacological interest. There are several other sites on the GABA$_A$ receptor where chemicals can modulate its function. For example, *barbiturates* and *benzodiazepines* have their own distinct sites on the GABA receptor. These medications by themselves do not open the GABA channel, but they can enhance the strength or frequency of the opening. Benzodiazepines plus

FIGURE 5.3 ● The GABA receptor showing other drugs that can modify and enhance the inhibitory effect of these receptors. GABA, γ-aminobutyric acid.

GABA results in more Cl^- entering the cell and a greater inhibitory effect.

Ethanol is another popular drug that enhances the function of the GABA receptor. Long-term use of ethanol decreases the expression of the GABA receptor, which may explain the tolerance that develops with alcoholism. Whether the receptor alterations contribute to the propensity for seizures when the alcohol is withdrawn remains unclear.

The steroid hormones can also modulate GABA receptors (sometimes called *neurosteroids* when they have effects on neurons) (see Figure 6.1). This may explain the psychiatric symptoms that develop at times when the sex hormones are reduced, for example, premenstrual syndrome, menopause, and chemical castration for men. Additionally researchers have found that some steroid hormone levels drop in patients who panic during an attack. Others have shown that medications such as olanzapine and fluoxetine—known to decrease anxiety—increase steroid hormone levels.

SLOW RECEPTORS: METABOLIC

Starting in the 1950s, researchers teased out the details of a second type of receptor—one that activates a cascade of biochemical events in the cytosol of the receptor cell that ultimately modifies the function of target proteins or the DNA. This type of receptor, called a *G-protein–coupled receptor*, is perhaps even more relevant to the effect of psychiatric medications than the transmitter-gated ion channel. G-protein is the short form for guanosine triphosphate–binding protein. Although there are many types of G-protein–coupled receptors, the basic style involves three steps:

1. A neurotransmitter binds to the receptor.
2. The receptor activates the G-protein, which moves along the intracellular membrane.
3. The G-protein activates the "effector" protein.

The activated "effector" protein can have a variety of functions including just opening traditional ion channels (not shown). However, the more interesting effector proteins are enzymes that trigger a process called a *secondary messenger cascade* (Figure 5.4). The neurotransmitter activates the G-protein, which slides along the membrane and stimulates the effector protein. The activated effector protein then converts adenosine triphosphate into cyclic adenosine monophosphate (cAMP): the secondary messenger, which will diffuse away into the cytosol where it can change the neuronal operations. With the exception of serotonin type 3 receptor (5-hydroxytryptamine3 [5-HT3]), all

TREATMENT ANTIEPILEPTIC DRUGS

The background about inhibitory and excitatory receptors helps one understand the major mechanisms of action of the antiepileptic drugs (AEDs). The goal of treatment with these medications is to modify the aberrant bursting properties, synchronization, and spread of abnormal firing without affecting ordinary electrical activity. These effects, although intended to control seizure disorders, have wide-ranging applications to other neuropsychiatric disorders such as bipolar affective disorder, anxiety, pain, and alcohol dependence, to name a few.

The major effects of the well-known AEDs fall into three categories and are shown in the table below. The first involves the voltage-gated sodium channel discussed in Chapter 3. Remember that these are the pores that allow rapid entry of sodium into the cell to propagate the action potential along the axon. Modulation of these channels is believed to account for some of the effectiveness of several AEDs. The second category involves the voltage-gated calcium channels, which are located on the terminals of the neuron and instigate the release of neurotransmitters into the synaptic cleft. Blockade of these channels decreases the neurotransmitter release and ultimately decreases excitability.

The final mechanism of action involves the GABA receptor and increasing inhibition, for example, barbiturates and benzodiazepines as mentioned above. Additionally, valproate and gabapentin increase GABA synthesis and turnover, with the net effect of increased activity of these inhibitory neurons. It is easy to understand the rationale for trying medications with different mechanisms of action when one medication fails to control the disorder.

The Mechanisms of Action for Some of the Well-Known Antiepileptic Drugs

	Sodium Channels $\geq$	Calcium Channels $\geq$	GABA System
Phenytoin	X	—	—
Carbamazepine	X	—	—
Lamotrigine	X	X	—
Valproate	X	X	↑ turnover
Gabapentin	—	X	↑ turnover
Phenobarbital	—	X	X
Benzodiazepines	—	—	X

GABA, γ-aminobutyric acid.

the monoamine receptors belong to the G-protein–coupled family—which means that most psychiatric medications deliver their punch through secondary messengers.

Serotonin Receptors

The original discovery of the serotonin receptor led to two subtypes: 5-HT1 and 5-HT2. Further discoveries, especially the application of molecular

POINT OF INTEREST

Autoreceptors reside on the cell body or terminal of the *presynaptic neuron*. They sense the presence of the neurotransmitter and provide negative feedback to the neuron. That is, if too much of the neurotransmitter is present, these receptors activate a second messenger and turn off further release of the neurotransmitter—and in some cases reduce synthesis of the neurotransmitter. The figure shows an example of this type of receptor using the 5-HT$_{1A}$ (anxiety-related) and 5-HT$_{1D}$ (migraine-related) receptors. Similar autoreceptors are known for other transmitters such as dopamine and norepinephrine. Blocking these specific receptors may provide unique ways to alleviate specific symptoms.

FIGURE 5.4 ● The initiation of the second messenger cascade starts with a neurotransmitter binding with the G-protein receptor and ends with the conversion of ATP into cAMP. ATP, adenosine triphosphate; cAMP, cyclic adenosine monophosphate; GTP, guanosine triphosphate; GDP, guanosine diphosphate.

cloning techniques, has resulted in multiple subdivisions of these two receptors and the addition of several more for a total of 14. Although the prospect of activating or blocking the various receptors for further refinement of psychopharmacologic treatment is an enticing possibility, the clinical results with a few exceptions have been limited.

The 5-HT$_1$ receptors make up the largest subtype with 5-HT$_{1A}$, 5-HT$_{1B}$, 5-HT$_{1D}$, 5-HT$_{1E}$, and 5-HT$_{1F}$. 5-HT$_{1A}$ has received the most interest and seems to play a prominent role in depression and anxiety. It is an autoreceptor on the cell body. Stimulation of this receptor reduces cell firing and curtails the release of serotonin. How this would improve mood is unclear, but blocking

this receptor has decreased the effectiveness of tricyclic antidepressants in rat models of depression. The anxiolytic buspirone (Buspar) is a partial 5-HT$_{1A}$ agonist, which suggests that 5-HT$_{1A}$ has some role in anxiety. The development and distribution of buspirone is an example of how a specific serotonin receptor is targeted for the development of a medication.

The 5-HT$_{1D}$ receptor is also an autoreceptor but is located on the nerve terminal at the synapse. Here it appears to function to sense the serotonin in the synaptic cleft and turn off release of more serotonin when stimulated. The 5-HT$_{1D}$ receptor is stimulated by the antimigraine drug sumatriptan (Imitrex), although the importance of this effect in the overall efficacy of the medication is unclear. Some researchers are exploring the effectiveness of a 5-HT$_{1D}$ receptor antagonist for the treatment of depression. The goal is to block the negative feedback mediated through the 5-HT$_{1D}$ receptor so that more serotonin is released into the synapse.

Some other important serotonin receptors for the psychiatrist are 5-HT$_{2A}$ and 5-HT$_{2C}$. The 5-HT$_{2A}$ receptor has been identified as playing an important role in the "atypicalness" of the second-generation antipsychotic agents (clozapine, risperidone, and olanzapine). These newer agents have a greater capacity to block 5-HT$_{2A}$ than the traditional agents such as haloperidol, and it is speculated that this results in the observed decrease in extrapyramidal symptom (EPS) and mediation of the negative symptoms of schizophrenia.

Dopamine Receptors

The dopamine receptors are involved in a wide range of functions including locomotion, cognition, psychosis, and even neuroendocrine secretion. It became clear after 1979 that there was more than one dopamine receptor: D$_1$ and D$_2$. More recently with molecular cloning they have identified three more receptors: D$_3$, D$_4$, and D$_5$. The D$_3$ and D$_4$ receptors are "D$_2$-like" and the D$_5$ receptor is "D$_1$-like." However, the D$_1$ and D$_2$ receptors remain the most important.

$$\text{"D}_1\text{-like"} = \text{D}_1 \text{ and D}_5$$

$$\text{"D}_2\text{-like"} = \text{D}_2, \text{D}_3 \text{ and D}_4$$

The D$_1$ and D$_2$ receptors have been distinguished by their differing affinity for binding with traditional antipsychotic agents such as haloperidol: The D$_2$ receptor has high affinity, whereas the D$_1$ receptor has low affinity. Increased D$_2$ receptor antagonism correlates with the therapeutic efficacy and EPS side effect with the traditional antipsychotics. There is great interest in the "D$_2$-like" receptors (D$_3$ and D$_4$) as possible alternative sites for therapeutic potentiation with antipsychotic agents, but as yet these receptors have failed to translate into clinically significant benefits.

The psychostimulants (cocaine, amphetamine, and methylphenidate) work in part by blocking the reuptake of dopamine and leaving more dopamine in the synapse to stimulate the dopamine receptors. The effects are increased energy, improved cognition, and even psychosis. The effects on reward and cognition seem to be more prominently mediated by the D$_1$ receptor. Augmenting D$_1$ and D$_2$

receptors (agonists) is the mainstay of treatment for Parkinson's disease.

Adrenergic Receptors

The adrenergic receptors are divided into three main subtypes α_1, α_2, and β. Each one of these has three subtypes: α_{1a}, α_{1b}, α_{1d}, α_{2a}, and so on. We focus on the three main subtypes. The α_1 receptor is believed to play a role in smooth muscle contraction and has been implicated in effecting blood pressure, nasal congestion, and prostate function. Although widely expressed in the central nervous system (CNS), the central role of the $\alpha 1$ receptor remains to be determined; locomotor activation and arousal have been suggested by some studies. Stimulation of the $\alpha 1$ receptor may synergistically increase the activity of the serotonin neurons in the raphe nucleus, although stimulation of the α_2 receptor may have just the opposite effect.

The α_2 receptor subtypes in the CNS inhibit the firing of the norepinephrine neurons through autoreceptors. This mechanism of action is believed to mediate the sedative and hypotensive effects of the α_2 receptor agonist clonidine. Additionally, stimulation of the α_2 receptors decreases sympathetic activity that may explain the therapeutic utility of clonidine for suppressing the heightened sympathetic state for patients in opiate withdrawal.

The β receptor subtypes are more famous for their part in slowing cardiac rhythm and lowering blood pressure. The functions of the β receptors in the CNS, although widely distributed, are not well understood. It is not uncommon to use a β blocker, for example, propranolol, for treating performance anxiety or antipsychotic-induced akathisia. Whether these benefits come from a central or peripheral blockage of the β receptor, or both, is not known.

Histamine Receptors

There are now four histamine receptors although H$_4$ is predominately in the periphery and only recently discovered. The H$_1$ receptor is the target for the classic antihistamines, which highlights its role in sedation and conversely arousal. Of great interest to psychiatrists is the role of H$_1$ in weight gain. Recent analysis has shown that the potential to gain weight with antipsychotic agents correlates with the antagonism for the H$_1$ receptor, for example, clozapine and olanzapine have the most affinity for weight gain, whereas aripiprazole and ziprasidone have the least.

The H$_2$ receptor is more traditionally associated with the gut. Blockade of the H$_2$ receptor has been a widely used treatment for peptic ulcer disease. The H₃ receptor functions as an inhibitory receptor on the histamine neurons as well as other nonhistamine nerve terminals. The role of this receptor is not clearly understood, but it may be involved in appetite, arousal, and cognition.

Cholinergic Receptors

It was with the cholinergic receptor that scientists first realized that one neurotransmitter (ACh) could have different receptors. The initial subtypes were identified and named after the drug that distinguished its effect. For example, nicotine will stimulate cholinergic receptors in skeletal muscle, but not in the heart. Conversely, muscarine will stimulate the heart, but has no effect on skeletal muscle. Therefore, the two receptors can be identified by the actions of different drugs and the receptors were named after those drugs: nicotinic and muscarinic. Unfortunately, it has been hard to find a drug with unique action on each receptor subtype, so we are stuck with designations such as 1A and 2B.

Many more subtypes of the nicotinic and muscarinic receptors have been identified since the early days of receptor delineation, but the significance of these various subtypes for the psychiatrist remains obscure. Clearly, ACh is important in cognition and memory as noted by the benefits of inhibiting acetylcholinesterase as a treatment for Alzheimer's disease. Likewise, the blockage of the muscarinic receptor by tricyclic antidepressants and antipsychotic medications results in troublesome dry mouth, constipation, and urinary hesitancy (which we generically call the anticholinergic side effects). However, the importance of one receptor subtype over another has not been shown.

DISORDER

Myasthenia gravis is an autoimmune disease in which the body produces antibodies to the nicotinic ACh receptor. Patients complain of weakness and fatigue in the voluntary muscles resulting from the interruption of the chemical signal at the neuromuscular junction. Muscarinic receptors in the heart and CNS are unaffected.

ACh, unlike the monoamines, is cleared from the synaptic cleft by an enzyme, acetylcholinesterase. One treatment for myasthenia gravis is with the acetylcholinesterase inhibitors such as edrophonium (Tensilon) that prolong the life of the released ACh.

SIGNALING THE NUCLEUS

After the neurotransmitter has stimulated the G-protein to slide across the membrane and activate an enzyme (which is the case with most of the catecholamines), a cascade of events with second messengers transpires to modify neuronal function. Neurons use many different second messengers as signals within the cytosol—two of which we have discussed: Ca²⁺ and cAMP. The secondary messengers regulate neuronal function by activating enzymes that will add a phosphate group (*phosphorylation*) to other proteins in the cell. The *protein kinases*, of which there are wide varieties, are the enzymes that add a phosphate group to other proteins. Protein kinase A and calcium/calmodulin protein kinase are two examples of this type of enzyme. Once proteins are phosphorylated, they are "turned on" and can execute a broad range of cellular functions such as regulating enzyme activity or ion channels.

Additionally, the protein kinases can induce our two favorite words—*gene expression*. The protein kinases can "turn on" the DNA and start the synthesis of messenger ribonucleic acid. This process takes longer but can have large and relatively stable effects on the cell, for example, upregulation of receptors or the production of growth factor proteins. Figure 5.5 shows an example of how two different types of receptors—a G-protein–coupled receptor and a transmitter-gated ion channel—can activate a second messenger that will stimulate the production of new proteins.

LONG-TERM POTENTIATION: A SUMMARY EXAMPLE

Understanding long-term potentiation (LTP) is a way to apply what has been discussed in the past few chapters to a topic of great relevance to neuroscience: learning and memory. LTP is a laboratory example of learning that was discovered accidentally. As we have seen, applying a single stimulus to a neuron generates an excitatory impulse (EPSP) in the cell. Applying high-frequency stimuli—hundreds of impulses within a second—generates a higher EPSP in the cell. What was found accidentally was that once a neuron has been exposed to high-frequency stimulation, something changes, and now a single stimulus will generate a high EPSP. This sort of change has been shown to last for several months if not longer. Figure 5.6 shows these three steps.

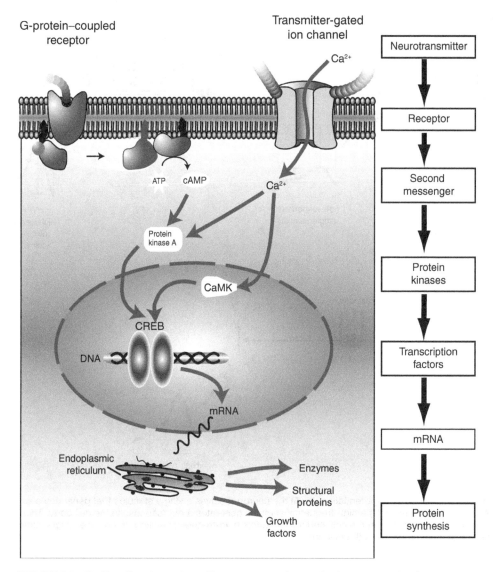

FIGURE 5.5 ● Signaling the nucleus. The neurotransmitters stimulate a cascade of events that ultimately leads to activation of the DNA (gene expression) and the synthesis of proteins that can modify the function of the cell. ATP, adenosine triphosphate; cAMP, cyclic adenosine monophosphate; CaMK, calcium/calmodulin protein kinase; CREB, cyclic adenosine monophosphate response element binding; mRNA, messenger ribonucleic acid.

LTP sounds like one of those topics that neuroscientists discuss ad nauseam, but which has little relevance to practicing clinicians. *Oh contraire*! LTP is a demonstration—although artificial—that neurons can incorporate lasting changes, which is an essential step to developing memories and skills. And what is life without memories? Unfortunately, some people are haunted by memories. LTP is an example, at the cellular level, of what

may happen for people who experience overwhelming trauma and develop posttraumatic stress disorder.

Furthermore, the changes brought about with LTP can be analyzed at the molecular level. Researchers have shown that both glutamate receptors (NMDA and AMPA) must be operational for the process to work. Likewise others have shown that calcium (a second messenger) and the kinases

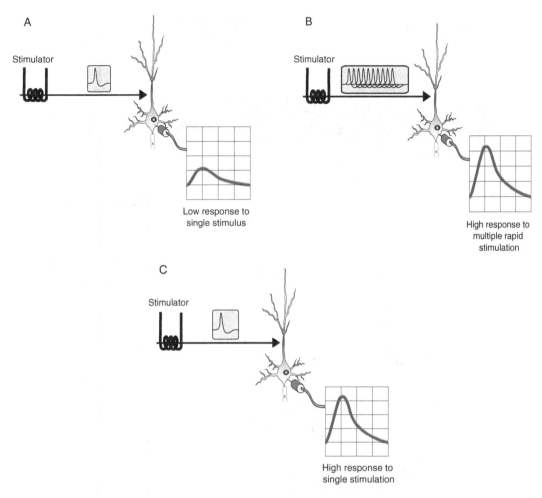

FIGURE 5.6 ● Long-term potentiation. In (**A**) the neuron receives a single stimulus that generates a small impulse in the cell body. In (**B**) a high-frequency stimulus generates a big response in the cell body. This process changes something in the cell, and following this high-frequency testing, the original single stimulus (**C**) generates a big response in the cell body.

are required for LTP. Of even greater interest is the demonstration that protein synthesis (gene expression!) is an essential part of the development of LTP. All the processes shown in Figure 5.5 are involved in LTP.

What happens inside the cell with the induction of LTP? Clearly there is some strengthening of the connection between the two cells that are communicating when LTP occurs. Figure 5.7 depicts the events that transpire when the presynaptic cell is hyperstimulated, the postsynaptic cell signals its nucleus, and the connection between the two cells is enhanced by the insertion of more glutamate receptors. Additional evidence has shown that a retrograde signal such as nitric oxide diffuses

back across the synaptic cleft and induces the presynaptic neuron to release more transmitters. The combined result is increased sensitivity and responsiveness at the synapse: more transmitters and more receptors resulting in a stronger signal.

Amazingly, the structural changes to the synapse can actually be seen under the right experimental circumstances. Engert and Bonhoeffer filled neurons from the hippocampus with fluorescent dye and then induced LTP. They captured the development of new spines on the postsynaptic dendrite as shown in Figure 5.8. This research is consistent with other data that suggest that the development of spines is possibly the structural manifestation of learning and memory.

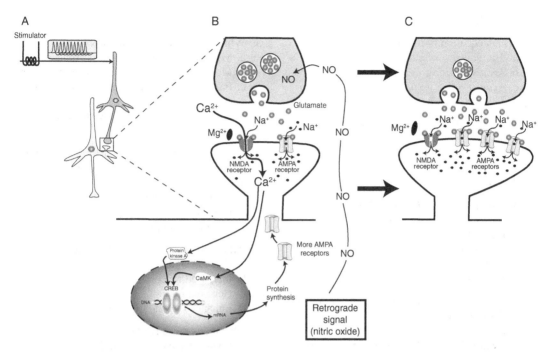

FIGURE 5.7 ● LTP inducing a change at the synapse. **A.** Hyperstimulation of the presynaptic neuron. **B.** The NMDA and AMPA receptors open, allowing the entry of the second messenger, calcium, which signals the nucleus to synthesize more receptors. **C.** The new AMPA receptors are inserted into the membrane, which has the effect of increasing the cell's responsiveness to future stimulation. LTP, long-term potentiation; NMDA, N-methyl-D-aspartate; AMPA, α-amino-3-hydroxy-5-methyl-4-isoxazole propionate.

TRANSCRANIAL MAGNETIC STIMULATION

LTP has not been established in humans for obvious ethical reasons. Repetitive transcranial magnetic stimulation offers a possible noninvasive method of stimulating conscious human subjects that can mimic the effects of LTP. The prospect of inducing long-lasting changes to the human cortex through noninvasive stimulation offers the prospect of a new kind of treatment applicable to a wide range of mental disorders.

Preliminary studies have demonstrated changes in motor skills consistent with changes seen with LTP when subjects receive continuous stimulation at the motor cortex. The changes lasted up to 60 minutes beyond the period of stimulation. Although the utility of a change lasting only 60 minutes is of little clinical value, the prospect of altering the function of the cortex without breaching the blood–brain barrier is an exciting possibility.

LTP demonstrates that electrical, molecular, and structural changes are involved in the process of storing information. It is a small leap to conclude that highly charged events in our lives—the emotional equivalent of high-frequency stimulation—leave enduring changes to neuronal connections in a manner similar to LTP.

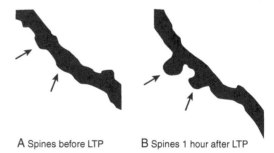

A Spines before LTP   B Spines 1 hour after LTP

FIGURE 5.8 ● With the induction of LTP in neurons from the hippocampus, new spines developed on the dendrite within an hour as shown by the *arrows*. LTP, long-term potentiation. (Adapted from Engert F, Bonhoeffer T. Dendritic spine changes associated with hippocampal long-term synaptic plasticity. *Nature*. 1999;399(6731):66-70.)

QUESTIONS

1. Which equation is correct?
   a. *Antagonist = stimulate.*
   b. *Agonist = block.*
   c. *Agonist = transmitter.*
   d. *Antagonist = endogenous ligand.*

2. Which is not a glutamate receptor?
   a. NMDA.
   b. cAMP.
   c. AMPA.
   d. Kainate.

3. The strength of the GABA inhibitory signal is enhanced by all of the following except
   a. Ethanol.
   b. Phenobarbital.
   c. Carbamazepine.
   d. Neurosteroids.

4. The AEDs exert their major effects through all of the following except
   a. Decreasing glutamate activity.
   b. Modulation of the voltage-gated sodium channels.
   c. Blockade of the voltage-gated calcium channels.
   d. Increasing GABA activity.

5. Which of the following is true?
   a. Mg^{2+} is a common second messenger.
   b. Most monoamine receptors are fast receptors.
   c. Fast receptors typically lead to gene expression.
   d. Autoreceptors give negative feedback to the neuron.

6. Gene expression stimulated by a neurotransmitter involves all of the following except
   a. Phosphorylation.
   b. Long-term potentiation.
   c. Protein kinases.
   d. G-protein–coupled receptor.

7. All of the following about LTP are true except
   a. Enhanced EPSP.
   b. Increased receptors.
   c. Gene expression.
   d. Enhanced ligand binding.

8. Which describes LTP best?
   a. It was discovered by accident.
   b. Neuroscientists love to pontificate on this topic.
   c. It is an example of learning.
   d. All of the above.

See Answers section at the end of the book.

CHAPTER 6

Genetics and Epigenetics

Woody Guthrie, the Depression-era folk singer ("This Land Is Your Land"), developed Huntington's disease late in his thirties. The disease is an autosomal dominant neurodegenerative disorder, which often is not expressed until middle age. Woody's son, Arlo Guthrie, who popularized the Vietnam era song about Alice's Restaurant, has not developed the disorder as he did not inherit the deviant gene from his father. Huntington's disease is an example of simple Mendelian genetics—one dominant gene leads to the disorder. With other simple Mendelian disorders, such as cystic fibrosis and sickle cell disease, the affected individual must inherit two recessive genes—one from each parent. (Single gene changes with large effects.)

Unfortunately, the genetic patterns of the common psychiatric disorders are not this simple. As a matter of fact, they remain incomprehensibly complex. We have yet to find a gene or a set of genes that can explain any major psychiatric disorder. Analysis of the human genome has revealed that the genetic mechanisms are more complex than we had imagined. Furthermore, events from the environment (toxins, abuse, isolation, etc.) can alter gene expression by changing the molecules **around** the DNA. The genetics of mental illness remains a mystery.

HERITABILITY OF MENTAL ILLNESS

There is no question that psychiatric disorders are genetically linked. The twin and adoption studies (Figure 1.1 and Table 1.1) show that behavioral traits and mental illness run in families. The DNA that puts individuals at risk for mental disorders is passed from parent to child. Geneticists use the term *heritability*, which they define as the proportion of observed variance in a group of individuals that can be explained by genetic variance. What does that mean? Well, heritability (h^2) of a trait is the total proportion of the total variance that is genetic ($h^2 = V_G/V_P$). Clear as mud. A better way to understand heritability is shown in Table 6.1.

Kenneth Kendler created the scale in Table 6.1 to correlate heritability percentages with common traits. Language and religion have zero genetic influence. Asian babies raised by American families speak English without an accent and vice versa. At the other extreme of the scale is height. In the absence of malnutrition or a pituitary tumor, height is almost completely determined by the genes inherited from the parents. Monozygotic twins rarely differ in height by more than half an inch.

The heritability of psychiatric disorders is placed next to this scale for comparison. We cannot think of any psychiatric condition that does not have some genetic influence. Even traumatic brain injury, which should be the result of a random accident, is probably linked to impulsive and risk-taking genes. The common

---

JARGON

The comedian Steve Martin said, "Those French...they have a different word for EVERYTHING!!!" At times, it seems like geneticists are speaking French, only without the passion. For example, gene is the term to describe a unit of heredity—a portion of DNA that codes for proteins or RNA. An allele is one of two or more forms of the DNA sequence for a gene. Such a gene is polymorphic. It gets worse. For example, the protein catechol-O-methyltransferase has a common polymorphism (Val158Met) at the chromosome 22q11.2. Ugh! We try to minimize the jargon and stick to simple terms. Sacré bleu!

TABLE 6.1

Benchmarks for a Scale of Heritability for General Traits and Psychiatric Disorders

Human Traits/Diseases	Heritability (%)	Heritability of Psychiatric Conditions
Language, religion	0	
Myocardial infarct, breast cancer	20–40	Anxiety, depression, and eating disorders
Cholesterol, blood pressure	40–60	Alcohol and drug dependence
Weight, intelligence	60–80	
Height	80–100	Schizophrenia, bipolar disorder, autism, and ADHD

ADHD, attention-deficit/hyperactivity disorder.

psychiatric disorders have moderate heritability, while the serious mental disorders have strong genetic components. The take-home message is clear—mental disorders are influenced by genes, although some more than others. But which genes are causing the problems? First, a word about the human genome.

HUMAN GENOME PROJECT

Genome is the term used to refer to the sum total of genetic information in a particular organism. The human genome is the entire DNA code contained in the chromosomes in each nucleated cell. The Human Genome Project was a large international scientific study focused on sequencing the nucleic acids (called base pairs) for the entire human genome. It was the Manhattan Project for biologists. They started in 1990 and completed the project in 2003. Important findings included the following:

- the human genome is made up of 3 billion base pairs,
- less than 2% of the DNA codes for proteins, and
- there are only approximately 23,000 protein-coding genes.

Although it is hard to find an example in which the Human Genome Project has advanced our medical treatment, it certainly has transformed our conceptualization of the storage of genetic information. The most shocking aspect is that we have so few protein-coding genes—just about 23,000. This is a bit unsettling especially when one considers that *Caenorhabditis elegans* (a flat worm ~1 mm in length) has about 20,000 protein-coding genes. The governor of South Carolina seems so much more intelligent than a flat worm, yet they have about the same number of protein-coding genes. How can this be? Clearly, there is more to complexity than the total number of protein-coding genes.

Protein-Coding Genes

For decades, the central dogma of biology purported that DNA makes RNA, which in turn makes proteins. Here is the key point: it was presumed that proteins orchestrate all the important functions in a cell—regulatory, metabolic, structural, etc. So, how can the governor of South Carolina and a flat worm have roughly the same number of protein-coding genes? The answer seems to be hidden in the other 98% of the genome that is not coding for proteins. This portion of the genome, which has been called "junk DNA," was presumed to be useless, inert DNA that was only there to connect the important sections together. In fact, the "junk DNA" is more active and more important than most people had imagined.

It's an RNA World

A new respect for the "junk DNA" developed after the mouse genome was sequenced and compared with the human genome. Mice and people share many of the same protein-coding genes—this was expected. However, much to everyone's amazement, the two species also share vast regions of "junk DNA." This was remarkable because the mouse and human lineage diverged over 75 million years ago. If large sections of "junk" DNA were preserved over that time, then they must be important for the function of the cell. Equally revealing, it appears that the complexity of an organism is related to non–protein-coding DNA. Figure 6.1

Percentage of genome that is non-protein coding

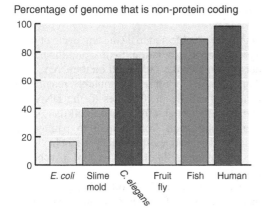

FIGURE 6.1 ● The percent of the genome that does not code for proteins increases as the complexity of the organism increases. This may explain why the governor of South Carolina is more complex than a *C. elegans*. (Adapted from Taft RJ, Pheasant M, Mattick JS. The relationship between non-protein-coding DNA and eukaryotic complexity. *BioEssays*. 2007;29:288-299.)

shows how the percent of non–protein-coding DNA increases with the complexity of the organism.

Further evidence of the importance of RNA comes from analysis of the transcriptional activity of the DNA. Even though less than 2% of the DNA codes for proteins, fully 85% of the genome is transcribed into RNA. The scientific literature has exploded with a dazzling array of various newly discovered non–protein-coding RNA molecules that differ from our old friend messenger RNA (see Figure 3.2). Molecules with such names as microRNA, long non-coding RNA, and small nucleolar RNA are examples of RNA that are transcribed throughout the genome. Even introns, the RNA spliced out of the protein-coding messenger RNA, seem to be functional. Figure 6.2 shows a schematic representation of the new conceptualization of the genome.

FIGURE 6.2 ● **A.** It used to be so simple. DNA made RNA, which made proteins. **B.** Now it appears that there are fewer protein-coding genes and much more non–protein-coding RNA.

A New Level of Gene Regulation

We know the cell would not expend energy transcribing the DNA into RNA if it was not beneficial. But what are all the non–protein-coding RNA molecules doing? Some of the functions that have been identified are as follows:

- Maintain DNA integrity,
- Transcriptional regulation,
- Post-transcriptional modification,
- Viral defense, and
- Epigenetic modification.

MicroRNA provides a good example of what the non–protein-coding RNA may be doing in the cell. MicroRNAs have the capacity to silence gene expression by blocking the messenger RNA. MicroRNAs have complementary nucleic acids that bind to the nucleic acids on the messenger RNA, effectively shutting down any translation of the mRNA into protein—like putting gum in a typewriter. Mechanisms such as this and others that are beyond the scope of this book enable non–protein-coding RNA to affect and influence gene expression.

This new view of the genome is relevant for mental illness because non–protein-coding RNA is highly expressed in the brain. Small changes in these RNA molecules can affect the expression of multiple genes and may underlie neurodevelopmental, neurodegenerative, and psychiatric disorders. Recent studies have shown that some microRNAs are downregulated while others are upregulated in schizophrenia.

AN RNA WORLD

The origins of life in the primordial world remain a mystery. The development of a mechanism to pass along the instructions for building, maintaining, and replicating the cell was an essential step for sustaining any life form. It has been assumed that life started with DNA. Yet, DNA requires proteins to build RNA, which in turn makes the required proteins. It is a chicken-and-egg dilemma. New thinking postulates that RNA was the original hereditary molecule. Lincoln and Joyce from the Scripps Research Institute recently created a self-replicating RNA that can, by itself, reproduce indefinitely. It is possible DNA was developed later in evolution as a more stable form of storage and proteins evolved as molecules more adapted to control the functions of the cell.

FINDING THE OFFENDING GENES

Our DNA is subjected to a constant cycle of damage and repair. Radiation, toxins, and the natural decay of molecules take a toll on the DNA. Most damage is irrelevant as it is quickly repaired or results in cell death. Changes to the DNA that endure can have an effect on the cell that occurs along a spectrum from benign to pathogenic. Finding the changes that affect the behavior of the organism is the Holy Grail of psychiatric genetics.

It is easier to find the offending genes if the pathophysiology of a disease is known. For example, an abnormal type of hemoglobin is known to be the cause of sickle cell anemia, and the errant gene has been identified down to the single altered nucleotide. The pathophysiologies of psychiatric disorders, however, remain obscure. For many years, the prevailing theories about psychiatric pathology developed from the effects of psychiatric medications—the monoamine hypothesis or dopamine hypothesis—what we call the "chemical imbalance" theories. However, analyses of genes that control for serotonin and dopamine or their receptors have failed to locate abnormalities that correlate with the frequency of the disorder. When such genes are identified, they are either too common in the unaffected population or fail to replicate in further studies.

Single Genes

Linkage Studies

Prior to the era of genome-wide studies, we used to read reports linking a specific gene or chromosomal region with a particular disease. This was done by analyzing families with an illness and searching for the genes. Figure 6.3 shows a pedigree for an Amish family with bipolar disorder. The heritability of the disorder is readily apparent. The location of the gene or genes causing the problem is much harder to find.

Researchers used linkage studies to narrow down the location of the problematic gene. Linkage studies are based on the understanding that genes are located on the arms of chromosomes and that during meiosis some swapping of genes occurs between the arms. The closer two genes are to each other on the chromosome arm, the more "linked" they are. Consequently, using known locations for various genes, and the co-occurrence with the disorder, researchers can estimate where the gene might be. In this situation, the gene was narrowed down to the tip of the short arm of chromosome 11. Unfortunately, and this is the problem

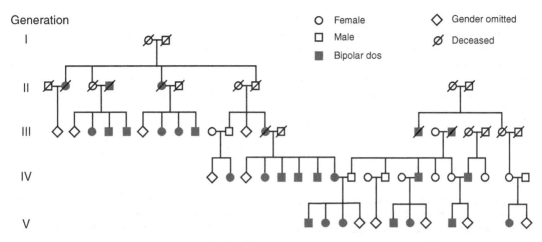

FIGURE 6.3 ● The high prevalence of bipolar disorder in this Amish family is shown in this pedigree. Linkage studies suggested a single gene located on chromosome 11. (Adapted from Law A, Richard CW 3rd, Cottingham RW Jr, Lathrop GM, Cox DR, Myers RM. Genetic linkage analysis of bipolar affective disorder in an Old Order Amish pedigree. *Hum Genet.* 1992;88:562-568.)

with most single gene studies, subsequent research failed to replicate the initial finding.

Few single gene linkage studies have yielded enduring results for mental illness. The apolipoprotein E gene is one exception. The E4 allele (there are three common alleles) is associated with late-onset Alzheimer's disease. People with two copies of the gene have 15 times the risk of developing the disease. People with any copies of the gene who sustain head trauma suffer more residual cognitive problems. Unfortunately, there are few other single gene linkage studies with such significant findings in our field. Furthermore, the Human Genome Project has transformed the search to identify the pathogenic genes.

Many Small Changes

Single Nucleotide Polymorphism

If single problematic genes do not cause the common psychiatric disorders, then maybe the disorders arise from many minor changes—not one big bang but the cumulative effect of many small hits. Small changes in the DNA are one-letter variations called single nucleotide polymorphisms (SNPs—pronounced "snips") (Figure 6.4). Genome-wide studies have identified that humans have numerous SNPs that seem to have little effect on observable characteristics (phenotype) of the person. For example, James Watson (of Watson and Crick fame) had his genome sequenced. They discovered he had 3.3 million SNPs. Of interest, 10,000 of the SNPs occurred in protein-coding genes, which

might have caused a malfunction in building an important protein—yet he won a Nobel Prize and is alive in his eighties.

Many of the common SNPs co-occur with various diseases. However, the majority of people who have a particular SNP do not develop the disease—that is, a particular SNP by itself has a

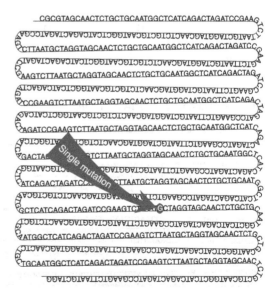

FIGURE 6.4 ● A hypothetical example of a single nucleotide polymorphism. In this single strand of DNA, a "C" has been replaced with a "G." This is roughly one nucleotide change in a strand of 1,000 nucleotides, which is about the difference between any two humans.

low predictive value of developing the disease. But maybe common diseases are caused when enough of the common SNPs show up in the same unlucky person. So, the natural next step has been huge studies with large numbers of subjects attempting to correlate numerous SNPs with the disease states. Unfortunately, the studies thus far have been a big disappointment. The results continue to have low predictive value.

Structural Variation

Copy Number Variation

It was not until 1956 that geneticists could identify and count the number of human chromosomes—called karyotyping. They were surprised to find 46 chromosomes instead of 48 as they had expected. Subsequently, curious clinicians looked at the chromosomes of children with inherited disorders. In

1959, Jérôme Lejeune, a French pediatrician and geneticist, karyotyped the chromosomes in children with Down syndrome—what was called mongolism at the time. Lejeune discovered that these children had an extra chromosome, which was later identified as chromosome 21 (Figure 6.5 A).

The presence of the extra chromosome in Down syndrome, or in some cases just an extra part of the chromosome, has profound effects on the cognition and physical development of the child. While it is not clear what molecular problems result from the additional DNA, we know something goes awry. It may be that the extra DNA results in excessive gene expression, which overwhelms the precise mechanisms of normal development—like having too many cooks in the kitchen.

Henry Turner, an endocrinologist in Illinois, first reported in 1938 a syndrome in girls of short

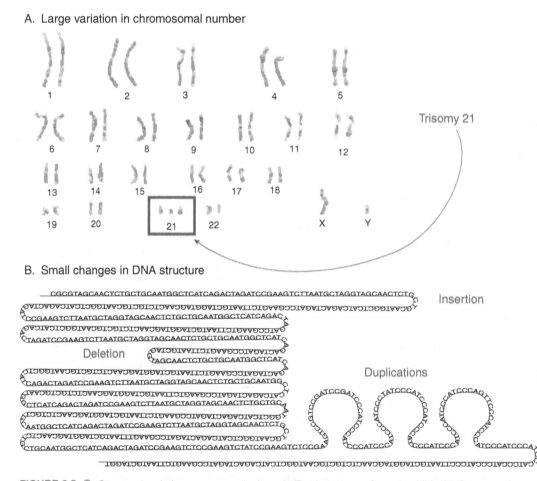

FIGURE 6.5 ● Structural variation—macro and micro. **A.** The karyotype of a male child with Down syndrome showing the addition of an extra chromosome. **B.** Copy number variations are smaller insertions, deletions, or duplications within the DNA strand.

stature and undeveloped secondary sexual characteristics. It was not until 1959 that the syndrome, which has since taken his name, was recognized as resulting from the absence of an X chromosome. Affected women have 45 chromosomes—only one X. Down syndrome and Turner syndrome are examples of genetic abnormalities at the macro level—large additions or deletions in the total quantity of DNA. SNPs, on the other hand, are at the other end of the spectrum—single-letter changes. There is a spectrum of alterations between these two extremes (whole chromosome additions/deletions and SNPs) and these are called copy number variations (CNVs).

CNV is a term that describes small insertions, deletions, or duplications within the DNA molecule (Figure 6.5B). CNVs range in size from hundreds up to millions of base pairs of DNA. Remarkably, they are harder to detect than SNPs because CNV detection requires microarray technology, which is different from the method used to sequence the genome. Recently, attention has turned to the role CNVs may play in mental illness. Many labs are comparing CNVs in normal populations with those in patients with disorders. Studies suggest that CNVs play a role in schizophrenia, autism, and attention-deficit/hyperactivity disorder (ADHD). The recent study in ADHD highlights some of the problems. Four hundred and ten children with ADHD were compared with 1,156 healthy, matched controls. Fourteen percent of the ADHD children had large rare CNVs, while only 7% of the controls had similar genetic deficits. While this is a significant difference, it is also disappointing for it shows that most children with ADHD do not have CNVs and many healthy controls do.

Missing Heritability
In spite of the technological advances in analyzing the genome, the genetic causes of the common medical and psychiatric disorders remain elusive. At this time, a good family history remains more clinically useful than expensive genetic sequencing. Where is the missing heritability? One answer is that the genetic mechanisms are more complicated than previously expected. Another answer may be that events from the environment can alter the genome, further complicating the picture. This is the topic of the next section.

EPIGENETICS
Every nucleated cell in the body contains a complete copy of the organism's genetic code. Cardiac cells, liver cells, and neurons all contain the same DNA. Yet, only a fraction of the genes in any particular cell are expressed. Most are literally switched "off," so that only the appropriate DNA is transcribed for any given cell line. During embryonic development, different cell lines emerge by turning on some genes (at the appropriate time) and turning off all the rest.

Understandably, transcription is under tight control in any cell. Having the correct "key" to a particular gene is one mechanism the cell uses to limit transcription. Each gene has a sequence of DNA called the promoter region that signals the starting point for RNA synthesis. Transcription factor proteins specific for that promoter, along with RNA polymerase, bind with the DNA and synthesize RNA (Figure 6.6). (Less is known about the control of transcription of non–protein-coding RNA.) Another mechanism to control gene expression is for a cell to limit access to the promoter region. Remarkably, events during the course of one's life can affect these mechanisms.

Unfolding the DNA
The DNA in each of our 46 chromosomes is one long strand of a double-helix fiber, which would measure approximately a meter if laid end to end. The cell must package these strands into the nucleus (Figure 6.7). This is accomplished by using dense proteins called histones—vacuum storage bags at the cellular level. The DNA, which is negatively charged, wraps around a series of positively charged histones. These "beads on a string" are then folded into a compact structure called chromatin. The chromatin is further coiled and folded to form the chromosome.

The histones do more than just package the DNA. They also regulate gene expression. DNA is inaccessible to regulatory signals when it is folded in its chromatin structure. Transcription factors cannot initiate gene expression when they cannot physically reach the promoter region of the DNA. Transcription of the gene requires the unfolding of the chromatin, the unwrapping of the histone, and the exposure of the promoter region.

Epigenetics
The attachment of other molecules to the DNA or histones can have a tremendous impact on gene expression. Epigenetics (literally meaning "above the genetics") has come to mean changes in gene expression that take place without a change in the sequence of A, T, C, and G nucleotides. In other words, the specific genetic code is not changed, but the accessory molecules hanging on the nucleotides

FIGURE 6.6 ● Transcription factors and RNA polymerase (A) must combine and lock onto the promoter region of the gene before the DNA can be transcribed into mRNA (B).

and/or histones may alter gene expression. In particular, the addition (or subsequent removal) of methyl or acetyl groups to the DNA or the histone proteins can alter access to the promoter region of the gene. Typically methyl groups decrease gene expression, while acetyl groups increase gene expression.

FIGURE 6.7 ● The DNA must be properly packaged to fit into the nucleus. For gene expression (transcription) to occur, the appropriate section must be unfolded and exposed.

Cytosine

FIGURE 6.8 ● **A.** Addition of a methyl to the cytosine nucleotide. **B.** Methylation of the promoter region of the gene prevents transcription factors from locking onto the DNA and prevents gene expression, which silences the gene.

DNA Methylation

DNA methylation is the best understood of the epigenetic alterations. DNA methylation involves the addition of a methyl group (CH_3) to one of the nucleotides—in this case cytosine (Figure 6.8). The methyl group is only a problem when it is added to cytosines found in the promoter region of genes. DNA methylation of the cytosine nucleotide in the promoter region effectively silences that gene by preventing the transcription factors from binding with the DNA. If transcription cannot get started, gene expression does not occur.

Chromatin Remodeling

Chromatin remodeling is another epigenetic mechanism regulating gene expression. The addition or deletion of various molecules to the histone proteins can affect the structure of the chromatin. The chromatin structure can be more tightly wrapped or more loosely exposed depending on which molecules are attached to the histone. Open chromatin structure allows greater access to the promoter region of a gene and enhances gene expression.

There are many molecules that can be attached to the histone, but the two most widely reported in behavioral studies are methyl and acetyl groups. The methyl groups tend to compress the chromatin structure and silence the gene. Acetylation, on the other hand, opens up the chromatin structure and allows the transcription factors greater access to the DNA and hence greater gene expression (Figure 6.9).

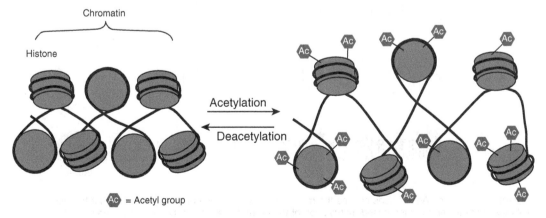

FIGURE 6.9 ● The addition of acetyl groups to the histones opens up the chromatin and allows greater access to the genes. The result is generally increased gene expression.

Environmental Events and Epigenetics

Now, this is where it gets really interesting! It turns out stimuli from the environment (toxins, radiation, trauma, etc.) can alter gene expression through epigenetic mechanisms. Physical or emotional events during one's life can literally alter gene expression through epigenetic mechanisms—without changing the genetic code. For example, smoking can increase the risk of cancer through epigenetic mechanisms. Smoking can turn off tumor suppressor genes. Without the tumor suppressor genes producing suppressor proteins, tumors can grow unimpeded. The individual's behavior has negative health effects through epigenetic mechanisms.

Epigenetics may also explain why identical twins do not always develop the same diseases—an issue broached in Chapter 1. Although genetically identical, the twins do not live identical lives and grow increasingly discordant for epigenetic markers as they age. Figure 6.10 shows chromosome 17 stained for methylation from two sets of twins—one 3 years old and the other 50 years old. The methylation pattern is practically identical in the young twins, but much more out of synch in the older twins. The events of one's life are recorded on the epigenome.

Agouti Gene

The Agouti gene in mice is a wonderful example of how environmental factors—in this case the mother's diet—can affect health through epigenetic changes. The Agouti gene is a problem. It not only turns the mouse's hair yellow but also predisposes

FIGURE 6.10 ● Color is used to show similar or discordant methylation patterns for each set of twins. The study suggests that epigenetic markers, similar when young, change over the course of one's life. (Adapted from Fraga MF, Ballestar E, Paz MF, et al. Epigenetic differences arise during the lifetime of monozygotic twins. *Proc Natl Acad Sci U S A.* 2005;102:10604-10609.)

it to diabetes, obesity, and cancer. Fortunately, the Agouti gene can be turned off if the promoter region in front of the gene is methylated—transcription factors cannot attach to the gene and it is silenced. This is good for the mouse. Figure 6.11 shows the results of a study by Waterland and Jirtle analyzing the methylation of the Agouti gene and the coat of the mouse. More methylation results in a browner, and healthier, mouse.

What is more remarkable is that a mother's diet when she's pregnant can affect the methylation of the Agouti gene in her pups. Mother mice fed a supplemental diet high in methyl groups (folic

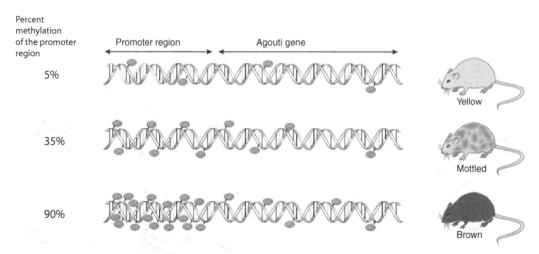

FIGURE 6.11 ● The Agouti gene causes the mouse to have a yellow coat and predisposes it to obesity, diabetes, and cancer. With increased methylation of the promoter region of the gene, the gene is not expressed and the mouse is brown and healthy.

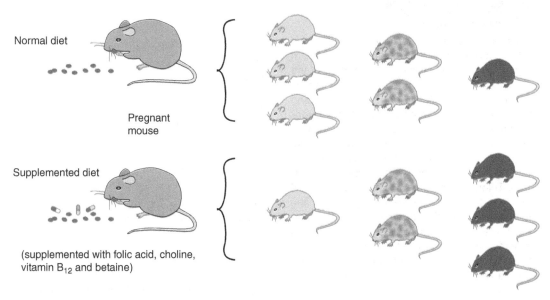

Normal diet

Pregnant mouse

Supplemented diet

(supplemented with folic acid, choline, vitamin B_{12} and betaine)

FIGURE 6.12 • Pregnant mice fed a supplemental diet high in methyl groups will produce more pups with a silenced Agouti gene due to increased methylation of the gene.

acid, vitamin B_{12}, choline, and betaine) will produce a greater percentage of brown, healthy pups (Figure 6.12). This study shows a clear connection between an environmental event (in this case diet) and subsequent epigenetic effects on physical appearance and health.

A fascinating study conducted in Sweden suggests that the diet of our **grandparents** has enduring epigenetic effects on our health. Researchers studied a small, isolated community in northern Sweden, which was subjected to periods of feast and famine in the 19th and early 20th centuries. People who enjoyed bountiful harvests during their preadolescent years had grandchildren who died younger. On the other hand, people who were underfed when they were between the ages of 8 and 12 sired grandchildren who lived longer. In other words, the diet of our grandparents during their preadolescent years may have epigenetic effects that are passed on to future generations. If this is true, what will the current epidemic of obesity in children have on future generations?

Epigenetics is of particular relevance in understanding mental illness. We know that environmental events (trauma, relationships, drugs, poverty, etc.) play a large role in the development of mental disorders. Epigenetic mechanisms may explain the link between events in the environment and gene expression. It is a topic that appears frequently in the coming chapters.

Perhaps one reason it is so hard to find the genes of mental illness is that epigenetic factors obscure the real culprits. If the genome is the hardware of inheritance, then epigenetics describes the software. A problem with *both* the hardware (the actual genetic code) and the software (the environment and how life events affect gene expression) would be especially difficult to identify.

Multifactorial

All mental disorders result from some problem with gene expression: too much or too little—either starting during embryonic development or beginning later in life. Yet, finding the genes involved remains hidden at this point. The genome has proved to be more complex than we imagined. Disorders are likely caused by hundreds of additions, substitutions, or deletions, each having a small effect. Epigenetic effects compound the difficulty of finding the offending genes. Furthermore, what appears to be one illness such as anxiety or schizophrenia could be many different conditions with a similar effect on a final common pathway behavior. This has been observed with the genetics of the different epilepsy syndromes. Clearly, the predisposition to a major mental illness is to some degree inherited, but the sources of the errors are too numerous and mysterious to identify with our current technology. The search continues.

TELOMERE

Telomeres are the molecular caps on the end of each strand of DNA. Like a knot at the end of a rope, they identify the terminal portion of the chromosome. This ensures that the enzymes that repair the DNA will not mistake the end for a break in the strand and attempt to connect it to some other free end—a process that normally preserves the DNA, but under these circumstances scrambles the genetic code.

Telomeres shorten with every cell division. Telomere shortening is an inevitable and unfortunate consequence of aging. As the telomeres grow shorter, the cells eventually reach the limit of their replicative capacity and progress to senescence or death (apoptosis). Consequently, telomere length can be considered a rough measure of cell age (see figure below).

Patients with mental disorders have been found to have accelerated shortening of their telomeres. Patients with mood disorders, schizophrenia, Alzheimer's disease, and a history of childhood abuse have shorter telomeres when compared with healthy controls. Exercise appears to preserve telomere length.

Adapted from Calado RT, Young NS. Telomere diseases. *N Engl J Med*. 2009;361:2353-2365.

Cancer is the result of cells that replicate continuously and without constraint. The telomeres—although small—are preserved. In many cancers, an enzyme called telomerase is produced that adds nucleotides back on to the end of the DNA and preserves the telomeres—and the cell. Actually every cell has the capacity to synthesize telomerase, but few do. Some people speculate that harnessing telomerase may be the fountain of youth.

THE NEUROSCIENCE MODEL

Up to this point in this book, we have been reviewing the basic parts of the brain. We started with the big organ and got increasingly small: from cortical structures, to cells, down to molecules. In this chapter, we have gone to the deepest level, the DNA—where it all begins. If you view this sequence of chapter in the opposite order, genes to molecules to cells to networks to behaviors and then the effects of the behaviors on the DNA, this is what we call the neuroscience model (Figure 6.13). It is the most up-to-date model for understanding normal behavior and mental illness.

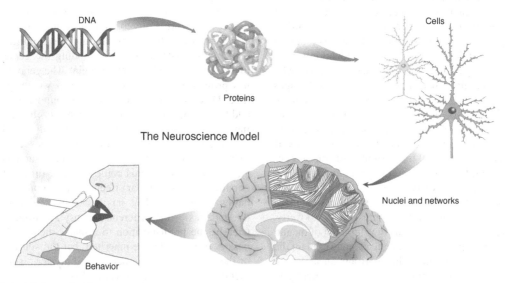

The Neuroscience Model

FIGURE 6.13 ● The neuroscience model. Although the term is not used, this is the prevailing model of understanding the physiology of normal behavior and mental illness.

QUESTIONS

1. Why does the governor of South Carolina have so few protein-coding genes?
   a. The governor believes protein-coding genes are another example of too much government control.
   b. The governor is closely related to *C. elegans.*
   c. The governor sold off the vast majority of protein-coding genes in an attempt to balance the state budget.
   d. Because much of the complexity of the human species is controlled by other parts of the DNA.

2. All of the following lead us to believe "junk DNA" is important except
   a. Non–protein-coding sections are highly expressed in the brain.
   b. RNA has more capacity to control functions in a cell than previously recognized.
   c. Defects in "junk DNA" have been identified in autism.
   d. Some microRNAs have been implicated in schizophrenia.

3. What has happened to the "chemical imbalance" theories of mental illness in the genomic era?
   a. Genome-wide studies fail to implicate genes that are associated with neurotransmitters or their receptors.
   b. Genes for the serotonin receptor have been identified in families with bipolar disorder in multiple linkage studies.
   c. The dopamine transporter gene on chromosome 11 is altered in most patients with childhood-onset schizophrenia.
   d. A significant number of patients with panic disorder lack the gene for the A section of the GABA receptor.

4. Understanding epigenetics helps us understand
   a. Why non–protein-coding sections are so highly expressed in the brain.
   b. How events in the environment can alter gene expression.
   c. The cognitive effects of trisomy 21.
   d. The increased potential for insertions, deletions, and duplications in the seriously mentally ill.

5. Which of the following is most accurate?
   a. Methylation increases gene expression and acetylation increases it.
   b. Methylation increases gene expression and acetylation reduces it.
   c. Methylation reduces gene expression and acetylation increases it.
   d. Methylation reduces gene expression and acetylation reduces it.

6. All of the following are true of the Agouti gene in mice except
   a. Methylation of the promoter region produces more brown pups.
   b. What the pregnant mothers eat can have enduring effects on the pups' DNA.
   c. Pups with less expression of the Agouti gene are healthier.
   d. A pregnant mother's diet high in polyunsaturated fats will silence the Agouti gene.

7. All of the following are true about telomeres except
   a. Identify the terminal end of a chromosome.
   b. They are altered by the diet of one's grandparents.
   c. Shorter with increasing replication.
   d. Are believed to correlate with some mental disorders.

See Answers section at the end of the book.

SECTION II

Modulators

CHAPTER 7

Hormones and the Brain

CHARACTERISTICS OF A HORMONE

In the preceding chapters, we reviewed the electrochemical connection between neurons. This is the predominant method of communication within the brain and the focus of much attention from psychiatrists. The next four chapters describe systems that modulate the electrochemical connections. We start with hormones—molecular messengers sent through the bloodstream.

Neurons and neurotransmitters can be compared with telephone wires connecting one phone to another. Hormones are like TV signals that are broadcast across the skies and only recognized by appropriate receivers. With the advent of cell phones and cable TV, the distinction between direct and broadcast communication has blurred. This blurring has also occurred in the brain—traditional neurotransmitters sometimes function as hormones and hormones sometimes function as neurotransmitters. For example, epinephrine can be a neurotransmitter, but functions as a hormone when released from the adrenal medulla with a signal from the sympathetic division of the autonomic nervous system (ANS).

Although they can act in a similar manner, hormones differ from neurotransmitters in several key ways. Hormones tend to do the following:

1. Effect behavior and physiology in a gradual manner over days and weeks.
2. Receive reciprocal feedback.
3. Secrete in small pulsatile bursts.
4. Vary the levels on a circadian rhythm.
5. Have different effects on different organs.

The last point (no. 5) is of great interest to us and will be a large part of the focus of this chapter.

The γ-aminobutyric acid (GABA) receptor provides an example of a hormone modulating an electrochemical communication. Steroid hormones, as well as other molecules, influence the GABA receptor (see Figure 5.3). Figure 7.1 shows how a progesterone metabolite enhances the influx of Cl⁻ ions through the GABA receptor. This will reduce the potential of the postsynaptic neuron to fire, effectively calming the neuron. This may explain the emergence of psychiatric symptoms with sex hormone fluctuations.

The difference between hormones and neurotransmitters is further blurred by the existence of *neuroendocrine* cells (sometimes called *neurosecretory cells*). Neuroendocrine cells are hybrids of neurons and endocrine cells (Figure 7.2). They receive neural signals, but secrete a hormone into the bloodstream. For example, the neuroendocrine cells of the hypothalamus receive electrical impulses from the cerebral cortex and then signal the pituitary through the bloodstream.

Classification

There are three types of hormones, which can be grouped by their chemical structure: (a) protein, (b) amine, and (c) steroid (Table 7.1). Protein hormones, such as neuropeptides, are large molecules composed of strings of amino acids. Amine hormones are small molecules derived from amino acids. Steroid hormones are composed of four interlocking rings synthesized from dietary cholesterol.

Effecting Target Cells

Hormones have two primary effects on target cells:

1. Promote differentiation and development.
2. Modulate the rate of function.

Hormones bind to specific receptors on or in the target cell in three ways. Most of the protein

73

FIGURE 7.1 ● The Cl⁻ current is enhanced when a progesterone metabolite is added to γ-aminobutyric acid (GABA). (Adapted from Rupprecht R, Holsboer F. Neuroactive steroids: mechanisms of action and neuropsychopharmacologic perspectives. *Trends Neurosci.* 1999;22(9):410-460.)

and amine hormones exert their effects by binding with receptors imbedded in the cell wall (as is the case with the classic neurotransmitters). The steroid hormones and thyroid hormones are

Neurotransmitter

Endocrine

Neuroendocrine

FIGURE 7.2 ● Chemical communication systems in humans.

TABLE 7.1

The Major Classes of Hormones

Protein Hormones
  Oxytocin
  Vasopressin
  Releasing Hormones
      Corticotropin-releasing hormone (CRH)
      Thyrotropin-releasing hormone (TRH)
      Gonadotropin-releasing hormone (GnRH)
      Growth hormone–releasing factor (GHRF)
Tropic Hormones
      Adrenocorticotropic hormone (ACTH)
      Thyroid-stimulating hormone (TSH)
      Luteinizing hormone (LH)
      Follicle-stimulating hormone (FSH)
      Growth hormone (GH)
      Prolactin
Amine Hormones
  Epinephrine
  Norepinephrine
  Thyroid hormone
  Melatonin
Steroid Hormones
  Estrogens
  Progestins
  Androgens
  Glucocorticoids
  Mineralocorticoids

lipophilic and can pass directly through the cell wall. They bind with receptors inside the cell. The steroid hormones bind with a receptor in the cytoplasm, which initiates protein synthesis when the complex couples with the DNA. The thyroid hormone receptor belongs to a family of nuclear hormone receptors. These receptors reside in the nucleus on the gene and suppress gene expression until activated by thyroid hormone (specifically T₃). Figure 7.3 shows these three different receptors.

   In all cases, the hormones change the function of the target cell by stimulating gene expression. This process is called a *genomic effect*. Some

FIGURE 7.3 ● The three types of receptors utilized by different hormones. CREB, cyclic adenosine monophosphate response element binding; cAMP, cyclic adenosine monophosphate.

hormones effect neurons without stimulating the transcription of genes by modulating ion receptors: a *nongenomic effect*.

CENTRAL NERVOUS SYSTEM AND HORMONES

The primary endocrine glands in the brain are the hypothalamus and the pituitary gland. The hypothalamus appears to be the command center that integrates information about the state of the brain and the body by way of neuronal projections and intrinsic chemosensitive neurons. The hypothalamus coordinates the actions of the pituitary gland to maintain homeostasis in response to changes in the body and environment. Some of the essential somatic functions controlled by the hypothalamus and pituitary gland are as follows:

1. Control of blood flow (e.g., drinking, blood osmolarity, and renal clearance).

2. Regulation of energy metabolism (e.g., feeding, metabolic rate, and temperature).
3. Regulation of reproductive activity.
4. Coordination of response to threats.
5. Control of circadian rhythms.

The remarkable number of functions governed by these relatively small glands is possible due to the diversity of neuronal projections sent to the hypothalamus from the brain, as well as up the spinal cord. Additionally, the hypothalamus and pituitary gland have a multitude of intrinsic chemosensitive neurons that respond to circulating levels of various hormones. The pituitary gland, as well as some areas of the hypothalamus, is an area of the brain not protected by the blood–brain barrier. This allows for quicker feedback about the current status of target organs.

Of particular interest to behavioral neuroscientists are the direct afferent projections the hypothalamus receives from areas of the brain with well-known psychiatric functions. Four of these important projections are as follows:

1. Corticohypothalamic fibers: frontal cortex.
2. Hippocampohypothalamic fibers: hippocampus.
3. Amygdalohypothalamic fibers: amygdala.
4. Thalamohypothalamic fibers: thalamus.

These afferent fibers play a large role in the stimulation, or lack of stimulation, to the hypothalamus and the pituitary gland that results in many of the endocrine abnormalities found during different behavioral conditions.

Figure 7.4 shows the complex relationship among the cortex, hypothalamus, pituitary gland,

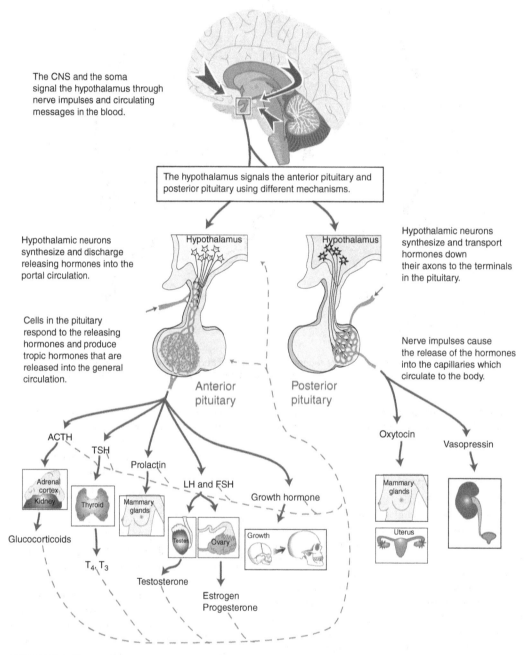

FIGURE 7.4 ● Information from the cerebral cortex and bloodstream converges on the hypothalamus, which instigates a cascade of actions and in turn responds to feedback from the target organs. CNS, central nervous system; ACTH, adrenocorticotropic hormone; TSH, thyroid-stimulating hormone; T₄, tetraiodothyronine; T₃, triiodothyronine; LH, luteinizing hormone; FSH, follicle-stimulating hormone.

Releasing hormones	CRH	TRH	PRH	GnRH	GHRH	Hypothalamus
Tropic hormones	ACTH	TSH	Prolactin	LH and FSH	Growth hormone	Anterior pituitary
Target organs	Adrenal cortex Kidney	Thyroid	Mammary glands	Testes Ovary	Growth	
Peripheral hormones	Gluco-corticoids	T_4, T_3		Testosterone Estrogen Progesterone		

FIGURE 7.5 ● The anterior pituitary. Releasing hormones excreted by the hypothalamus stimulate the release of tropic hormones from the anterior pituitary. The tropic hormones then stimulate the target organ to change or release its own hormone. CRH, corticotropin-releasing hormone; TRH, thyrotropin-releasing hormone; PRH, prolactin-releasing hormone; GnRH, gonadotropin-releasing hormone; GHRH, growth hormone–releasing hormone; ACTH, adrenocorticotropic hormone; TSH, thyroid-stimulating hormone; LH, luteinizing hormone; FSH, follicle-stimulating hormone; T_4, tetraiodothyronine; T_3, triiodothyronine.

and target organs for the neuroendocrine system. The figure illustrates the central location of the hypothalamus, the two sides of the pituitary, the variety of target organs affected, and the feedback mechanisms. Figure 7.5 shows most of the hormones associated with the anterior pituitary gland, particularly the releasing hormones excreted by the neuroendocrine cells of the hypothalamus, which stimulate the release of the tropic hormones.

While most of the hormones affect the brain in one way or another, we only focus on the two systems most relevant to mental illness: the hypothalamic-pituitary-thyroid (HPT) axis and the hypothalamic-pituitary-adrenal (HPA) axis.

THYROID: THE HYPOTHALAMIC-PITUITARY-THYROID AXIS

Thyroid hormones are involved in maintaining optimal metabolism in nearly every organ system and are integral to the temperature regulation of the body. The secretion of thyroid hormones is controlled by the HPT axis shown in Figure 7.6. The neuroendocrine cells in the hypothalamus secrete thyrotropin-releasing hormone (TRH) into the portal circulation of the pituitary. TRH binds with receptors on the thyrotroph cells of the anterior pituitary and stimulates the release of thyroid-stimulating hormone (TSH). The hypothalamic

neuroendocrine cells also synthesize and release somatostatin, which inhibits the release of TSH (as well as growth hormone).

TSH stimulates the synthesis and release of two thyroid hormones from the thyroid gland: triiodothyronine (T_3) and tetraiodothyronine (T_4). T_4 is the predominant form of thyroid released by the gland, but T_3 is the more biologically potent form. T_4 is converted into T_3 by the target organs as well as the brain.

In humans, congenital hypothyroidism causes severe structural and functional neurologic abnormalities known as cretinism. This disorder is easily corrected, but a disaster if missed. It is one of the few medical conditions routinely screened for in the newborn nursery.

The role of thyroid hormones in the maintenance of the mature brain is less understood. The brain maintains tight control over the level of thyroid hormone in the central nervous system (CNS), and thyroid nuclear receptors are highly expressed throughout the brain, particularly within the hippocampus. Clinical features of hypothyroidism and hyperthyroidism, including significant neuropsychiatric symptoms, are described in Table 7.2.

Additionally, clinical studies have shown that the T_3 hormone can augment other medications used to treat patients with treatment-resistant depression, as well as accelerate the response

FIGURE 7.6 ● The hypothalamic-pituitary-thyroid axis showing the complex relationship between the brain and thyroid hormones. The important point is that tetraiodothyronine (T_4) and triiodothyronine (T_3) have direct effects on the brain as well as the body. CNS, central nervous system; TRH, thyrotropin-releasing hormone; TSH, thyroid-stimulating hormone.

TABLE 7.2

Common Clinical Features of Abnormal Thyroid Function

	Physical Symptoms	Psychiatric Symptoms
Hyperthyroidism	Tachycardia	Anxiety
	Weight loss	Irritability
	Heat intolerance	Trouble in concentrating
	Sweating	Emotionally labile
		Psychomotor agitation
Hypothyroidism	Fatigue	Depressed mood
	Weight gain	Decreased libido
	Cold intolerance	Psychomotor retardation
	Dry skin	Poor memory
		Severe forms: delusions and hallucinations

to antidepressants when initiating treatment for depression. However, meta-analysis of augmenting and accelerating studies found the trials to be small in number and not uniformly positive. The efficacy of liothyronine augmentation was compared with lithium augmentation as the third step for treatment-resistant depression in the STAR*D study. Both groups showed only modest remission rates (liothyronine 24.7% vs. lithium 15.9%) and were not statistically significantly different.

Thyroid hormones are important for the function of the adult brain, but the underlying molecular mechanism by which the HPT axis influences neuropsychiatric conditions remains unclear. Many authors in psychiatry postulate that the cognitive and emotional symptoms associated with thyroid disorders are related to changes in serotonin, norepinephrine (NE), and dopamine. Indeed, studies on rats have found increased serotonergic transmission concomitant with decreased 5-hydroxytryptamine (5-HT)$_{1A}$ sensitivity and increased

5-HT$_{2A}$ sensitivity with exogenous thyroid. With regard to NE, Gordan et al. have demonstrated anterograde transport of T$_3$ from the cell bodies in the locus coeruleus to the nerve terminals in the hippocampus and cerebral cortex. They believe that T$_3$ functions as a cotransmitter along with NE. This suggests that sufficient T$_3$ is needed for proper NE activity.

An alternative explanation for the influence of thyroid hormones on the psychiatric status of the mature brain revolves around their role with nerve growth factors. Nerve growth factor genes are activated by T$_3$ during development, although growth factors, such as brain-derived neurotropic factor (BDNF), are unaltered by thyroid hormone in the adult brain. Recently, Vaidya et al. established that 5-HT$_{1A}$ stimulation with chronic T$_3$ administration altered the production of BDNF in the hippocampus, although neither did so alone. They postulate a synergistic relationship between 5-HT$_{1A}$ receptors and thyroid hormones in the expression of BDNF (see Chapter 21 for more on the role of BDNF in depression).

The most compelling explanation for the correlation between mood disorders and thyroid hormones appears to be related to the general effect that thyroid has on brain metabolism, much like the effect on peripheral metabolism. Positron emission tomography studies on patients with hypothyroidism show global reduction in brain activity and as much as a 23% reduction in cerebral blood flow compared with controls. In a remarkable study at the National Institutes of Mental Health,

MOOD DISORDERS

Although it is clear that thyroid disorders cause neuropsychiatric symptoms and that adding thyroid hormone can accelerate and augment the treatment of mood disorders, relatively few psychiatric patients have thyroid disease. Two analyses of clinical patients with depression found a 2% to 2.5% incidence of thyroid disease. The researchers concluded that routine screening for thyroid disease was not justified. Furthermore, although some patients with affective disorders can have mild laboratory changes, often referred to as *subclinical thyroid disease*, almost all anomalies resolve with effective treatment of the psychiatric disorder.

ANOREXIA NERVOSA

Women with anorexia nervosa, when purging and undernourished, often have symptoms that resemble hypothyroidism (cold intolerance, bradycardia, low resting metabolic rate, etc.). Thyroid studies of patients in this condition have found low normal T_4, low T_3, and normal TSH. Additionally, reverse T_3, the metabolically inactive enantiomer of T_3, is increased. This thyroid profile is called *euthyroid sick syndrome*. It can be produced by starvation in normal volunteers and is corrected with weight gain.

This decrease in active T_3 thyroid profile seems like a physiologic adaptation to malnutrition, with the goal of preserving calories and limiting the expenditure of energy. Some patients with eating disorders will surreptitiously take exogenous thyroid to stimulate their metabolism and try to lose weight.

Marangell et al. examined TSH in medication-free patients with mood disorders, none of whom had overt thyroid disease. The study found an inverse relationship between TSH and global cerebral blood flow: TSH was up when cerebral blood flow was down. The areas with the greatest reduction in blood flow were the areas of the brain associated with depression: left dorsolateral prefrontal cortex (PFC) and medial PFC.

One can postulate that the hypothalamus responds to the reduced metabolism of the PFC (by way of the afferent fibers) as a result of the depression and reacts by stimulating the release of TSH. In essence, the HPT axis is seeking to correct the brain disorder.

HYPOTHALAMIC-PITUITARY-ADRENAL AXIS AND STRESS

The HPA axis controls the synthesis and release of the corticosteroids. The corticosteroids are derived from dietary cholesterol in the adrenal cortex and include the mineralocorticoids, sex hormones, and glucocorticoids (Figure 7.7). The mineralocorticoid aldosterone assists in the maintenance of the proper ionic balance by stimulating the kidney to conserve sodium and excrete potassium. The sex hormones are secreted in negligible amounts, but have physiologic significance, and are covered in more detail in Chapter 16. The hormone of greatest interest to the mental health community is the glucocorticoid cortisol.

Cortisol is of interest because it mobilizes energy (by promoting catabolic activity) and increases cardiovascular tone. At the same time, cortisol suppresses anabolic activity, such as reproduction, growth, digestion, and immunity. The release of cortisol varies throughout the day, with maximal secretion in the early morning hours to effectively prepare the brain and body for the rigors of the day. Cortisol also plays a large part in acute and chronic stress, which we discuss subsequently.

The secretion of the adrenal cortex is controlled by the hypothalamus (Figure 7.8). The hypothalamus, with input from the cortex and feedback through the blood, synthesizes and releases corticotropin-releasing hormone (CRH) into the portal circulation of the pituitary, which in turn stimulates the release of adrenocorticotropic hormone (ACTH) from the anterior pituitary. The input to the hypothalamus from the cortex includes inhibitory signals from the hippocampus and activating signals from the amygdala. In other words, a healthy hippocampus turns down the HPA axis, while an active amygdala turns it up. This is important in understanding the endocrine role in depression and anxiety.

POINT OF INTEREST

CRH is an example of a hormone that has multiple functions. The primary role of CRH is the stimulation of ACTH, but CRH receptors can be found throughout the brain, not just on the anterior pituitary, suggesting other, as yet unknown, effects for this hormone.

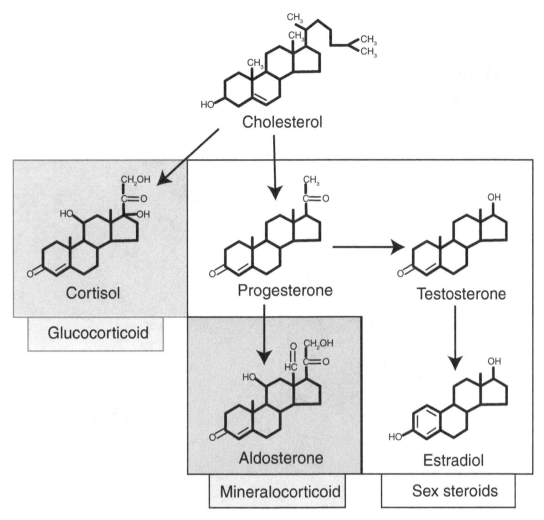

FIGURE 7.7 ● The corticosteroids are built from the sterol backbone of cholesterol by the addition or removal of side groups.

ACTH is released into the systemic circulation from the anterior pituitary. ACTH starts as a large propeptide precursor that is cleaved into smaller segments, some of which (such as ACTH) are biologically active (see Figure 16.13). ACTH stimulates the release of cortisol from the adrenal cortex. This has a variety of physiologic effects, including changes in the CNS. The high incidence of psychiatric symptoms in patients with primary endocrine disorders, such as Cushing's disease and Addison's disease, is supportive evidence of the direct effects of cortisol on the brain.

Stress

In his book *Why Zebras Don't Get Ulcers*, Sapolsky uses a clever example to illustrate the difference between the acute physical stress that a zebra experiences when running from a lion and the chronic psychological stress that many people experience in modern industrial societies. The acute response is the biologic equivalent of mobilizing troops to handle a perceived threat. The sympathetic activation by the ANS and the liberation of cortisol bring the body and brain to an alert, fight-or-flight orientation. Cortisol has the effect of mobilizing energy, increasing cerebral glucose, and turning down the nonessential functions (i.e., erections and digestions). Ultimately, the brain becomes more focused and vigilant.

The body and brain pay a price for maintaining a heightened state of alertness when the stress persists and the person cannot adapt. As seen with Addison's and Cushing's diseases, too little or too

FIGURE 7.8 ● The hypothalamic-pituitary-adrenal axis. Note that adrenocorticotropic hormone (ACTH) releases an array of hormones with a diurnal variation. As with all hormones, there are direct effects on the cerebral cortex. CNS, central nervous system; CRH, corticotropin-releasing hormone.

DISORDER ADDISON'S AND CUSHING'S DISEASES

Addison's disease, first described by Thomas Addison in 1855, results from a loss of cortisol and aldosterone secretion due to the near total or total destruction of both the adrenal glands. Classic symptoms include anorexia, nausea, and hypotension, along with neuropsychiatric symptoms of apathy, fatigue, irritability, and cognitive impairment.

Cushing's disease is named after neurosurgeon Harvey Cushing, who in 1932 linked adrenal hyperplasia and hypercortisolemia with a pituitary adenoma. The somatic effects of excessive cortisol include easy bruising,

truncal obesity, muscle atrophy, osteoporosis, and impaired immune response. The psychiatric symptoms are similar to endogenous depression: irritability, depressed mood, insomnia, and trouble with memory/concentration. Patients can also experience euphoria and even hypomania, as well as psychosis. However, these symptoms are more common in patients taking glucocorticoid medications. With both Addison's and Cushing's diseases, most psychiatric symptoms remit with the resumption of normal endocrine status.

much cortisol is pathologic. The benefits of cortisol can be graphed as an upside-down "U." Moderation is best.

Chronic stress is best defined as an adverse experience that induces heightened arousal over which one has little control. One of the effects of chronic stress is that the brain is unable to turn down the HPA axis, which exposes the brain and body to excess glucocorticoids. Although most of the data come from patients on glucocorticoid medications with Cushing's disease or from laboratory animal studies, the adverse consequences are believed to be similar to that of the harried stressed-out individual.

Pathologic consequences of heightened sympathetic activity and HPA activation are hypertension, formation of atherosclerotic plaque, diabetes, ulcers, and impaired immune function. In the brain, the most dramatic negative effect involves the hippocampus, a structure with ample glucocorticoid receptors and afferent fibers to the hypothalamus. The hippocampus is well known for its role in memory, and excess glucocorticoids have indeed been shown to have the following effects:

1. Impair memory performance.
2. Disrupt long-term potentiation (LTP).
3. Induce atrophy of hippocampal dendrites.
4. Shrink the hippocampus.
5. Decrease neurogenesis (next chapter).

These cognitive changes do not develop without an active amygdala. The amygdala, well known for its role in anxiety, is stimulated by glucocorticoids, which in turn potentiates the hippocampus (see Figure 7.9). Chronic stress increases the dendritic arborization of neurons in the basolateral amygdala, which may be a reason people have trouble forgetting traumatic events.

Cushing's Disease

Excessive glucocorticoid levels, for any reason, have been shown to cause impairments in declarative memory as well as hippocampal atrophy. In a remarkable analysis of patients with Cushing's disease who underwent neurosurgical resection, Starkman et al. showed that decreasing urinary cortisol correlated with increase in the hippocampal

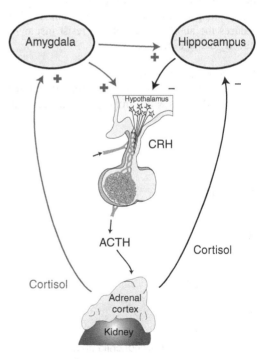

FIGURE 7.9 ● A schematic representation of the connections and feedback between the hypothalamic-pituitary-adrenal axis and the amygdala and hippocampus. CRH, corticotropin-releasing hormone; ACTH, adrenocorticotropic hormone.

volume. In a follow-up study, they showed that a greater improvement in memory (word list learning) was associated with greater increase in the hippocampal volume.

Aging

There is evidence that glucocorticoids may contribute to age-related neuronal atrophy and cognitive decline. An essential aspect of a healthy, adaptive stress response is the ability to shut off the system when the threat has passed. Studies on rats have shown that the HPA axis is slower to turn off as the animal ages. With age, it is exposed to more continuous high levels of glucocorticoids. In humans, the ability to turn off the HPA axis and the sympathetic nervous system in tranquil times is a variable trait. Some people are able to do this more effectively than others. Possibly this is a feature of being more resilient.

Lupien et al. followed up 51 healthy volunteers over 6 years and annually measured 24-hour plasma cortisol. They assessed memory and hippocampal volume in subgroups of those with high levels of cortisol and compared those findings with the groups with lower levels of cortisol. They found greater impairments in memory and a 14% reduction in the volume of the hippocampus in the group with high cortisol levels. This suggests that prolonged exposure to glucocorticoids either reduces the ability of neurons to resist insults or directly damages the neurons.

Depression and Anxiety

There is a long history of correlating alterations in the HPA axis with anxiety and depression.

A few recent studies demonstrate the application of new research to this correlation. One research group in the Netherlands has analyzed glucocorticoid receptor number before military deployment and then assessed psychiatric symptoms upon return from combat. Glucocorticoid receptors were indirectly measured from the dexamethasone binding capacity of peripheral leukocytes. In separate studies they found greater numbers of glucocorticoid receptors, predeployment, in those individuals who developed depression and PTSD. With PTSD, they found that with an increase of every 1,000 glucocorticoid receptors, the risk of developing the disorder increased 7.5-fold.

Another group at Emory University analyzed polymorphisms of the CRH receptor, history of child abuse, and depression as an adult (Figure 7.10). A greater incidence of child abuse predicted higher adult depression scores. However, genetic differences of the CRH receptor influence the subsequent depressed mood. In this case, and there were other genetic changes with similar results, having the two base pairs AA at this location protected the abused person from developing depression. The CRH receptor, child abuse, depression connection is an example of the current understanding of mental illness. That is, disorders develop in genetically vulnerable people who are exposed to detrimental environmental events.

Although the HPA axis seems to play an important role in psychiatric disorders, attempts to alter the HPA axis, for example, CRH blockers, have not yet proven to be effective treatments.

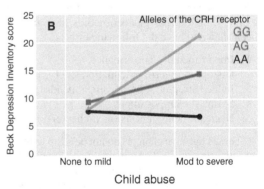

FIGURE 7.10 ● **A.** More incidence of abuse as a child led to increased depressive symptoms as an adult. **B.** Single nucleotide polymorphism of the corticotropin-releasing hormone (CRH) receptor alters the propensity of an abused individual to develop depression.

QUESTIONS

1. The primary mechanism by which the estrogen molecule stimulates the cell is?
   a. Binding to a protein receptor imbedded in the cell wall.
   b. Activating a G-protein-coupled receptor.
   c. Binding with a receptor in the cytoplasm.
   d. Coupling with a receptor in the nucleus.

2. Which of the following is true?
   a. Thyroid hormone can enhance the GABA current.
   b. Protein hormones bind a receptor on the DNA.
   c. Hormones are used for fast signals.
   d. Neuroendocrine cells excrete directly into the circulation.

3. Which of the following is correct?
   a. GnRH → LH → estrogen.
   b. GHRH → LH → testosterone.
   c. TRH → TSH → prolactin.
   d. CRH → TSH → cortisol.

4. Possible explanations for the role of thyroid hormone in mood disorders include all of the following except
   a. Changes in brain metabolism.
   b. Effects on growth hormones.
   c. Changes in glucocorticoid receptors.
   d. Effects on 5-HT receptors.

5. Women in the acute phase of anorexia nervosa exhibit a thyroid profile called "euthyroid sick syndrome," which includes all of the following except
   a. Low T_3.
   b. Low reverse T_3.
   c. Low to normal T_4.
   d. Normal TSH.

6. The triad of hippocampal atrophy, hypercortisolemia, and cognitive impairment has been found with all the following except
   a. Cushing's disease.
   b. Addison's disease.
   c. Alzheimer's disease.
   d. Major depression.

7. All of the following go together except
   a. Amygdala atrophy.
   b. Hippocampal atrophy.
   c. Memory deficit.
   d. LTP disruption.

See Answers section at the end of the book.

CHAPTER 8

Adult Development and Plasticity

In a video produced in 1996 by Robert Sapolsky for the Teaching Company entitled *Biology and Human Behavior*, Dr. Sapolsky stated

> To the greater extent you've got all the neurons you're ever going to have to deal with by the time we're 4 or 5 years old and, unfortunately, all you do from there is lose them.

Until recently this belief—stated by Dr. Sapolsky such a short time ago—was shared by almost all clinicians and neuroscientists. We are not criticizing Dr. Sapolsky, whose outstanding contributions to the field were cited in the previous chapter. Rather, we wish to show that even astute Stanford professors once believed the brain was a static organ. The authors of this book were no more enlightened at that time.

Additionally, an abundance of new research has established that the brain is not the fixed structure we used to envision. Our brains have more plasticity (or ability to change) than we previously imagined. Although the rate of change is especially prominent early in life, altering the structure of the brain in response to environmental factors remains a feature across the entire life span.

The almost unbelievable prenatal development of the central nervous system (CNS) is a topic we briefly touched on in Chapter 2. The fundamental miracle of the brain is that a single fertilized egg ultimately develops into 100 billion neurons with 100 trillion connections. In utero, this process is largely genetically driven. After birth, interactions with the environment play a greater role in determining the direction of development.

PHASES OF DEVELOPMENT

The cellular events can be divided into four phases:

1. *Neurogenesis*: The production, migration, and development of distinct new cell types—nerve or glial—from undifferentiated stem cells.
2. *Cell expansion*: The branching of axons and dendrites to make synaptic connections.
3. *Connection refinement*: The elimination of excessive branching and synaptic connections.
4. *Apoptosis*: Programmed neuronal cell death.

Neurogenesis

The cells of the intestinal epithelium are turned over every 2 weeks, whereas skin cells are replaced every 1 to 2 months. The adult brain is not nearly this prolific, but is not barren either. In 1998 unequivocal newborn neurons were identified in the hippocampus of elderly subjects whose brains were examined shortly after death. We now know that undifferentiated neural stem cells remain in the CNS and continue to divide throughout life (Figure 8.1). Neural stem cells can develop into neural precursors that grow into neurons or support cells. However, they must migrate away from the stem cell's milieu before they can differentiate, and only about half the cells successfully move and transform.

The locations and potential for division of stem cells in the adult human brain is a hot, controversial topic. Clear evidence for adult neurogenesis has been established in two areas of the brain: the subgranular zone (SGZ) in the hippocampus and the subventricular zone (SVZ) of the lateral

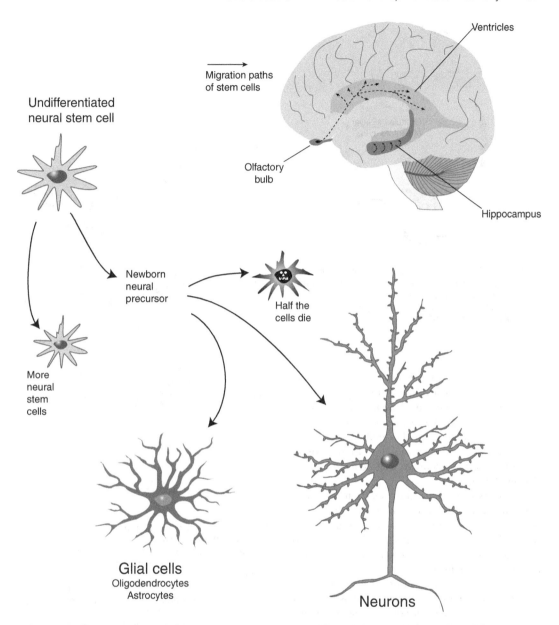

FIGURE 8.1 ● The process of neurogenesis starts with an undifferentiated neural stem cell that has the capacity to migrate and transform into functioning nerve cells. (Adapted from Gage FH. Brain, repair yourself. *Sci Am*. 2003;289(3):46-53.)

ventricles (Figures 8.2 and 8.3). Newborn cells are identified by tagging them with a molecule such as bromodeoxyuridine (BrdU), a thymidine analogue that can be incorporated into newly synthesized DNA. A florescent antibody specific for BrdU is then used to detect the incorporated molecule and thereby indicate recent DNA replication.

The SGZ is part of the hippocampus. The utility of creating new neurons in the hippocampus remains a mystery, but may facilitate the stabilization of new memories. The cells born in the SVZ, on the other hand, primarily migrate to the olfactory bulb. This might be helpful for a dog, but it is hard to imagine how this benefits the human brain. However, in 1999, Gould et al. identified newborn nerve cells in the neocortex (prefrontal, temporal, and parietal) of adult monkeys. They established that neural stem cells migrated through the white matter and differentiated into neurons and extended axons

FIGURE 8.2 ● The granule cell layer of just under the dentate gyrus (called the subgranular zone) is the most studied location of neurogenesis. (Adapted from Gage FH. Mammalian neural stem cells. *Science.* 2000;287(5457):1433-1438.)

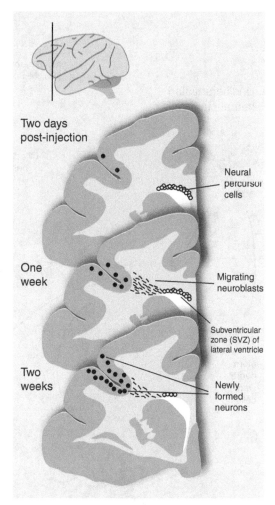

FIGURE 8.3 ● Adult macaque monkeys were injected with bromodeoxyuridine and sacrificed 2 hour, 1 week, and 2 weeks later. These sections from the prefrontal cortex show the development and migration of neural precursor cells from the subventricular zone (SVZ), through the white matter to the neocortex. Additional tests established that some of the cells were newly formed neurons. (Adapted from Gould E, Reeves AJ, Graziano MS, et al. Neurogenesis in the neocortex of adult primates. *Science.* 1999;286(5439):548-552.)

Figure 8.3). Unfortunately, the number of new cells is less than that found in the hippocampus or olfactory bulb and is inadequate for significant CNS repair. Future neurological treatments may come from finding methods (medications, exercise, magnetic stimulation, etc.) to invigorate the limited primate neurogenesis so as to replace damaged tissue.

A remarkable recent study seems to establish that adult neurogenesis does *not* generate new neurons that become working cells in the gray matter. Researchers utilized a remnant of the cold war to determine the age of neurons and nonneural brain cells in postmortem cortical biopsies.

Throughout the history of life, the amount of ^{14}C carbon in the atmosphere remained almost constant until above-ground nuclear bomb testing during the 1950s and 1960s resulted in an explosive increase in ^{14}C. The carbon isotope rapidly spread around the globe and was incorporated into any new organic molecules. Since the 1963 Test Ban Treaty, the amount of ^{14}C in the atmosphere has steadily decreased.

The amount of ^{14}C in a cell can be used to give an accurate date of the cell's birth when plotted on the known curves of ^{14}C available in the atmosphere over the last 50 years. For example, the ^{14}C in rings in a tree will match the ^{14}C in the atmosphere at the time that ring was formed. The neuroscientists in Sweden used this technique to determine the age of brain cells in seven individuals who died suddenly.

The researchers were able to separate nuclei of neurons and non-neuronal cells from various regions of the cortex. Then the DNA was extracted, analyzed for ^{14}C, and plotted on the known levels of ^{14}C in the atmosphere. The results are shown in Figure 8.4. These results seem to establish that all the adult human neurons in the *neocortex* were created perinatally and none since birth. Non-neuronal brain cells continued to form and were born, on average, 5 years after the birth of the individual. One limitation of this study is the exclusive use of healthy brains. We still do not know if new neurons replace damaged cells after trauma or ischemia.

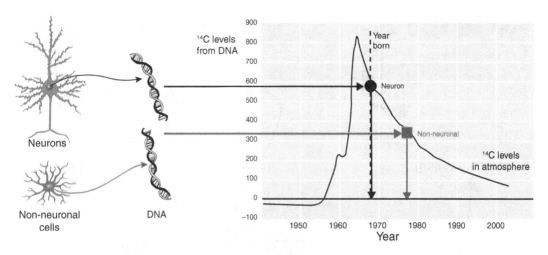

FIGURE 8.4 ● Postmortem analysis of ^{14}C levels in DNA from neurons and non-neuronal brain cells shows that the neurons were created at the time of this individual's birth. (Adapted from Bhardwaj RD, Curtis MA, Spalding KL, et al. Neocortical neurogenesis in humans is restricted to development. *Proc Natl Acad Sci U S A*. 2006;103(33):12564-12568.)

In summary, it appears that neurons are born in the SGZ and the SVZ throughout the life of mammals, but after birth they are not inserted as functional neurons into the cerebral cortex—at least in healthy brains. So why is it that the brain continues to make new neurons until we die?

Rate of Neurogenesis

The rate of neurogenesis is modulated by various factors. It is known that enriched environments and exercise will increase neurogenesis (Figure 8.5). Additional research suggests that gonadal steroid hormones may also enhance new cell production. For example, testosterone will stimulate nerve cell production in songbirds (and possibly middle-aged men seeking to recapture the vigor of their youth). The point is that various factors may promote neurogenesis and could be utilized as a part of treatment for neurological disorders.

POINT OF INTEREST

The studies establishing an increase in neurogenesis with enriched environments for mice have also documented increased size of the dentate gyrus of the hippocampus. Additionally, the mice showed improved memory performance on hippocampal-dependent memory tasks (water maze). These findings validate the link between neurogenesis, neuronal growth, hippocampal size, and memory.

Stress, on the other hand, has an inhibitory effect on neurogenesis. Extended maternal separation is a well-characterized model of early life stress for a rodent. As adults, such rodents will show protracted elevations of corticotropin-releasing factor, adrenocorticotropic hormone, and corticosterone (cortisol equivalent in a rat), as well as behavioral inhibition in response to stress. Work from Gould's laboratory has shown that rats exposed to prolonged maternal separation will have an enduring blunting of neurogenesis. When the corticosterone is experimentally lowered, the neurogenesis rebounds to normal levels—suggesting that hypersensitivity to corticosterone may be the mechanism of action that suppresses neurogenesis.

The relationship among early stress, the hypothalamic-pituitary-adrenal (HPA) axis, and neurogenesis is particularly interesting because of the role of the hippocampus in modulating the HPA axis. We can conceptualize that a healthy hippocampus is necessary to put the brakes on an activated HPA axis after the stressful event dissipates. The above research suggests that early stress (an unavailable mother) leads to a smaller hippocampus due to insufficient neurogenesis, which results in an overactive HPA axis and all those secondary problems discussed in the previous chapter.

Stem Cells

One potential way to rebuild a damaged brain is to implant human embryonic stem cells that have been isolated from a very immature embryo (only

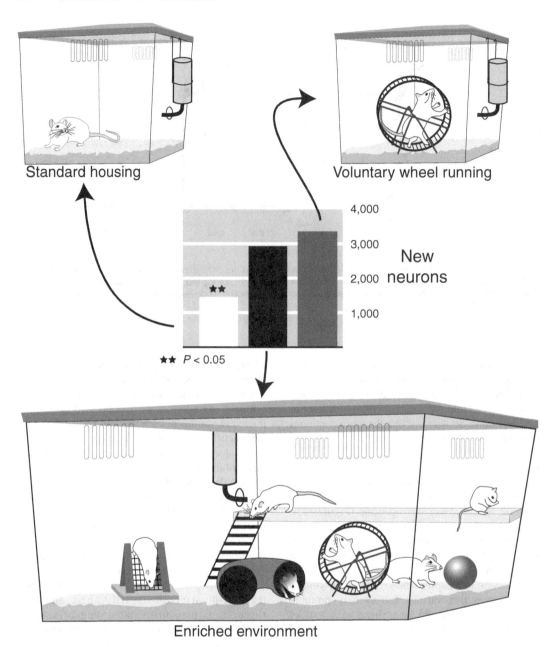

Standard housing

Voluntary wheel running

4,000

3,000

New

2,000 neurons

1,000

★★

★★ *P* < 0.05

Enriched environment

FIGURE 8.5 ● A study by Brown et al. showed that an enriched environment and physical exercise stimulated neurogenesis in the hippocampus but not in the olfactory bulb in mice. (Graph adapted from Brown J, Cooper-Kuhn CM, Kempermann G, et al. Enriched environment and physical activity stimulate hippocampal but not olfactory bulb neurogenesis. *Eur J Neurosci*. 2003;17(10):2042-2046.)

100 to 200 cells). So far it has been difficult to get these immature cells to differentiate into functioning neurons outside the olfactory bulb and hippocampus. The problem may be the absence of biochemical signals that normally prompt the developing stem cell to migrate and differentiate.

Parkinson's disease involves the loss of dopamine neurons. Stem cells offer a potential source for cell replacement therapy. A group in Japan reported a successful treatment in monkeys with chemically induced Parkinson's disease. The important difference may have been a "cocktail" of several growth factors that coaxed the undifferentiated cells to develop into neurons and then into authentic dopamine neurons. These cells were injected into the bilateral putamen of the "Parkinsonian" monkeys.

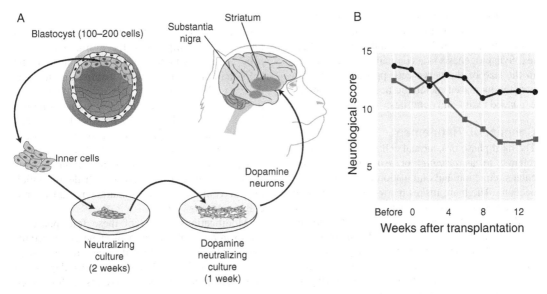

FIGURE 8.6 ● **A.** Harvesting embryonic stem cells, stimulating the development of dopamine neurons in several cultures, and injecting them into a monkey with chemically induced Parkinson's disease. **B.** Improved neurological scores over 14 weeks. (Adapted from Takagi Y, Takahashi J, Saiki H, et al. Dopaminergic neurons generated from monkey embryonic stem cells function in a Parkinson primate model. *J Clin Invest.* 2005;115(1):102-109.)

Figure 8.6 shows a diagram of the procedure and some results. Unfortunately, studies with humans have been disappointing and this potentially exciting intervention remains a dream.

Cell Expansion

The second phase of neuronal growth, often called *synaptogenesis*, describes the extensive growth of axons and dendrites to make synaptic connections—a process that primarily occurs early in life. The tips of axons and dendrites have *growth cones* that appear to reach out with fingerlike structures, *filopodia*, and literally pull the growth cone to its destination. The axons are guided in a specific direction by chemical signals that attract and repel the growth cone, that is, *chemoattractants* and *chemorepellents*.

In a comprehensive postmortem analysis, Huttenlocher determined synaptic density across the life span in two regions of the human brain from 14 individuals. Using an electron microscope and special stains, he counted synaptic connections from thin sections taken from the visual cortex and prefrontal cortex. The results, displayed graphically in Figure 8.7, show that the greatest synaptogenesis takes place shortly after birth and occurs

FIGURE 8.7 ● **A.** Schematic representation of changes in synaptic density. **B.** Measured synaptic densities in visual and prefrontal cortex from 14 individuals who died of non-neurological diseases. (Adapted from Huttenlocher PR, Dabholkar AS. Regional differences in synaptogenesis in human cerebral cortex. *J Comp Neurol.* 1997;387(2):167-178.)

sooner for the visual cortex. Maximum synaptic density is reached before the first year in the visual cortex, but not until 3.5 years in the prefrontal cortex. Synaptogenesis is accompanied by an increase in the size of the nerve cell, presumably to support the increased metabolic needs created by the expanded axons and dendrites.

Connection Refinement

The third phase of neuronal cell development often referred to as *pruning*, or *synaptic elimination*, entails retraction and elimination of excessive connections. The brain makes many more connections than are needed and the weak ones (or those not used) regress. As with synaptogenesis, the pruning proceeds at different rates for different regions of the brain, based on need. For example, sensory and motor areas go through refinement before the regions devoted to executive functions. Clearly, moving and seeing are more essential than writing a poem.

The late and extensive reduction of the frontal cortex correlates with psychological tests measuring improved executive function. It is paradoxical that the maturing process that our adolescents struggle through is actually a refinement and reduction of the gray matter and not growth. We (the authors) have teenage children. Studies suggest they have more gray matter than we do, but we dominate when it comes to wisdom and smarts. The point is this: less is more. This is not the usual pattern in nature. Typically bigger is better. But then elephants and whales, with the largest brains, do not rule the planet like humans.

Disordered pruning may be the pathological basis for such conditions as autism and schizophrenia. A consistent finding in patients with autism is greater total brain volume, which is not present at birth but develops during the first few years of life. It has been suggested that this is due to abnormal connectivity and a lack of pruning. Schizophrenia, which typically develops in late adolescence and is associated with a loss of gray matter, may be the result of excessive pruning.

POINT OF INTEREST

Mark Twain said, "When I was a boy of 14, my father was so ignorant I could hardly stand to have the old man around. But when I got to be 21, I was astonished at how much he had learned in 7 years." With this clever statement, Twain captures the refinement of the adolescent prefrontal cortex that a teen experiences but does not recognize.

Apoptosis

Programmed cell death, *apoptosis*, is the final phase of the sculpting of the brain. It is called *programmed*, which reflects the fact that the cells actually carry genetic instructions to self-destruct. Neurotrophins, discussed next, save the neuron by turning off the genetic program. When the intracellular "self-destruct button" has been activated, apoptosis proceeds in a characteristic process: cell shrinkage, fragmentation, and phagocytosis of the cellular remnants. This is distinguished from necrotic cell death, which results from trauma and is characterized by rapid cell membrane lysis.

Modifications of any of these four phases—for example, enhancing neurogenesis or retarding apoptosis—are potential targets for treatment interventions for such conditions as depression and Alzheimer's disease. Active research for such treatments is going on.

Brain Imaging Studies

The postmortem studies by Huttenlocher provided an in-depth analysis of synaptic connections, but were limited by the total number of brains that he could analyze. Brain imaging technology, on the other hand, allows the noninvasive examination of a larger number of subjects, in real time, with the potential to be repeated as the subjects age. Unfortunately, brain imaging does not have the resolution to the level of the synapse, so studies follow the trajectory of larger structures, such as gray matter thickness or volume.

The noninvasive magnetic resonance imaging technology has allowed extensive studies of brain development beginning in childhood and progressing into adulthood. One study, shown in Figure 8.8A, scanned 145 healthy subjects, 99 of whom had at least two scans. Gray matter development proceeded on a trajectory of growth until 10 to 12 years of age followed by a decrease in adolescence—consistent with the pattern of synaptogenesis followed by connection refinement. The age of maximal volume (an indirect measurement of development) varies by brain region.

NEUROTROPHIC GROWTH FACTORS

Neurotrophic factors—literally growth factors for nerve cells—are best defined as any molecule that affects the nervous system by influencing the growth or differentiation of neurons or glia. Neurotrophic factors, affectionately called "brain fertilizers," are the stimulus behind neurogenesis and

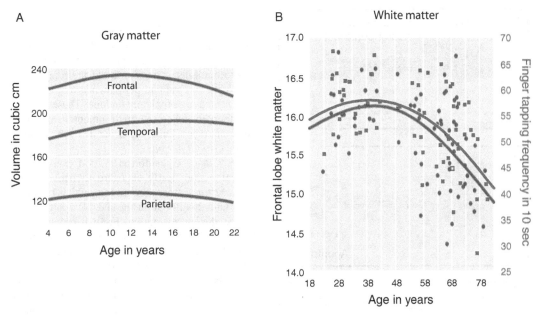

FIGURE 8.8 ● **A.** MRI analyses from 145 healthy subjects showing the changing gray matter volumes for different regions of the brain for males. **B.** Myelination of the frontal lobes correlates with motor speed and peaks in at 39 years of age. (**A** Adapted from Giedd JN, Blumenthal J, Jeffries NO, et al. Brain development during childhood and adolescence: A longitudinal MRI study. *Nat Neurosci.* 1999;2(10): 861-863. **B** Adapted from Bartzokis G, Lu PH, Tingus K, et al. Lifespan trajectory of myelin integrity and maximum motor speed. *Neurobiol Aging.* 2010;31:1554-1562.)

synaptogenesis (Figure 8.9). Rita Levi-Montalcini et al. accidentally discovered the first growth factor 40 years ago (see Figure 1.9). They were able to isolate a protein from a mouse sarcoma that stimulated the growth of nerve cells as well as increased the size and branching of the cells. Although called *nerve growth factor* (NGF)—implying that it stimulates all nerve cells—this particular neurotrophin only affects sympathetic neurons and some sensory ganglion cells. Several decades of research have established four principles regarding the cells affected by NGF.

1. NGF mediates cell survival.
2. Cells that do not receive enough NGF die.
3. Target organs produce NGF.
4. Specific NGF receptors are present on innervating nerve terminals.

Because NGF is specific for a limited subset of peripheral nerves, it was assumed for many years that there were a host of other neurotrophic factors following similar rules waiting to be discovered. Unfortunately, the fortuitous discovery of NGF has not been repeated with other factors. Identifying and purifying factors that are excreted in such minute quantities has turned into an arduous task. Several factors have been discovered and are being

studied, such as neurotrophin-3, glial cell line–derived neurotrophic factor, and insulinlike growth factor, to name a few, but the one that is of most interest to the mental health community is brain-derived neurotrophic factor (BDNF).

The actions of neurotrophins such as BDNF are mediated primarily through Trk (for tyrosine kinase) receptors on the nerve cell membrane. The extracellular portion of the receptor binds with the neurotrophic factor, which in turn initiates an intracellular cascade that leads to gene expression. As yet, there are no small molecule agonists or antagonists for these receptors, which hinders a better understanding of the action of the neurotrophic factors.

Signaling the Trk receptor can lead to changes in three aspects of the cell state:

1. Cell survival or death.
2. Synaptic stabilization or elimination.
3. Process growth or retraction.

The effect is determined by the specific neurotrophic factor, the combination of receptors signaled, and the intracellular pathways expressed in that cell. Disruption of the neurotrophic factor signaling is presumably an explanation (and possible treatment) for some neurodegenerative

FIGURE 8.9 ● Neurotrophic factors mediate cell proliferation and elimination by promoting cell growth, stimulating synaptogenesis, and preventing apoptosis.

diseases, for example, Huntington's, Parkinson's, and Alzheimer's diseases. Likewise, the enduring symptoms resulting from substance abuse may be the result of inappropriate neurotrophic factor synthesis.

TREATMENT NEUROTROPHINS

Medicating with neurotrophins or stimulating their increased production is an exciting prospect for future neuropsychiatric treatment. Some studies suggest that this may be the mechanism by which lithium, electroconvulsive therapy, and antidepressants resolve depression (see Chapter 21). If this is true, future treatments for depression will focus on more effective ways to stimulate growth factors. Other researchers have examined the therapeutic benefits of growth hormones for such disorders as amyotrophic lateral sclerosis and multiple sclerosis. The biggest difficulty is finding effective yet unobtrusive methods to deliver the neurotrophins to the CNS.

CRITICAL PERIODS

As we have said before, genes control development in utero, but the environment influences the direction after birth. Early interactions during the time of great cellular expansion mold the brain's anatomy with an ease and permanence that can never be repeated or completely undone. These stages in development when the environmental input is so crucial to determining the structure of the brain are called *critical periods.*

Language acquisition is a good example of a critical period. Early exposure to native sounds has a lasting impact on speech, which is hard to alter later in life. Johnson and Newport demonstrated this by examining English proficiency in Korean and Chinese speakers who arrived in the United States between the ages of 3 and 39. They found that subjects who arrived in the United States before the age of 7 had equivalent fluency to native speakers, whereas those who arrived after the age of 7 had a linear decline in performance until puberty (Figure 8.10).

The development of the visual cortex provides another example of a critical period. David Hubel and Torstern Wiesel (who later received the Nobel Prize for this work) established the importance of normal visual experience early in life for proper development of the visual cortex in cats and monkeys. In a series of experiments, they sutured one eyelid shut in kittens and later monkeys for short lengths of time during various weeks after birth. They established, down to the level of the neuron, the profound effect of visual deprivation at critical periods of development.

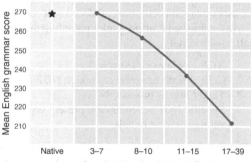

FIGURE 8.10 ● Language acquisition as measured by English grammar tests for native speakers compared with Korean and Chinese immigrants. (Adapted from Johnson JS, Newport EL. Critical period effects in second language learning: the influence of maturational state on the acquisition of English as a second language. *Cognit Psychol.* 1989;21(1):60-99.)

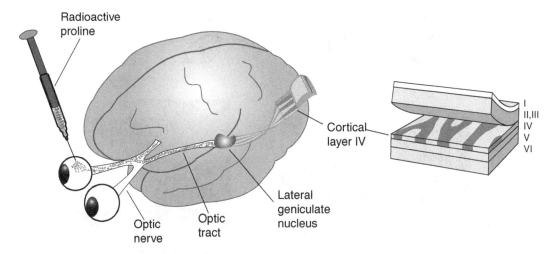

FIGURE 8.11 ● Injecting radioactive proline into an eye allows visualization of the cortical innervation in layer IV from that eye when the animal is sacrificed several weeks later. (Adapted from Bear MF, Connors BW, Paradiso MA, eds. *Neuroscience: Exploring the Brain*. 3rd ed. Baltimore, MD: Lippincott Williams & Wilkins; 2007; Purves D, Augustine GJ, Fitzpatrick D, et al. *Neuroscience*. 5th ed. Sunderland, MA: Sinauer; 2011.)

Figure 8.11 shows how the experiments by Hubel and Wiesel were conducted. Radioactive proline was injected into an eye where it was absorbed and transported down the axons to the lateral geniculate nucleus (LGN) of the thalamus. Some of the labeled proline that spilled out of the terminal would be taken up by the LGN neurons and transported to the visual cortex. The location of the radioactive molecules can be visualized using autoradiography.

Figure 8.12 shows the results—both real and schematic—of suturing one eye shut for differing periods of time early in life. The autoradiographs in the B row show a normal cat compared with a cat whose eye was closed from 2 weeks until 18 months. This demonstrates—as do the drawings in the C row—how the neurons from the occluded eye regress and the neurons from the good eye expand. The D row shows the terminal branching, *arborization*, of the LGN neurons in the visual cortex for a normal eye and one that was occluded for just 1 week at 30 days of age. Hubel and Wiese have estimated that the critical period for ocular deprivation in a cat is 3 to 4 months.

In humans, the critical period for vision extends out to 5 or 6 years of age. For example, children with congenital cataracts can have substantial and permanent visual deficits if the occluded lens is not corrected early enough. However, adults with cataracts regain their preexisting visual acuity when the lens is replaced because occlusion past the critical period does not damage the cortex.

Strabismus, often called *lazy eye*, is a misalignment of the eyes due to improper control by the eye muscles. Children with this condition experience double vision. The response of the brain to receiving two images is to suppress the input from one eye. This can result in low acuity or even blindness in the suppressed eye due to developmental impediments during the critical period. One form of treatment is to patch the good eye and force development in the cortical regions connected to the lazy eye.

ADULT NEUROPLASTICITY

Plasticity is defined as the capability to be formed or molded. Neuroplasticity describes the brain's ability to adapt to environmental factors that cannot be anticipated by genetic programming. The description of critical periods described above

DISORDER PERSONALITY

Extrapolating these studies to behavior, one wonders about critical periods and personality development. For example, what is the effect of early exposure to TV? Recent studies suggest that too much time in front of the TV leads to attentional problems for children, poorer academic achievement, and increased aggression. What neuronal connections fail to develop when children spend too much time watching TV?

Normal development

One eye sutured shut

A

B

Looking down on cortical layer IV

One eye occluded from age
2 week until 18 month

C

Cortical layers

II
III
IV

D

Cortical layers

III
IV
V

Terminal axons and dedritic
branching in visual cortex
from lateral geniculate nucleus

One eye occluded for 1 week
1 month after birth

E

Percentage of neurons

Ocular dominance group

FIGURE 8.12 ● A–E. Comparing the normal development of the visual cortex on the left with development on the right when one eye has been sutured shut for varying lengths of time. E. Electrodes inserted horizontal to the cortex show distinctive patterns of ocular dominance depending on which eyes developed properly. (B. From Wiesel TN. Postnatal development of the visual cortex and the influence of environment. *Nature*. 1982;299(5884):583-591. D. From Antonini A, Stryker MP. Rapid remodeling of axonal arbors in the visual cortex. *Science*. 1993;260(5115):1819-1821. Reprinted with permission from the AAAS.)

Sensory cortical map

Before rotation

Rotation of disk

After rotation

FIGURE 8.13 ● The expansion of cortical representation of the dorsal fingers of a monkey before and after several weeks of controlled hand use. (Adapted from Jenkins WM, Merzenich MM, Ochs MT, et al. Functional reorganization of primary somatosensory cortex in adult owl monkeys after behaviorally controlled tactile stimulation. *J Neurophysiol.* 1990;63(1):82-104.)

suggests a bleak picture for plasticity in the adult brain, but there is more hope for your old cortex than one might think. For example, the organization of the representation of the sensory input in the cortex (called cortical maps) is continually reshaped by experience.

Studies with monkeys have shown a startling capacity of the cortical maps to change in response to sensory input. In one classic study, animals were taught to rotate a disk using only digits 2, 3, and sometimes 4 to receive banana-flavored pellets. After several weeks of practice, the cortical regions (the cortical map) used by fingers 2, 3, and 4 were enlarged (Figure 8.13). Practice literally changed the brain.

In another experiment by the same group, the researchers measured the representation of the fingers on the cortex before and after amputation of the middle finger. Figure 8.14 shows how the cortex adapted to the change. Neurons deprived of their normal sensory input from the middle finger switch to responding to stimulation from the closest finger. Similar changes have been observed with humans after medical amputation. For some patients, when their face is scratched, they "feel" a sensation as though it was coming from their amputated lower arm—a phantom sensation. Functional imaging scans performed during such stimulation have shown activation of the somatosensory region for both the face and where the lower arm was. It appears that the sensory neurons in the brain do not die when input ceases. Rather, they shift their focus.

The Musician's Brain

Learning to play a musical instrument is a complex task requiring practice, practice, practice. Musicians' brains serve as a model of

Before amputation

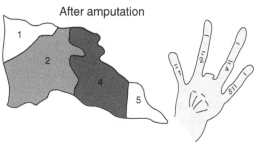

After amputation

FIGURE 8.14 ● After amputation of a monkey's finger, the cortical neurons reorganize. The neurons formally responding to stimulation of the third finger now respond to stimulation from the second and fourth fingers. Similar "re-mapping" also occurs in the thalamus. (Adapted from Merzenich MM, Nelson RJ, Stryker MP, et al. Somatosensory cortical map changes following digit amputation in adult monkeys. *J Comp Neurol.* 1984;224(4):591-605.)

neuroplasticity. Figure 8.15 shows the enhanced signals from the somatosensory and auditory cortex for highly skilled musicians compared with controls. Figure 8.15A shows the representation of the cortical signal from the little finger on the left hand for string musicians and controls when the fingers were stimulated. This difference did

FIGURE 8.15 ● Musicians (*black arrow*) and controls (*white arrow*) show differences in the somatosensory (**A**) and auditory (**B**) cortex. (Adapted from Pantev C, Engelien A, Candia V, et al. Representational cortex in musicians. Plastic alterations in response to musical practice. *Ann N Y Acad Sci.* 2001;930:300-314.)

not exist for the thumb or the fingers on the right hand. In Figure 8.15B, the musicians had a 25% greater neuronal excitation for the piano tones than the controls. In both cases, the musicians who had started playing at the youngest age displayed the largest signal.

Taken in total, these studies suggest that starting early is best, but even the late bloomers can change their brains and develop new skills. Clearly, as anyone who has tried to learn a new language, instrument, or sport knows, it requires work and diligence to master the task—or literally to change the brain. Fortunately, it appears that even an old cortex can adapt. Hubel and Wiesel described a monkey who had one eye occluded between days 21 and 30. Initially the monkey appeared blind in the deprived eye. Remarkably, 4 years later he had an estimated acuity of 20/80 in the bad eye and 20/40 in the normal eye.

Maladaptive Neuroplasticity

Prolonged practice has its dark side. Approximately 1% of professional musicians will develop a condition called *focal dystonia*: loss of control of skilled movements in the performing hand. It is usually a career-ending disorder and is believed to result from maladaptive neuroplasticity stimulated by long hours of repetitive movements. Neuroimaging studies show a fusion of the digital representations in the somatosensory cortex (Figure 8.16). It is almost as though the neurons are attempting to move two fingers when they should be only moving one. Consequently, individual finger movement is no longer possible.

Cellular Changes

The cellular mechanisms that accompany the cortical changes seen with monkeys rotating disks and musicians playing instruments (and hopefully readers of this book) are poorly understood. Some similar processes that may play a role in the dynamics of the neocortex were discussed in earlier chapters of this book. A good model is long-term potentiation (LTP). Figure 5.8 shows an example of new spine development induced with LTP. Such spine development along with branching of the dendrites is seen with enriched environments (Point of Interest Chapter 3). It is tempting to speculate that successful learning

---

TREATMENT   STROKE

After a stroke, many patients will avoid using the affected limb and preferentially use the intact limb. Functional imaging studies of stroke patients have shown contraction of the cortical representation of the affected limb, which is how the brain responds when it is not used. A new kind of rehabilitation for stroke patients called *constraint-induced movement therapy* corrects this problem and improves function even in chronic conditions. Patients have their good limb restrained with a mitt or harness and are forced to use their impaired limb. Controlled trials have shown this treatment to improve motor skills as well as increase the cortical activity in the affected area. The brain has the capacity to change, but it must be exercised.

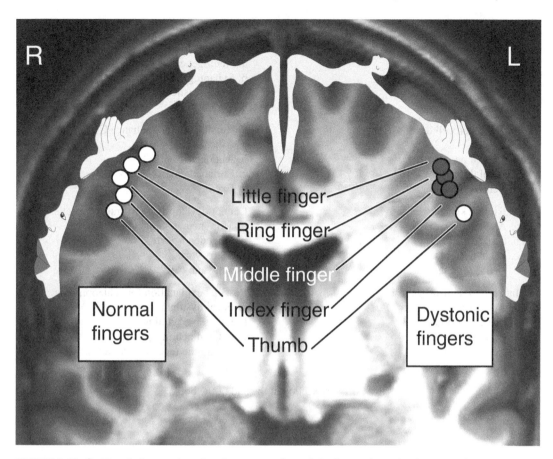

FIGURE 8.16 ● The circles are functional representations of the fingers from the right and left hands of a musician with focal dystonia of the left hand. The response from the somatosensory cortex is superimposed on a MRI. Note the fusion of the representations for the fingers from the affected left fingers that is not seen with the separated fingers from the right hand. The thumb—a digit not requiring as much movement when playing— is unaffected. (Adapted from Elbert T, Candia V, Altenmuller E, et al. Alteration of digital representations in somatosensory cortex in focal hand dystonia. *Neuroreport*. 1998;9(16):3571-3575.)

involves production of growth factor proteins that stimulate arborization of dendrites in the cortex, resulting in bigger, bushier neurons.

Adult Nerve Regeneration

Why is it that the nerves in the peripheral nervous system (PNS) can regenerate while those in the CNS cannot? Likewise, why can amphibians regrow long nerve connections, but mammals cannot? How come the most complex organ in the universe is less capable of repair than more primitive organs? It appears that the brain responds to injuries with actions that are intended to preserve the complex connections, but this ultimately also prevents regeneration.

Oligodendrocytes and astrocytes respond to CNS injury by forming what is called a *glial scar*. This scar is part of the inflammatory response and limits cellular damage by isolating and protecting the injured area. Unfortunately, the glial scar is full of molecules (not found in the PNS) that inhibit the growth cone and prevent regeneration. But more on this in the next chapter when we discuss immunity and inflammation.

QUESTIONS

1. Brain fertilizer
   a. Apoptosis.
   b. Critical period.
   c. Focal dystonia.
   d. Neurotrophins.

2. Programmed cell death
   a. Apoptosis.
   b. Critical period.
   c. Focal dystonia.
   d. Neurotrophins.

3. Maximum synaptogenesis
   a. Apoptosis.
   b. Critical period.
   c. Focal dystonia.
   d. Neurotrophins.

4. Inappropriate neurogenesis
   a. Apoptosis.
   b. Critical period.
   c. Focal dystonia.
   d. Neurotrophins.

5. Not one of the phases of development
   a. Neurogenesis.
   b. Synaptogenesis.
   c. Neuroplasticity.
   d. Pruning.

6. Factors that do not enhance CNS neurogenesis
   a. Amputation.
   b. Antidepressants.
   c. Enriched environments.
   d. Exercise.

7. Cannot develop from neural stem cells
   a. More neural stem cells.
   b. Oligodendrocytes.
   c. Astrocytes.
   d. Schwann cells.

8. Possible explanation for schizophrenia
   a. Focal dystonia.
   b. Excessive pruning.
   c. Altered neurotrophins.
   d. Dopamine receptor apoptosis.

See Answers section at the end of the book.

CHAPTER 9

Inflammation and Immunity

Up to this point, we have discussed a number of mechanisms that may explain how the mentally ill brain is different from the normal brain. The immune system is increasingly being viewed as a possible culprit. The body's reaction to foreign invasion (or mistaken foreign invasion) and the resulting inflammatory response may contribute to the development of some psychiatric disorders.

For a long time, there have been indications of subtle links between mental illness and the immune system. The first antidepressants were developed in the 1950s when it was noted that the antitubercular medication *iproniazid* had a positive effect on mood. When treated with this medication, even some terminally ill patients became more cheerful, physically active, and hopeful. Ultimately this antibiotic was refined and transformed into the first effective antidepressant: the monoamine oxidase inhibitors.

In 1929 the Swiss psychiatrist Tramer reported an increase in schizophrenic births during the months from December to May. Tramer noted that children born during the winter/spring months were more likely to develop schizophrenia as adults. It is postulated that the seasonal fluctuation is influenced by exposure to infections during the perinatal period, which are more common during the winter months—more on this topic later in the chapter.

Perhaps the oldest link between infection and psychiatric disorders lies with syphilis. This microbe was the cause of about 20% of the hospitalizations for mental illness at the beginning of the last century. In 1910 it was Paul Ehrlich's "magic bullet," compound 606, that became the first effective medication for syphilis—the beginning of psychopharmacology. The microbe that causes syphilis, *Treponema pallidum*, provides a good example of the immune response and the problems this response causes.

THE IMMUNE RESPONSE

The body's immune system is poised to recognize and attack foreign invaders—anything that is nonself: splinters, bacteria, Fox News, etc. The attack is conducted by a confusing array of cells and proteins—some of which stand guard at all times, while others remain dormant until the alarm is sounded. All the components interact with each other through a litany of signals to rally the defenses when a microscopic terrorist is identified. Likewise the defenses must be turned off when the coast is clear. For the purposes of this book, we can simplify the immune response down to four major components:

1. Cellular—white blood cells (leukocytes)
2. Humoral—antibodies
3. Complement—little torpedoes
4. Cytokines—the molecular signals

All four of these components come into play when the syphilitic bacteria *T. pallidum* invades the body.

Syphilis

Syphilis is a sexually transmitted disease caused by the corkscrew shaped bacteria *T. pallidum* (Figure 9.1). When a contagious individual has sex with an uninfected partner, there is about a 30% chance the disease will be transferred. The body's first line of defense against infection is the skin. *T. pallidum* spirochete penetrates the dermal barrier by twisting through microabrasion.

The body's next line of defense is the complement system (Figure 9.2A). The complement system is made up of numerous proteins circulating in the blood poised to coalesce into little torpedoes. When activated by foreign proteins, such as those found on bacteria, the complement molecules lock on to the bacteria. As more and more of these proteins accumulate on the bacteria, the complement can literally drill a hole in the cell wall. This allows fluid to pore in and the bacteria explodes. The trick is to limit the attack to the foreign invaders—to avoid attacking host cells.

Also standing ready to fend off foreign invaders are a variety of white blood cells (leukocytes). Two of these, the macrophage and the neutrophil, are frontline defenders. The macrophage patrols the perimeter of the skin and mucus membranes cleaning up debris and searching for bad guys. (They also are one of the cells that will present foreign antigens to T cells to start the production of antibodies.) Neutrophils circulate in the blood ready to come to the aid of defenseless tissue. They aggressively attack *T. pallidum* but generally also make a mess of the healthy tissue. The initial physical sign of syphilis—the chancre that develops on the genitalia at the site of the infection—is in large part due to neutrophils. Pus is predominantly dead neutrophils—suicide bombers at the cellular level.

FIGURE 9.1 ● The bacteria that causes all the problems of syphilis is this annoying spirochete *Treponema pallidum* seen here in an electron micrograph. (From Centers for Disease Control and Prevention.)

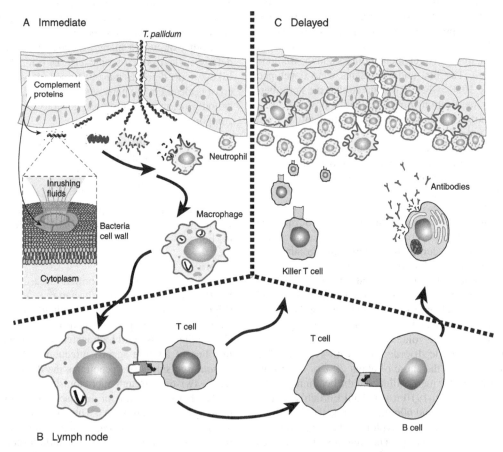

FIGURE 9.2 ● **A.** When bacteria invade the body, complement, macrophages, and neutrophils are the first defenders. **B.** Antigen presenting cells take pieces of the bacteria (antigens) to lymph nodes when the B cells and T cells are activated. **C.** T cells and B cells, specifically matched to the antigens of the bacteria, follow the cytokines to the site of the injury.

Syphilis Continued

After the first phases of syphilis, most people enter a latency phase—usually within 6 months. During this phase, they do not have signs or symptoms of the illness and are not contagious. However, microbes remain hidden within the body and laboratory studies are still positive. Remarkably, the *T. pallidum* can quietly live undetected in the host for years. How is this possible?

The best explanation for the stealth capabilities of *T. pallidum* is the relative inertness of the outer membrane. The proteins that protrude through the phospholipid bilayer cell membrane wall (called integral proteins) are few and far between in *T. pallidum*. It is these proteins that killer T cells and antibodies grab when they attack the bacteria. In comparison, *T. pallidum* has only 1% of the integral proteins compared with *Escherichia coli*. So, this bacteria can remain hidden, under the radar so to speak, and not be recognized as different—like little terrorist sleeper cells.

If left untreated, approximately one-third of the people infected with syphilis will cure themselves, another third will remain in the latency phase until they die, and the last third will develop tertiary syphilis—the most serious phase of the infection. Of particular interest for us is neurosyphilis. Neurosyphilis includes inflammation of the meninges, cerebral vasculature, or neural tissue of the brain and/or spinal cord. Although animal studies have shown that *T. pallidum* can find their way to the central nervous system (CNS) within 18 hours after the initial infection, the serious manifestations of neurosyphilis do not develop for 10 to 50 years.

The important point is this: once the immune system catches up with syphilis in the CNS, it is the inflammatory response—not the bacteria per se—that damages the brain. *T. pallidum* does not produce a toxin nor directly attacks the cells of the nervous system. It is the overexuberant cellular response to *T. pallidum* that blocks the vascular support and kills the neurons. The military calls this collateral damage. The incessant neural loss once the immune system is activated leads to personality changes, psychosis, and dementia as well as paralysis, seizures, and death.

Inflammation

The inflammatory response is the body's overall reaction to foreign invasion. The signs are swelling, redness, heat, and pain. The mechanisms that cause the inflammation are engorgement of the blood vessels, movement of fluid into the tissue, and, above all, attraction of leukocytes to the infected area. The signals that start the inflammatory process and coordinate the response are the cytokines. (More on the cytokines later in the chapter.)

Adaptive Immunity

A large part of the success of the mammalian defense system results from the capacity of the system to proliferate and attack specific and unique molecular features of the invader. This adaptive immunity commences when pieces of the destroyed bacteria are taken to the lymph nodes and presented to T cells—essentially shopped around to find a good match (Figure 9.2B). When a close match is found, the T cells multiply and head off to attack that specific remnant of the invader, but not before activating the B cells. The B cells with a similar match will start producing antibodies. Antibodies are the "Y"-shaped proteins that can lock on to the specific foreign molecules of the bacteria, virus, or infected cell. Antibodies attached to a foreign cell serve as a signal to other leukocytes, essentially saying that this cell is ready for demolition (Figure 9.2C).

The important points to grasp are the varied mechanisms the body uses to defend against foreign invasion and the need for numerous checks and balances to keep the response under control, that is, to avoid damaging the host cells. As with any battle, "civilian casualties" are unavoidable. War, even at the microscopic level, is a dirty business.

IMMUNITY IN THE BRAIN

The immune response inside the brain is less aggressive than the response normally seen in the rest of the body. Constraining the response is essential because the rejuvenating capacity of the brain is limited and the effects of collateral damage from inflammation are more serious. White blood cells are rarely seen in the CNS. But the brain is not defenseless. Although once thought to be "immune

---

TREATMENT COCAINE VACCINE

Cocaine dependence is a major health problem. There is no Food and Drug Administration (FDA)–approved pharmacotherapy. One research group has developed a vaccine that stimulates the immune system to produce anticocaine antibodies. These antibodies can sequester circulating cocaine and prevent the substance from entering the brain and quelling any euphoria. Early studies have found reduced cocaine intake for addicts whose body produced sufficient antibodies. Future research is focused on eliciting a stronger and more sustained immune response in more patients.

privileged"—that is, able to tolerate the presence of an antigen without eliciting an inflammatory response—the brain is now recognized to have a unique but muted immune response to invaders.

The brain has three layers of protection against foreign invasion.

1. The blood–brain barrier—physical barrier to isolate the brain.
2. Microglia—the macrophage of the brain.
3. Leukocytes infiltration reserved for serious damage.

The distinguishing feature of the CNS immune system is the microglia. The microglia, although considered a nerve cell, actually originate from a different cell line. While neurons, oligodendrocytes, and astrocytes develop from cells of neuroectodermal origin, the microglia come from mesenchymal stem cells (bone, cartilage, and blood cells). Microglia move in and take up residence among the neural cells very early during embryonic development.

The microglia are most closely related to the macrophage and are the central component of the brain's innate immune system. Like the macrophage, they are dormant until activated, can migrate to the battle zone, and attempt to gobble up whatever should not be there. The microglia respond to chemical signals of danger, emit pro-inflammatory cytokines, and can function as

antigen presenting cells—similar to the macrophage. In addition, microglia can also release cytotoxic substances such as hydrogen peroxide to damage the invader. Unfortunately, the hydrogen peroxide also kills neurons.

Neural Prostheses

The protagonist of the 1970s television series *The Six-Million Dollar Man* was a NASA astronaut whose injured body was rebuilt with mechanical parts. Oh, if only it was this easy. Forty years later, real researchers are still struggling with the basics. A device that could restore simple movements for people with spinal cord injuries would be of great value to those confined to a wheelchair. While still very much in the experimental stages, the goal is to capture the individual's neural signals generated in the motor cortex and turn them into useful movements (Figure 9.3).

Electrodes implanted directly into the gray matter of the motor cortex are an intrusive element needed to determine the person's intentions. The electrode captures the electrical activity as the neurons generate action potentials and the signals are sent to a computer. The computer—after substantial training—decodes the signals and moves the external device—in this case a mechanical arm. Problems develop as the brain's immune system produces a sustained reaction against the foreign body electrode.

Digitalize neural signals

Digital signals converted to mechanical movements

FIGURE 9.3 ● Electrodes in the motor cortex capture the neural activity of purposeful movement. The signals are digitalized and the computer learns to turn the impulses into movements of the mechanical arm.

Indwelling Electrodes

The gray matter of the cortex is dense with blood vessels. Invariably as the electrodes are pushed into the brain, the vasculature is ruptured. This breaches the blood–brain barrier and allows the entry of inflammatory proteins as well as macrophages, neutrophils, and T cells. In short, the wound healing process is initiated and neurons—the ones the electrode needs to record—can be damaged or destroyed. While the bloodborne inflammatory response is the most serious, microglia and astrocytes become activated regardless of the vascular damage (Figure 9.4).

Microglia, in their resting state, look like stars with elaborate branching structure. When they sense trouble, they multiply and morph into rounder structures. They also increase their production of cytokines and growth factor proteins. In this activated state, they engulf and digest the cellular debris generated by the injury—acting like their macrophage cousins from the periphery.

Astrocytes usually support the neurons and maintain the integrity of the blood–brain barrier. In response to injury they too become activated. Their main function in response to trouble is to isolate the problem. They produce and release a fibrous substance that plays an essential role in forming a physical barrier around the injury. This barrier is commonly called the glial scar. This is a problem for the whole contraption, since the scar impedes contact between neurons and the electrode.

Glial Scar

Reactive gliosis, the formation of the glial scar, helps to isolate the injury, prevent overwhelming inflammation, and limit cellular degradation. The importance of gliosis was established in mice whose astrocytes were depleted. Small stab wounds in their spinal cords resulted in greater blood–brain barrier disruption, larger leukocyte infiltration, increased neural loss, and more motor deficits than comparable mice with normal astrocytes.

Clearly, the glial scar is essential to limiting CNS damage after trauma. Unfortunately, there is a price to pay. Neurons of warm-blooded animals will not regenerate through the glial scar. This is why patients with severed spinal cords remain paralyzed. The axons on either side of the injury are prevented from reconnecting by the glial scar. Treatments in the future may dissolve the scar once the injury is stabilized, thus allowing axons to regenerate.

CYTOKINES

Cytokines are known as the "hormones of the immune system." These chemical messengers orchestrate the direction, magnitude, and duration of the inflammatory response. Virtually all the immune cells produce cytokines, although the type and function vary. First discovered in the late 1960s, the number of known cytokines has exploded fills large, small fonted tables. Reasonable readers avoid such material. Suffice it to say that the major cytokines are interferon (IFN), interleukin (IL), and

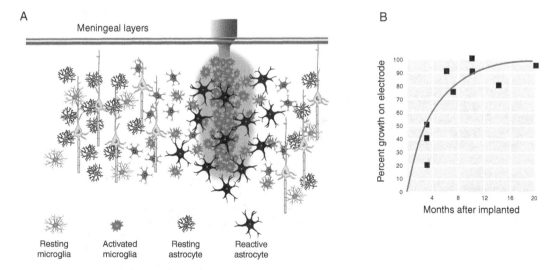

FIGURE 9.4 ● **A.** Electrodes implanted in the gray matter elicit an inflammatory response. Activated microglia and astrocytes produce a "scar" that isolates the electrode. **B.** Within 6 months, 75% of the electrode is surrounded by glial cells. (Adapted from Rousche PJ, Normann RA. Chronic recording capability of the Utah Intracortical Electrode Array in cat sensory cortex. *J Neurosci Methods.* 1998;82:1-15.)

tumor necrosis factor (TNF), although each type has numerous variants designated with numbers or Greek letters.

Cytokines coordinate the entire response to an infection—from generating a fever to promoting wound healing. However, the primary functions are activating and guiding immune cells. Some of the cytokines activate the white blood cells—induce the cellular feeding frenzy. Other cytokines, in the presence of an antigen, activate T cells and B cells to multiply and go find the pathogen.

Cytokines play an essential role in guiding the immune cells to the battlefield. Activated cells follow the "scent" of the cytokines to their destination (Figure 9.5). Endothelial cells in the blood vessels respond to cytokines by expressing adhesion molecules that "grab" immune cells floating by in the blood. The cells then transform, squeeze through the blood–brain barrier, and follow the scent of the cytokines to find the pathogen.

An essential feature of fighting any infection is the ability to turn off the inflammation when the job is done in order to limit injurious side effects. Cytokines are turned off in several ways. First, cytokines have a short half-life and quickly dissipate anyway. Second, production of cytokines is reduced as the offending antigens disappear. Finally, some cytokines are actually anti-inflammatory and are produced to turn down the immune response.

Neural Plasticity

Cytokines have important functions outside of their role coordinating the immune response. Some of the cytokines of the IL-6 family are known to have signaling functions during development of the normal brain and in response to brain injury. Studies have shown that these cytokines can

- induce differentiation of neural stem cells,
- promote axonal regeneration,
- promote maturation and survival of oligodendrocytes, and
- influence synaptic plasticity.

These unexpected discoveries have generated interest in potentially manipulating cytokines to prevent illness or promote healing. But which cytokines need to be neutralized and which ones enhanced is not easy to determine.

Neurogenesis provides an example of the complexity of manipulating cytokines to promote CNS healing. After a stroke, theoretically it would be beneficial to accelerate neurogenesis. The formation, migration to the site of the injury, and the differentiation into functioning neurons hold great potential as a means to help people recover after cerebral ischemia. Unfortunately, the inflammatory response, also occurring after a stroke, blocks neurogenesis. Consequently, controlling the inflammatory response has been one target postulated for enhancing neurogenesis and recovery. But, here is where it gets complicated; some of the cytokines (such as IL-4 and IFN-γ) also released as part of the inflammatory response actually induce neurogenesis.

The studies with traumatic brain injury (TBI) and stroke highlight the current dilemma with cytokines. They not only contribute to long-term damage but also facilitate healing. Interventions in the future will likely neutralize some cytokines while allowing others to work their magic.

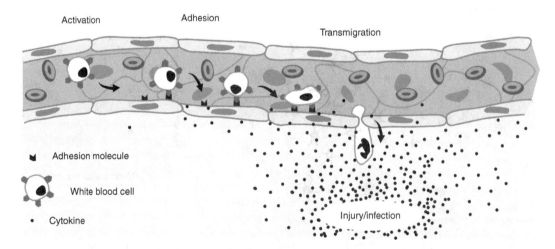

FIGURE 9.5 ● White blood cells in the capillaries are attracted to the site of an injury. Cytokines released at the injury activate a process that enables leukocytes to adhere to the endothelial cells and then migrate to where they are needed.

Mental Illness

The pathophysiology of most mental disorders remains a mystery. Dysfunctions of the mono-amines, the hypothalamic-pituitary-adrenal (HPA) axis, and the neurotrophins have been discussed as possible mechanisms. Infections and inflammation many also play a role in the development of psychiatric disorders. The capacity of cytokines to affect neural plasticity may contribute to psychiatric illness as collateral damage from a normal immune reaction or some autoimmune activation. If this mechanism is culpable, it opens a whole new avenue for treatment interventions. The most compelling evidence is found with depression and schizophrenia.

Depression

Interferon alpha (IFN-α) for the treatment of hepatitis C makes the most impressive connection between depression and cytokines. Hepatitis C is the major cause of chronic liver disease in the Western world. Only about 15% of people infected with this evasive virus can cure themselves. Of those who develop the chronic infection, 20% to 30% will develop cirrhosis within several decades—2.5% develop hepatic cancer.

The IFN cytokines have anti-viral effects and work in conjunction with T cells to clear viruses. IFN-α was approved for the treatment of hepatitis C in the United States in 1992 and, when given with ribavirin, yields a sustained response rate of about 55%. However, a significant proportion of patients treated with IFN-α develop psychiatric symptoms. About 30% to 50% will develop depression, fatigue, anxiety, irritability, and even hypomania. Prophylactic treatment with antidepressants reduces the psychiatric morbidity in patients receiving IFN-α.

A different example connecting cytokines and depression comes from analyzing the blood of depressed people. Compared with healthy controls, patients with depression typically have higher levels of circulating cytokines. In a meta-analysis of similar studies, the pro-inflammatory IL-1 and IL-6 were elevated in depressed patients. One study found that high levels of C-reactive protein (a nonspecific measure of inflammation) preceded the development of depression in an elderly population. Finally, there is some evidence that high inflammatory markers are predictive of treatment-resistant depression.

What about treating depression with anti-inflammatory medication? One would think that with all the anti-inflammatory medications on the market (prednisone, aspirin, etc.) some bright clinician would have noted positive benefits on

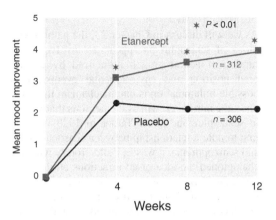

FIGURE 9.6 ● The TNF inhibitor etanercept significantly improved depressive symptoms in patients with psoriasis as measured by the Beck Depression Inventory. (Adapted from Tyring S, Gottlieb A, Papp K, et al. Etanercept and clinical outcomes, fatigue, and depression in psoriasis: double-blind placebo-controlled randomised phase III trial. *Lancet*. 2006;367:29-35.)

mood from one of these medications. Remember, this is how the first antidepressants were serendipitously discovered. So, the lack of a robust effect with the prevalent anti-inflammatory medications is a bit disconcerting. However, there are some studies showing positive effects on mood with anti-inflammatory interventions, which suggest that controlling inflammation may improve mood.

One impressive study was with the TNF inhibitor etanercept in a large placebo-controlled trial for psoriasis. Etanercept is a monoclonal antibody that attaches to and neutralizes the pro-inflammatory cytokine TNF. In this phase III trial, the researchers followed symptoms of depression and fatigue in patients who were ostensibly being treated for psoriasis. Figure 9.6 shows the results for depressive symptoms. Fatigue also improved with active treatment.

TREATMENT	ANTI-INFLAMMATORY ANTIDEPRESSANTS

It turns out that antidepressants as well as mood stabilizers have anti-inflammatory properties. For example, bupropion (Wellbutrin) actually inhibits TNF synthesis! What is the effective component of these medications: increasing monoamines in the synapse, or anti-inflammation, or both?

Schizophrenia

As we will discuss in Chapter 23, the pathophysiology of schizophrenia appears to involve a disruption of neural growth influenced by genetic predisposition and environmental events. It is possible inflammation is one mechanism that may upset the normal growth of the neurons that results in schizophrenia. While Tamer in 1929 was the first to note a relationship between seasonal births and schizophrenia, it was E. Fuller Torrey who has championed the idea of an infectious etiology. In 1973, Dr. Torrey published a paper in *Lancet* entitled "Slow and Latent Viruses in Schizophrenia." His theories were not well received at the time. Now there seem to be several articles on the topic every week.

Initially, the research focused on finding the specific microbe that might cause schizophrenia—cytomegalovirus or *Toxoplasma gondii*, for example. In the past decade, as with depression, the focus had shifted to inflammation and cytokines. A meta-analysis of 62 studies comparing cytokine levels in 2,200 schizophrenics and 1,800 healthy controls found an increase in three cytokines and a decrease in one in the schizophrenic patients. This analysis suggests that inflammation plays a role in maintaining schizophrenia. However, a more convincing explanation may be the detrimental effect inflammation has on the brain during critical developmental spurts.

An inflammatory reaction when the neurons are sprouting or pruning, such as during the first trimester or adolescence, may discombobulate normal neural growth. One research group has used Finnish medical records from 1947 to 1990 to look at the effect of infection during pregnancy. They located women who were hospitalized in Helsinki with upper urinary tract infections (pyelonephritis) while they were pregnant. Pyelonephritis is a serious infection but one in which the microbe is not transmitted to the fetus—only the mother's inflammatory response crosses the placenta.

The authors compared the psychiatric outcome in adulthood for the 9,596 children who were exposed to pyelonephritis in utero with 13,808 siblings who were not. As an added variable, they organized the adults according to family history of psychosis. The results are seen in Figure 9.7.

Figure 9.7 shows graphically the additive effect of infection and genes on the development of schizophrenia. The authors wrote, "38% to 46% of the individuals who developed schizophrenia in our sample did so as a result of the synergistic action of prenatal exposure to infection and positive family history." This study captures what many people believe about schizophrenia and infection—that

FIGURE 9.7 ● Mothers who had pyelonephritis while pregnant and have a family history of psychosis are almost five times more likely to have children who develop schizophrenia as adults. (Adapted from Clark MC, Tanskanen A, Huttunen M, et al. Evidence for an interaction between familial liability and exposure to infection in the causation of schizophrenia. *Am J Psychiatry*. 2009;166:1025-1030.)

schizophrenia develops in genetically vulnerable individuals exposed to an infection at a vulnerable time for the brain.

Duality of the Inflammatory Response

One gets the impression that if we could just turn off inflammation we would all live longer, richer, happier lives. If only it were true! TBI provides a good example of the duality of the inflammatory response.

Many people suffer enormous long-term disability after TBI. Increasingly, we are recognizing the profound and enduring effects of minor TBI, particularly in soldiers within close proximity to explosions or professional athletes with multiple concussions. Brain damage following trauma is the result of immediate tissue injury from the impact and secondary injury from the inflammatory response. Considerable damage to the neural structures is caused by edema, cytokine release, and leukocyte infiltration after the initial impact.

Studies with animals have established that limiting the inflammatory response can reduce some long-term deficits from TBI. But not all studies are positive. In one interesting study, brain trauma was inflicted on mice genetically engineered not to express TNF-α (knockout mice). Initially, the knockout mice showed less behavioral impairment than wild-type mice. However, after several weeks, the knockout mice remained significantly impaired while the wild type recovered. It appears, at least with TNF-α, that the inflammatory response is also involved with healing. This may be due to the beneficial effects the cytokines have on neural plasticity.

TREATMENT ANTI-INFLAMMATORY DIET

If one searches "inflammation" in Amazon.com, the screen quickly fills with books extolling the advantages of the anti-inflammatory diet. Is there such a thing? Most people would agree that the Western diet is a catastrophe, causing an epidemic of obesity, heart disease, and diabetes.

There is substantial evidence that a Mediterranean diet (rich in fruits and vegetables, nuts, olive oil, legumes, and fish; moderate in alcohol; and low in red meat, processed meat, refined carbohydrates, and whole-fat dairy products) is healthier for the body. A recent prospective study in Spain found a smaller incidence of depression in subjects with stricter adherence to the Mediterranean diet. OK, but is it anti-inflammatory?

Well, the omega-3 polyunsaturated fatty acids (commonly called fish oils) can reduce the magnitude of the inflammatory response.

A prospective analysis of inflammatory markers in post-myocardial infarction survivors compared adherence with the Mediterranean diet to inflammatory markers (C-reactive protein and IL-6; see figure). While the results are not overwhelming, they do suggest that diet may influence the inflammatory system.

AUTOIMMUNE DISEASE

Multiple sclerosis (MS) is the quintessential autoimmune disease. The immune system is designed to tolerate self and attack foreign bodies. Sometimes mistakes are made. MS patients have T cells that react to a protein in the myelin sheath. In theory, this alone should not be a problem. The T cells are in the periphery, while the myelin sheaths are protected behind the blood–brain barrier in the CNS. Additionally, the T cells are no threat as long as they are not activated. But for some people, all these safeguards fail and the T cells go after the myelin in the CNS.

It is likely that a viral infection initiates the process in genetically vulnerable individuals. A closely matching viral infection activates the aberrant T cells and the presence of inflammation allows the leukocytes to slip into the CNS where they attack the myelin. The loss of the myelin and axonal damage can result in a variety of unusual symptoms that wax and wane. Prior to the routine use of brain scans, it was not uncommon for a woman with ambiguous neurological symptoms to be diagnosed with conversion disorder or hysteria before it was recognized months or years later that she actually had MS. (A lesson to remember before we too quickly diagnose patients with personality disorders.)

The development of magnetic resonance imaging (MRI) has changed the way the illness is followed. The focal demyelination in the white matter is easy to identify on MRI. Furthermore, many lesions are clinically silent—meaning the patient is unaware of the problem because the lesion occurs in an area of the brain that does not produce a physical symptom. Figure 9.8 shows how lesions come and go over several months for one patient.

There seem to be different phases of MS. The first phase is one of demyelination with focal symptoms followed by remyelination and recovery. The second phase is one of increasing and unremitting disability due to axonal loss and whole brain volume shrinkage. How quickly one moves from the relapsing/remitting phase to the secondary progressive phase varies from one individual to the next. Of greater relevance to treatment interventions, the first phase appears to have more of an inflammatory component while the secondary progressive phase does not. This becomes apparent in the treatment response.

Prior to 1993, there were no licensed treatments for MS. Now several treatment options exist that focus on reducing symptoms (such as unstable bladder or fatigue) or limiting the inflammatory response. Even more exciting are the beta IFNs—naturally occurring cytokines. They have been reported to reduce relapses by 30%. Unfortunately, long-term follow-up suggests that they have limited effect on the only outcome that really matters: accumulation of disability.

FIGURE 9.8 ● Serial MRI scans at the same level for the same patient with multiple sclerosis show how lesions appear and recede over the course of 1 year.

Monoclonal antibodies are a new treatment option being developed for MS. Genetically engineered mice are raised to produce antibodies that target specific molecules on the T cells. When injected, these antibodies latch onto the problematic T-cell molecule, which results in destruction of the cell and reduced immune cell activity. Is that not incredible? In a phase II trial, the monoclonal antibody alemtuzumab reduced relapses by 75% compared with a beta IFN. Early studies suggest that alemtuzumab is most effective in the early phases of MS, but did not change the progression of the illness for those already in the secondary progressive phase—further evidence that the latter phases of MS may have different mechanisms of action.

NEURAL REGULATION OF IMMUNITY

Until now we have been discussing the effects the immune system has on the brain, but actually the influence is bidirectional. The CNS has the capacity to regulate the immune response as well. Generally speaking, the CNS tends to dampen the immune response in order to restore homeostasis and prevent excessive inflammation.

The process starts when cytokines are released by white blood cells and travel to the brain in the plasma (Figure 9.9). The CNS responds through the autonomic nervous and endocrine systems. The sympathetic and parasympathetic branches of the autonomic nervous system modulate the immune response through innervation of the individual immune organs such as the spleen and lymph nodes. The endocrine system exerts its control through the release of sex hormones, thyroid hormone, and, most importantly, cortisol.

In 1950, the Nobel Prize was awarded for the discovery of cortisol. Its extraordinary anti-inflammatory properties were quickly recognized and put to use for rheumatoid arthritis and other inflammatory diseases. Endogenous cortisol provides the most powerful feedback loop through which the CNS modulates the inflammatory response. The importance of cortisol to inhibit an excessive immune response has been demonstrated in animal studies. When animals have their adrenal glands removed and then are inoculated with an infectious agent, they show increased mortality from shock. The unrestrained cytokine and pro-inflammatory responses overwhelm the animal—too much inflammation is detrimental. One of the jobs of the CNS is to keep the immune response from getting out of control. The brain puts the brakes on the immune response by releasing adrenocorticotropic hormone, which in turn stimulates the adrenal release of cortisol (Figure 9.9).

Stress-Induced Immune Dysfunction

Folk wisdom has long recognized that psychological stress takes a toll on one's physical health. Many years of research support this belief. Studies with new military recruits, anxious medical students, and caregivers of spouses with Alzheimer's disease have shown the ill effects of stress on the body.

Stress affects the CNS, which in turn alters the signals sent to the body through the endocrine and autonomic systems. Figure 22.1 shows a good example of the endocrine response to the acute stress of learning to parachute. These endocrine and autonomic signals gently suppress the immune response, which in turn puts the subject at greater risk for illness.

This connection between stress and poor healing is eloquently shown in animal studies. Mice are stressed by placing them in a restraining tube—

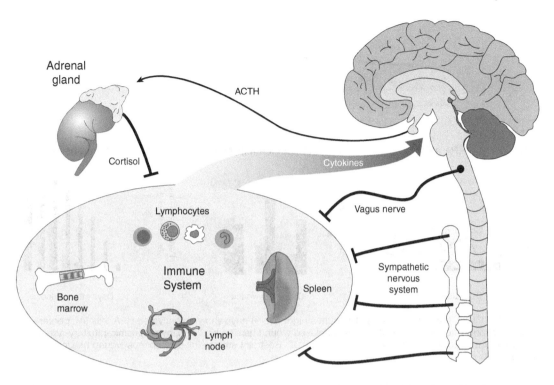

Adrenal gland

ACTH

Cortisol

Cytokines

Vagus nerve

Lymphocytes

Immune System

Spleen

Bone marrow

Sympathetic nervous system

Lymph node

FIGURE 9.9 ● The central nervous system restrains the immune response by way of the autonomic nervous system and endocrine system. ACTH, adrenocorticotropic hormone. (Adapted from Sternberg EM. Neural regulation of innate immunity: a coordinated nonspecific host response to pathogens. *Nat Rev Immunol.* 2006:6;318-328.)

overnight, when they are usually most active. In this particular study, the mice were restrained for 12 hours a night for 8 days in a row. On the third day, a small skin wound was opened. Figure 9.10 shows the results of this study for restrained mice compared with controls. The stressed mice had increased corticosterone (cortisol in a mouse), delayed leukocyte movement into the wound, and delayed wound healing.

Studies with humans have shown similar results—particularly patients with depression. Figure 21.3 shows the increased cortisol in depressed patients, suggesting an activated HPA axis. Furthermore, patients with diabetes, cancer, stroke, and myocardial infarction, who also are depressed, are at greater risk for death than similar patients without depression. Is the increased mortality secondary to impaired immunity?

Whitehall Study

The Whitehall study is one of those remarkable large epidemiologic studies that established with hard data what previously had been conjecture. The study followed almost 20,000 male British civil servants for 25 years and correlated the employment

grade with health. Simply looking at death, there is a dose–response association between employment grade and mortality (Figure 9.11A). A similar pyramid is seen regardless of whether the death is from for heart disease, neoplasm, stroke, or respiratory disease. Likewise, in one of the many side studies that came out of this project, measures of immune status also correlated with employment status. That is, men at the bottom of the employment pyramid had a more activated immune response as measured by C-reactive protein and circulating white blood cells (Figure 9.11B). Men in the lower employment grades were presumably more "stressed out," had poorer health, and showed greater immune activity.

Fatigue

Persistent fatigue is a frequent complaint with a long history. In 1869, the neurologist George Beard named the condition neurasthenia—a term that was in DSM-II in the neuroses section but was dropped from psychiatric nomenclature in 1980 with the publication of DSM-III.

In the mid-1980s, two practicing internists near Lake Tahoe, Nevada, generated considerable

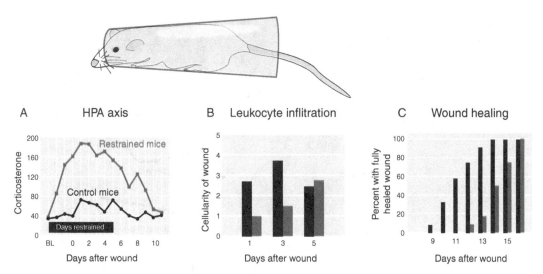

FIGURE 9.10 ● Mice restrained for 12 hours a night over 8 days show an activated HPA axis (**A**), poorer cellular response to the wound site (**B**), and delayed wound healing (**C**). HPA, hypothalamic-pituitary-adrenal. (Adapted from Padgett DA, Marucha PT, Sheridan JF. Restraint stress slows cutaneous wound healing in mice. *Brain Behav Immun.* 1998;12:64-73.)

excitement when they reported an epidemic of persistent fatigue associated with elevated titers of the Epstein-Barr virus (EBV). Ultimately, the Centers for Disease Control and Prevention (CDC) disproved EBV as a cause of the illness, but this was the start of what became chronic fatigue syndrome.

Chronic fatigue syndrome captured the attention of patients and clinicians. Many patients, who would never see a psychiatrist, were thrilled to be treated by infectious disease specialists. Researchers, likewise, raced to find the cause. However, all the findings have remained "soft." While immunologic abnormalities can be found, they are difficult to reproduce and are not diagnostic. Periodically, a new infectious agent is identified by one group only to have other labs

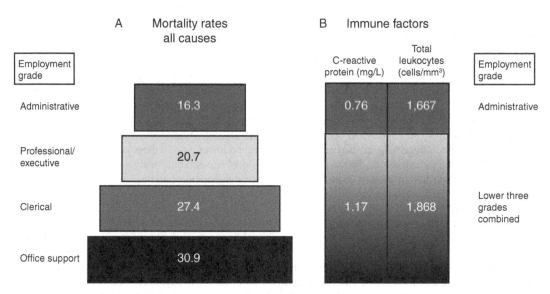

FIGURE 9.11 ● The Whitehall study showed that employment grade correlated with mortality (**A**) and immune activation (**B**) in British civil servants. Men in upper ranks had lower mortality and a more settled immune system.

fail to duplicate the results. The XMRV retrovirus is the current example.

Many clinicians see chronic fatigue as a psychiatric disorder with similarities to depression. Indeed, antidepressants, cognitive-behavioral therapy, and exercise are effective treatments for depression and chronic fatigue. In general, the medical community has gradually placed chronic fatigue back into a psychosomatic category. However, this chapter should attest to the interplay between the infectious/immunologic and the neuro/psychiatric, which raises the question: Is Chronic fatigue syndrome a stress-induced immunologic deficiency or a psychiatric disorder caused by an infection?

QUESTIONS

1. *Treponema pallidum* damages the brain
   a. Within 18 hours of infection.
   b. By targeting pyramidal neurons in the cortex.
   c. By releasing a toxin.
   d. By inducing an inflammatory response.

2. A cocaine vaccine
   a. Reduces immune activation.
   b. Stimulates anticocaine antibody production in the CNS.
   c. Reduces euphoria.
   d. Stimulates anticocaine leukocytes.

3. Cytokines are involved in all of the following except
   a. Neural plasticity.
   b. Turning off the inflammatory response.
   c. Mental illness.
   d. Identifying *Treponema pallidum*.

4. All the following are true of MS except
   a. Responds to TNF inhibitors.
   b. Can be confused with hysteria.
   c. Is a T-cell problem.
   d. Induces silent lesions.

5. The CNS reduces the inflammatory response through all of the following except
   a. Parasympathetic nervous system.
   b. Sympathetic nervous system.
   c. Cytokines.
   d. Adrenal gland.

6. An activated immune system
   a. Can be used to diagnose chronic fatigue syndrome.
   b. Complicates neural development.
   c. Occurs in the latent phase of syphilis.
   d. Promotes healing.

See Answers section at the end of the book.

CHAPTER 10

The Electrical Brain

MORE THAN CHEMISTRY

One of our favorite illustrations in this book is Figure 3.9, which highlights the electrochemical configuration of neural communication. Unfortunately, many mental health professionals view psychiatric disorders as exclusively chemical in nature. The term "chemical imbalance" is part of our cultural lexicon, a perspective that misses the rapid signals passed over long distances before any chemicals are released.

Electricity is the currency of the brain. It is not just chemistry—the brain is an electrical organ. This is not new information, but rather a different, newer, and more nuanced way to view the brain. The brain uses enough electricity to power the 20 W light in your refrigerator—if it was possible to harness the electricity in your brain. That is a significant amount of electrical energy! Merely keeping our brains running requires about 20% of all the calories we consume, and higher amounts when we concentrate (as opposed to watching TV).

We believe the electrical side of the electrochemical signal has been ignored for too long. This chapter—new to the second edition—has been added to correct the inequity. Probably the real impetus is not so much an attempt to be fair, but our reaction to the explosion of research on the effects of electrical manipulation of the brain.

History of Electrical Stimulation

Before it was possible to produce electricity on demand, the ancient Greeks and Romans reportedly used fish—electric eels or rays—to stimulate the brain as a treatment for intractable headaches. Of course the ancient physicians did not know they were using electricity and the clinical effectiveness of electrical eels for headaches is unknown. However, it is relevant to note that eNeuras Therapeutics is seeking the Food and Drug Administration (FDA) approval for a handheld device that delivers a

brief electromagnetic pulse (transcranial magnetic stimulation—more on this later) to the back of the head to "short circuit" an impending migraine. So, maybe an electric ray could actually have stopped an ancient headache. (If someone tries out the eel headache therapy, please write us and let us know of the outcome. [We certainly aren't recommending that you try this.])

In the first chapter we mentioned Luigi Galvani who in 18th century Italy demonstrated that electrical sparks could induce movement in an amputated frog's leg. He was the first to propose that the brain generates intrinsic electricity that spreads down through the nerves to the muscles. He believed electricity was the mysterious "vital force" controlling the body. His nephew Giovanni Aldini (1762–1834) spent many years conducting further research and promoting the beliefs of his uncle. Using primitive batteries developed by Volta, Aldini applied electrical stimulation to mammals and eventually even humans. He demonstrated throughout Europe—part science, part carnival—the effects of applying electrical stimulation to human cadavers. In London in 1803 at the Royal College of Surgeons, Aldini applied electrical stimulation to a freshly hung criminal and awed his audience with facial and body movements in the deceased human. Aldini's work was an inspiration for Mary Shelley's novel *Frankenstein*.

Of even greater interest were Aldini's efforts to treat the mentally ill with electrical stimulation. He is reported to have treated an Italian farmer suffering from melancholy madness with stimulation applied to the patient's shaved, damp head (Figure 10.1). After several weeks of treatment, the patient was well enough to return to his family. Later, Aldini met the famous French psychiatrist Philippe Pinel—the man who removed the chains from the insane—and applied his "galvanic" treatment to several patients at La Salpêtrière Hospital,

FIGURE 10.1 ● A patient receiving a crude form of direct current brain stimulation in 1803. As the brain is an electrochemical organ, it can be changed and manipulated with externally applied electricity. (Adapted from Parent A. Giovanni Aldini: from animal electricity to human brain stimulation. *Can J Neurol Sci*. 2004;31(4):576-584.)

but with limited success. We do not fully understand the doses and actual current that Aldini used, but today a different version of this type of treatment is called transcranial direct current stimulation (tDCS). While not FDA approved or even in regular use, tDCS is being studied as a possible intervention for Parkinson's disease, tinnitus, post-stroke deficits, and, you guessed it, just like Aldini demonstrated, melancholy (depression). tDCS involves passing a small (2 mA) direct current through the brain for 20 to 30 minutes. The brain regions under the anode become excited, and it takes less energy for that region to carry out its normal function.

Wilder Penfield is another one of the great figures that pioneered the use of electricity to study the brain. Penfield crossed paths with some of the leading neuroscientists mentioned in the first chapter. As a Rhodes scholar, he studied in Sherrington's lab at Oxford and later collaborated with Ramón y Cajal in Madrid. However, Penfield was a practicing neurosurgeon in Canada who studied the brain while he was treating patients. He perfected what came to be called the Montreal Procedure: the surgical removal of the site of the brain causing intractable seizures—still the most effective treatment for disabling epilepsy.

The unique aspect of the Montreal Procedure was the exploration of the patient's brain while they remained awake. Using local anesthesia, the patient's skull was opened and their brains exposed. Penfield gently stimulated the cortex around the

lesion with an electrode. Patients remained alert so they could identify what they felt or moved as Penfield applied the electricity. The goal was to identify the pathological tissue, but preserve as much of the healthy brain as possible. (Interested readers can see reenactments on YouTube by searching for "Wilder Penfield.")

While Penfield was treating these patients, he was also mapping out the sensory and motor cortex. For each patient he would record the location where different body parts were represented on the cortex. For example, Figure 10.2A shows the location of facial and eye sensations and movements for a number of patients. Figure 10.2B shows average location for the motor cortex compiled from data on almost 400 patients over 20 years. We now know the sensory and motor homunculus are not static, but are capable of reorganization after injury or with frequent use as we discussed in Chapter 8.

Penfield is best known in popular culture for awakening memories with electrical stimulation of the temporal lobes. This has led to the perception that memories are a fixed neural network (or engram) that can be repeatedly elicited when stimulated. The reality is not so impressive. It turns out that only about 8% of people whose temporal lobes were stimulated reported any memory. Of those that did "remember," most reported experiences similar to the aura that preceded their seizure or described something more like a hallucination. Furthermore, modern studies have failed to find clear memories that reproduce with each stimulation. A memory engram remains elusive.

In the late 1930s, around the time Penfield was refining the Montreal Procedure, Ugo Cerletti, an Italian physician, began using electricity to induce seizures as treatment for the seriously mentally ill. Although this may seem like an extreme intervention to us, it was actually a logical step in the progression of physical treatments of mental illness. Psychiatrists had been inducing convulsions with metrazol—a γ-aminobutyric acid (GABA) antagonist that increases neural excitability—but it was difficult to control. Cerletti saw an electrically induced seizure as a cleaner procedure: easier to induce and terminate—no residual metabolite to complicate the recovery. Cerletti's intervention has developed into electroconvulsive therapy (ECT) and remains the most effective treatment for depression.

The last historical figure we choose to discuss is Robert Heath, a psychiatrist and neurologist who in the late 1950s coordinated the placement of electrodes into the brains of patients with serious mental illness. He was influenced by the work of Olds and Milner (see Figure 12.2) and was hoping that small frequent doses of electricity applied directly

⊖ Eye sensation   E Eyelid movement
O Face sensation   + Face movement
H Head sensation

A

B

FIGURE 10.2 ● Actual recordings of sensation and movement for the eyes and face of patients examined by Wilder Penfield (**A**) compared with the cumulative motor homunculus for the average patient (**B**). (Adapted from Penfield W, Boldrey E. Somatic motor and sensory representation in the cerebral cortex of man as studied by electrical stimulation. *Brain*. 1938;60:389-443.)

to deep sectors of the brain might improve their mental condition. He conceptualized his intervention as an emotional pacemaker. (Interested readers can view actual clips of one patient by searching "Robert Heath" on YouTube.) The results were disappointing and his approach was controversial. However, Heath's work was the forerunner of deep brain stimulation (DBS), now a common intervention for Parkinson's disease—and something of great interest to many as a possible treatment for intractable depression.

BIOELECTRICITY

All living cells maintain a negative electrical charge. That is, they are more negative inside relative to the extracellular space. Nerve cells utilize this property to communicate with one another—a process that through millions of years of evolution has transformed the speed by which biological organisms sense and respond. Without bioelectricity, we would all be slower than slugs.

The negative charge inside a cell is the product of competing forces within the cellular realm. First and foremost, the cellular wall creates a boundary that limits the movement of charged substances into or out of the cell. The primary negative charge created in a cell is contained on the negatively charged organic molecules within the cell, for example, amino acids. These large molecules, too large to escape through the cell wall, provide the bulk of the negative charge inside the cell.

The negative charge inside the cell is reduced by the movement of positive ions, such as potassium

(K^+) and sodium (Na^+), into the cell. The positive ions are attracted to the negative charge inside the cell: remember, opposites attract in love and electricity. However, the movement of each ion is different. The K^+ ions flow freely into the cell until they reach a point at which the forces of the **concentration gradient** start to pull some K^+ back into the extracellular space. The propensity of ions to evenly diffuse within a contained space is called the concentration gradient. Ultimately, the amount of K^+ inside the cell is a product of the pull of the **electrostatic forces** into the cell and the push of the concentration gradient back out to the extracellular space.

The Na^+ ions, on the other hand, are actively removed from the intracellular space. Using what is called the **sodium–potassium pump**, the neurons pump out Na^+ ions that have leaked into the cell. Expelling Na^+ ions requires considerable energy, as the ions must be forced out of the cell against the concentration gradient and against the electrostatic pressure. Running the sodium–potassium pump is one of the primary reasons the brain is such an energy hog. The final concentrations within and outside of the cell are shown below. The result is an electrostatic charge of about −60 mV.

	Na^+	K^+	Large Organic Molecules
Intracellular	50	400	Many
Extracellular	440	20	Few

Nerve cells utilize a rapid and brief change in the polarization as a signal that can be quickly transmitted from one end of the cell to the other. In Chapter 3, we briefly described how nerve cells communicate—how the signal from incoming neurons depolarize or hyperpolarize the neuron (Figures 3.6 and 3.7)—and when the electrical charge at the axon hillock reaches the threshold (–40 mV), an impulse is sent down the axon (Figure 3.8). We have not discussed the transmission of the electrical impulse down the axon. The voltage-gated channel is the secret, but first a word about normal wave movement.

Usually waves diminish in size as they move away from the source. Think of throwing a pebble in a pond and watching the waves decay as they spread out. The 2011 tsunami in Japan provides a real world example of wave progression. Along the coast of Japan, the waves were estimated to be

almost 39 m tall, while they were only 2 m by the time they reached Hawaii 7 hours later. The action potential, on the other hand, does not diminish in size as it shoots down an axon—the amplitude remains constant.

It is **voltage-gated sodium channels** that maintain the amplitude of the action potential, which in humans may stretch for over a meter in length. (The recurrent laryngeal nerve in the giraffe, which descends into the thorax before climbing back up the neck to the larynx, may be as long as 15 feet. Fortunately for the giraffe, the signal at the larynx is just as robust as the one that left the brain.) The voltage-gated channel is triggered when it is depolarized—reaches its threshold. It then opens and ions—in this case Na^+—flood into the axon. This in turn depolarizes the next voltage-gated channels and the process repeats itself on down the axon (Figure 10.3).

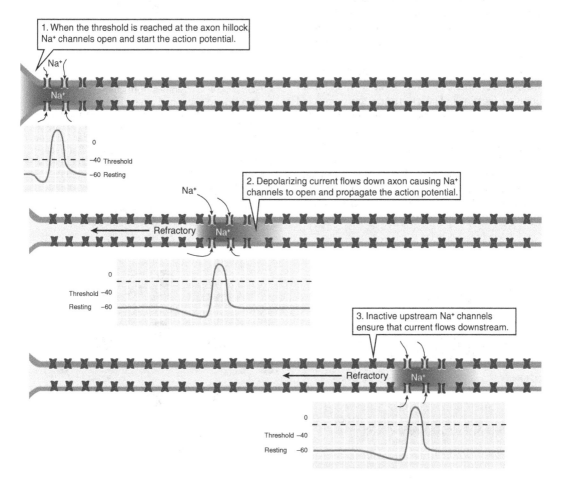

FIGURE 10.3 ● The rapid opening and closing of the Na^+ channels sends an electrical signal down the axon. The refractory period after the passing of an action potential keeps the signal moving in the correct direction. Note that the electrical tracing is proceeding from the right to the left, which is opposite of how it is usually shown (see Figure 1.7 for comparison).

ELECTROENCEPHALOGRAM

Sensitive instruments can detect the electrical signals generated by the nervous system. As early as 1875, recordings captured electrical activity from an exposed monkey brain. However, it was not until 1929 that an Austrian psychiatrist, Hans Berger, first recorded electrical tracing from the scalp of an awake human. Called electroencephalogram or EEG, Berger was able to show that different states of mind produce different rhythms. The EEG remains a useful tool to analyze sleep and epilepsy.

Synaptic activity at the dendrite generates a tiny electrical charge (Figure 10.4). When thousands of other cells contribute their small voltage, a signal becomes strong enough to be detected by the EEG electrode at the scalp. The EEG measures the sum of the electrical activity from the large pyramidal neurons. When the neurons fire in unison, large electrical waves are recorded on the EEG. Small waves, typically when one is alert and focused, reflect the chatter of asynchronous neurons. Figure 15.3 shows EEG recordings for different states of consciousness.

EEG recordings are generally made through two-dozen electrodes affixed to the scalp in predetermined locations. The electrodes are connected to amplifiers and continuous recordings are noted between 16 standard electrodes. Small voltage changes are measured between pairs of electrodes. Usually the voltage fluctuations are only a few tens of microvolts in amplitude. During deep sleep and seizure activity, large waves develop. Figure 10.5 shows actual EEG recordings for a patient with absence seizures.

FIGURE 10.4 ● Signals from afferent neurons (in this example just one afferent neuron) release a neurotransmitter at the synapse. The movement of positive ions into the pyramidal neuron leaves a slightly negative charge in the extracellular fluid. As the current spreads and escapes out of the deeper parts of the neuron, those extracellular sites become slightly positive. The EEG detects the cumulative charge between two scalp electrodes. (Adapted from Bear MF, Connors BW, Paradiso MA, eds. *Neuroscience: Exploring the Brain.* 3rd ed. Baltimore, MD: Lippincott Williams & Wilkins; 2007.)

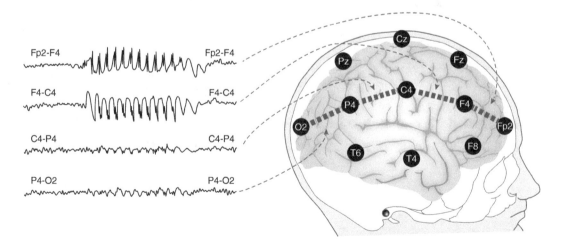

FIGURE 10.5 ● The EEG records electrical activity between two electrodes. This example of an absence seizure (also called petit mal seizure) shows just four tracings from the right brain. You do not have to be a neurologist to recognize that the seizure activity emanates from the frontal lobes.

Excessive or Insufficient

In this section of the book, we have been reviewing modulating factors on the brain—hormones, growth factor proteins, immunity, and now electricity. In each case, the modulation can be too much or too little, for example, too much cortisol or not enough and excessive or insufficient brain-derived neurotrophic factor. The question here is, does this paradigm apply to electricity in the brain?

Excessive Electrical Activity

A seizure is a clear example of excessive electrical activity in the brain. Recognized 3,000 years ago by the ancient Babylonians, epilepsy is, by definition, excessive abnormal neuronal electrical activity. The Epilepsy Foundation reports that 3 million Americans have the disorder. There are many different types of seizures, but broadly there are two types: focal seizures, when the electrical activity remains in a limited area of the brain, and generalized seizures, which affect the whole brain.

Every brain has the capacity to have a seizure. Psychiatrists can use ECT to induce a seizure in anyone. Various problems predispose the brain to erupt in a seizure, for example, fever, trauma, tumors, illicit drug use, and infections, to name a few. But some people appear to have a lower seizure threshold for no obvious reason, and they have spontaneous seizures. Some research suggests abnormalities of neural growth in which abnormal networks connect back on themselves and lead to self-excitation. Other research has identified abnormalities of receptors, in particular the voltage-gated sodium channel. Numerous mutations of the sodium channels have been identified that are believed to predispose the cortical neurons to electrical instability and spontaneous activity.

Kindling is a model for seizure activity and epilepsy that is of great interest to biological psychiatrists. (The concept is similar to the process shown in Figure 5.6.) Repeated subconvulsive stimulation (kindling) of the amygdala or hippocampus with an irritant or stimulant (cocaine) leads over time to an enhanced response and eventually cocaine-induced seizures and then finally spontaneous seizures. Although more theory than fact, this model gives one explanation for the development of some forms of epilepsy.

Some psychiatrists have latched on to the theory of kindling as a model for what might be happening with bipolar and unipolar depression, where first or second affective episodes early in life are often associated with life stresses or triggers, but later episodes appear to be spontaneous and not environmentally triggered. They see the gradual decline in some patients with repeated episodes of

WITHDRAWAL SEIZURES

Alcohol has been used for centuries to calm the brain. Since Librium was introduced in 1960, the benzodiazepines have become popular alternatives for stressed-out people. The brain reacts to the chronic use of sedative hypnotics by decreasing GABA activity and increasing the excitatory glutamate activity. Sudden withdrawal from alcohol or benzodiazepines unmasks the new balance, which results in too much accelerator and not enough brake. In such an overexcited state, seizures can develop.

the disorder as a kindling process. The effectiveness of the anticonvulsants in mood disorders is also suggestive of electrical aberration as a driving cause of mood disorders. However, the antidepressants actually lower the seizure threshold. One would think they would exacerbate a mood disorder, instead of improving the mood, if the pathophysiology was due to excessive electrical activity.

Insufficient Electrical Activity

If the epilepsies are a clear example of the brain having too much electrical activity, are there examples where the brain has simply too little electricity? Like a fire that won't light because the wood is damp, are there conditions in which the brain has become too sluggish and the electricity isn't flowing? Certainly it feels this way some mornings!

There are obvious examples of insufficient electrical activity in the brain—coma is one, intoxication is another. In the intensive care unit when an unresponsive person exists solely on life support, establishing the absence of electrical activity in the brain is how brain death is distinguished from a persistent vegetative state. These are overt examples of insufficient electrical activity associated with significant altered mental status. However, are there conditions we see in mental health that are a product of inadequate electricity in the brain?

The short answer is No! We do not know of any psychiatric disorders that are caused by insufficient electrical activity. Although it appears that some depressive symptoms and the negative signs of schizophrenia, for example, are produced by sluggish electrical connections, in all likelihood the absence of activity is more a product of insufficient neuronal metabolism. However, there is great interest in treatments that can awaken the glutamate neurons. In the next section, we briefly look at interventions that electrically stimulate the brain as treatment of mental disorders.

STIMULATING THE BRAIN

Focally stimulating the brain is a way of hijacking or using the brain's natural method of communicating (electrical flow through axons and neurons). Because the methods are applied directly to the brain, they do not have systemic side effects like oral medications, which have to pass through the body before entering the central nervous system. Another advantage of electrical stimulation is the absence of residue. When the electricity is turned off, there is nothing left to be cleared away.

Interested readers are referred to our other book for an in-depth review of this area, but it is helpful here to outline some of the more important methods. ECT is used to purposefully create a seizure in the prefrontal cortex and is the most effective treatment available for acute depression or mania. It is also used to treat catatonia and can help with Parkinson's symptoms and can even stop status epilepticus. New advances in the type of electricity used (pulse width) and electrode locations have improved outcomes while reducing, but not entirely eliminating, cognitive side effects (see Figure 18.12).

Transcranial magnetic stimulation involves placing a small electromagnet on the scalp and turning it rapidly on and off. This creates a powerful, and transient, magnetic field, which travels unimpeded through the scalp and into the brain, inducing an electrical current in brain cells just at the surface of the brain. Repeatedly stimulating the prefrontal cortex every day for 4 to 6 weeks is now an FDA-approved treatment for acute depression. It has also shown promise in treating pain (see TMS, PFC, and Postoperative pain box in Chapter 11).

Vagus nerve stimulation involves wrapping an electrode around the vagus nerve in the neck and connecting the nerve to a pacemaker implanted under the skin in the chest. Repeated current through this nerve has been shown to treat epilepsy and the device is approved for medication-resistant epilepsy patients. It is also FDA approved as a long-term treatment for patients with treatment-resistant depression.

DBS involves placing a wire directly into the brain through a burr hole in the skull and connecting the wire to small generators implanted in the chest wall. DBS in the basal ganglia can immediately treat tremors in Parkinson's disease and is FDA approved for that indication. There is much interest in whether DBS could treat depression, and clinical trials are underway.

Finally, tDCS, mentioned at the start of this chapter, involves a relatively simple system of passing direct current through discrete brain regions. It is being investigated heavily in a variety of disorders, with no clear therapeutic indications yet.

Priming the Pump

A potential emerging use for brain stimulation may be the benefit of adding electrical stimulation to standard treatment. The best example involves the treatment of anomia or aphasia after a stroke. Anomia is impaired word retrieval or, simply, the inability to find the right word. This is a common problem after strokes and the standard treatment is speech therapy. However, a number of clever researchers have used tDCS to add electrical stimulation to speech therapy as a way of enhancing the treatment. Figure 10.6 illustrates this procedure. Four cathodes and one anode are placed on the

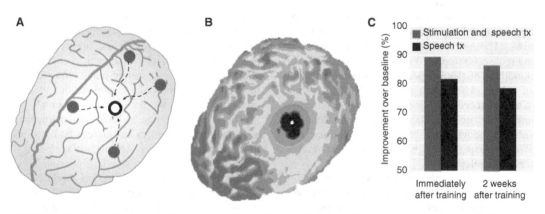

FIGURE 10.6 ● Electrical stimulation enhances speech therapy. **A.** Schematic of electrode placement. **B.** Functional imaging of actual stimulation. **C.** Stimulation plus speech therapy improved naming objects in patients with anomia after stroke. (**B** Adapted from Datta A, Bansal V, Diaz J, Patel J, Reato D, Bikson M. Gyri-precise head model of transcranial direct current stimulation: improved spatial focality using a ring electrode versus conventional rectangular pad. *Brain Stimul.* 2009;2:201-207. **C** Adapted from Flöel A, Meinzer M, Kirstein R, et al. Short-term anomia training and electrical brain stimulation. *Stroke.* 2011;42:2065-2067).

brain. The current moves from the cathodes (brown circles) toward the anode (white circle with black outline) (Figure 10.6A). Functional magnetic resonance imaging shows the activation of the brain during this kind of stimulation (Figure 10.6B). In a separate study, 12 patients with chronic anomia from left hemisphere strokes practiced naming different sets of objects with and without electrical stimulation. In this study, the stimulation was conducted over the right temporoparietal cortex—an area associated with long-term memory (see Figure 18.9) Both immediately and 2 weeks later, the objects learned with stimulation were more accurately named by the patients.

The key feature of using brain stimulation in this manner is that the person must be doing the exercise when the electrical stimulation is added. Simply adding current to the brain is not beneficial. But electrically stimulating the brain while the activity is being practiced seems to enhance learning. Could this intervention expedite learning a foreign language? Would psychotherapy be more effective if the brain was mildly stimulated at the same time? Clearly more studies are needed.

One advantage of tDCS is the simplicity of the procedure. Most new technologies in medical care are expensive and require trained personnel to operate the machinery. tDCS is inexpensive and easy to use: a few pads and a 9 volt battery. If tDCS can enhance learning, we may be on the cusp of a new treatment modality in mental health.

Consciousness

Let us end this chapter with one of the most important questions regarding the brain. What is consciousness? Is it related to the electrical energy flowing in the brain? Do we have less electrical activity in the brain when we sleep, or are unconscious? The answer is a complicated one maybe. In certain stages of sleep, such as rapid eye movement (REM), our brains are just as active as during the day when we are awake. However, in other non-REM stages, it appears as if different parts of the brain isolate themselves from the rest of the brain, and the brain is less connected. When we are unconscious, less electricity is flowing from any given brain region to all others. The brain is compartmentalizing when we are unconscious. This "connectedness as consciousness" theory is being used by some researchers as a way to explain what it means to be conscious (brain regions fully connected and passing electricity freely) or unconscious (brain regions disconnected). Why the brain needs to do this during sleep is still not clear.

QUESTIONS

Match the columns

1. tDCS

2. Preserves the action potential

3. Transcranial magnetic stimulation (TMS)

4. Deep brain stimulation (DBS)

5. The seizure is the treatment

6. Currency of the brain

7. Insufficient electrical activity

8. Prone to seizure activity

a. FDA indication for depression

b. Electricity

c. Voltage-gated sodium channels

d. Coma

e. 9 volt

f. Insufficient GABA

g. Robert Heath

h. ECT

See Answers section at the end of the book.

SECTION III

Behaviors

CHAPTER 11

Pain

Pain and pleasure are the major driving forces of human behavior. We cover pain in this chapter but are ever so looking forward to discussing pleasure in the next chapter.

ACUTE PAIN

Acute pain, as we all have experienced, starts in the periphery, is relayed to the spinal cord, and then passes up to the brain where it produces a negative reaction (Figure 11.1). Pain-producing stimuli are detected by specialized afferent neurons called *nociceptors*. The nociceptors are free nerve endings—not an identifiable structure as we have for touch and vibration. These cells respond to a broad range of physical and chemical stimuli, but only at intensities that are capable of causing damage.

Peripheral Tissue

The nociceptors in peripheral tissue are activated by injury or tissue damage that results in the release of bradykinins, prostaglandins, and potassium (Figure 11.2). These molecules in turn cause the secretion of substance P from other branches of the axon, which stimulates the release of histamine and promotes vasodilation.

Aδ and C fibers send the signal to the dorsal horn of the spinal cord by way of the dorsal root ganglion. The Aδ fibers are myelinated axons that quickly send the first, sharp signals of pain. The C fibers are unmyelinated and send a slower, dull pain signal (Figure 11.3). It is the duller, slow pain signal of the C fibers that becomes so troublesome in chronic pain conditions (see box).

Spinal Cord

The nociceptive afferent nerve fibers synapse in the dorsal horn of the spinal cord. Information about tissue injury is passed on to the next neurons, which then cross to the contralateral side and ascend to the brain.

The signal can be modified at this point by descending fibers (discussed later) or from simultaneous activity by nonpain neurons (mechanoreceptors: Aβ fibers). The Aβ fibers can dampen the pain signal in what is called the *gate theory of pain*. Figure 11.4 shows how a signal from the larger mechanoreceptor activates an inhibitory interneuron in the dorsal horn, which results in a smaller signal conveyed to the brain. The gate theory explains why rubbing an injury seems to reduce the pain and is the rationale for the use of transcutaneous electrical nerve stimulation.

Ascending Pathways

There are a variety of ways to describe the different nociceptive pathways that ascend to the brain in the spinal cord. Unfortunately, there is no consensus on the proper nomenclature for these tracts and no two authors seem to use the same terms. Recently, the perception of pain—and the areas participating, in the central nervous system (CNS)—has been divided into two prominent domains: **sensory-discriminative** and **affective-motivational**. This dichotomy (summarized in Table 11.1) is a convenient way to understand the ascending pathways.

Sensory-Discriminative

The sensory-discriminative domain encompasses the traditional sensory pathway taught in the first year of medical school. The signal travels up the *spinothalamic tract*, synapses in the lateral thalamus, and proceeds to the somatosensory cortex. Figure 11.5 is a diagram of this pathway. This type of pain allows the subject to become aware of the location of the pain and answer the question, "where does it hurt?" However, the perception of pain is much more than just identifying the location of a noxious sensation and withdrawing the injured limb.

FIGURE 11.1 ● The somatosensory cortex receives the negative sensation of pain from the peripheral nerves by way of the spinal cord.

Affective-Motivational

Other ascending sensory signals communicate the intensity of a noxious stimuli. There are several tracts that transport these signals, such as the *spinoreticular tract* or the *spinomesencephalic tract*—just to name a few. The important point is that all the signals travel in the anterolateral region of the spinal cord and terminate in different locations such as the reticular formation, periaqueductal gray (PAG)

matter, and the amygdala. The rest of the signals synapse in the medial thalamus before proceeding to other areas of the cerebral cortex (Figure 11.6).

The affective-motivational signals communicate the unpleasantness of the sensation and answer the question, "how much does it hurt?" In the cortex, these signals activate areas associated with emotional feelings, such as the anterior cingulate cortex (ACC), insular cortex, and prefrontal cortex—as

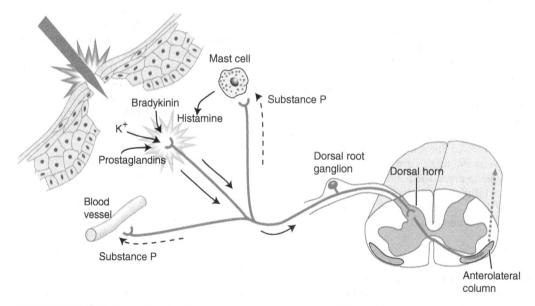

FIGURE 11.2 ● Peripheral nociceptive responses to acute trauma. (Adapted from Kandel ER, Schwartz JH, Jessell TM, eds. *Principles of Neural Science*. 4th ed. New York: McGraw-Hill; 2000.)

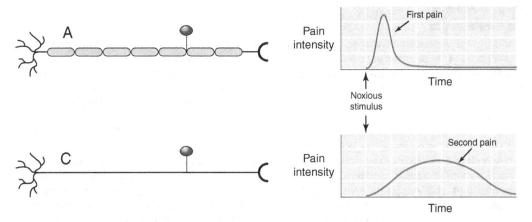

FIGURE 11.3 ● Aδ and C fibers transmit pain signals at different rates. (Adapted from Bear MF, Connors BW, Paradiso MA, eds. *Neuroscience: Exploring the Brain*. 3rd ed. Baltimore, MD: Lippincott Williams & Wilkins; 2007.)

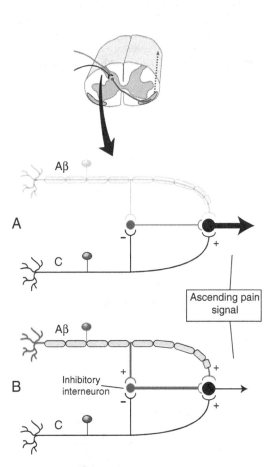

FIGURE 11.4 ● Gate theory of pain in the dorsal horn of the spinal cord. **A.** Without input from Aβ fibers a large signal is transmitted to the brain. **B.** A smaller signal is transmitted with input from Aβ fibers.

well as the amygdala. Functional brain imaging studies over the past two decades have documented activity in these areas during pain perception—areas we typically associated with mood, attention, and fear. Activity in these regions of the brain helps us understand the concomitant depression, hyperfocus, and anxiety we see with patients in pain.

Figure 11.7 shows drawings of some of the areas that become active with acute pain. In this study, subjects were scanned at rest and later with a hot probe (approximately 50°C) applied to the upper right arm. Note the diverse areas that become active with acute pain—thalamus, ACC, prefrontal cortex, and insula, as well as others. The experience of pain is more than just identifying where it hurts.

It is also important to note that some of the activation is on both sides of the brain. This shows that there is more to the processing of pain signals in the CNS than implied by our simplified Figures 11.5 and 11.6.

TABLE 11.1

The Two Afferent Pathways Bringing Pain Signals from the Periphery to the CNS

Sensory-Discriminative	Affective-Motivational
Where does it hurt?	How much does it hurt?
Lateral thalamus	Medial thalamus
Somatosensory cortex	ACC, insula, PFC, amygdala

ACC, anterior cingulate cortex; PFC, prefrontal cortex.

Over 20% of American adults struggle with chronic pain. The pharmaceutical industry is actively searching for an effective analgesic devoid of narcotic side effects or addictive potential. The transient receptor potential vanilloid 1 (TRPV1) receptor is one potential target. Found primarily on small diameter sensory neurons such as C fiber neurons, the TRPV1 receptor responds to a variety of noxious chemical and physical stimuli—including capsaicin, the active component of chili peppers. Animal studies suggest that blocking this receptor reduces the aching quality of chronic pain while preserving the sensations of touch and proprioception. The National Institutes of Health and several pharmaceutical giants are studying the effect of blocking the TRPV1 receptor in humans.

One concern regarding TRPV1 is the role the sensory neurons play in modulating inflammation. Activation of the TRPV1 receptor leads to the release of pro-inflammatory cytokines. Not surprisingly, animal studies have shown that TRPV1 disruption can impair bacterial clearance, cytokine response, and ultimately mortality from sepsis—another reminder that pain and protection are intimately connected.

CONGENITAL INSENSITIVITY TO PAIN

Congenital insensitivity to pain, a term used to describe rare genetic conditions in which people lack the ability to sense pain, initially sounds like a blessing but is actually a nightmare. Individuals with this condition fail to identify or respond to noxious, injuring stimuli and suffer excessive burns, fractures, and soft tissue damage. Ultimately, the unrecognized injuries and secondary complications lead to an early death.

The spectrum of congenital insensitivity to pain provides an example of the distinction between sensory and affective components of pain. Subjects with frank congenital insensitivity to pain are without the peripheral Aδ and C fibers. These patients

FIGURE 11.5 ● Spinothalamic tract transmitting the sensory-discriminative pain signal from the periphery to the somatosensory cortex.

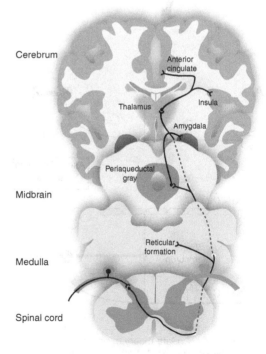

FIGURE 11.6 ● Affective-motivational pain tracts.

FIGURE 11.7 ● PET scans showing activity in the brain with acute pain. ACC, anterior cingulate cortex; Thal, thalamus; Cb, cerebellum; Ins, insula; PMv, ventral premotor cortex. (Adapted from Coghill RC, McHaffie JG, Yen YF. Neural correlates of interindividual differences in the subjective experience of pain. *Proc Natl Acad Sci U S A*. 2003;100(14):8538-8542.)

lack the sensory-discriminative as well as affective components of pain and are the most at risk for harm and premature death.

A milder condition, termed *congenital indifference to pain*, is found in individuals who can distinguish sharp and dull pain, but are indifferent to the sensation. They lack the emotional responses and normal withdrawal movements; they can feel the pain, but are not concerned. Subjects with this disorder have normal peripheral nerve fibers but seem to have an as yet unidentified central impairment of the affective-motivational component of pain.

Congenital insensitivity to pain with anhidrosis is a specific rare autosomal recessive disorder characterized by absence of pain (along with inability to sweat, unexplained episodes of fever, and mental retardation). Patients with this condition have a mutation in the gene for the Trk receptor—the receptor that binds with nerve growth factor. As we saw in Chapter 8, nerves need nerve growth factor proteins to survive. Cells lacking the receptor are unable to incorporate the growth factor and wither away (or fail to develop). The patient lacks pain fibers and therefore does not experience pain.

Pain Tolerance Spectrum

People have different abilities to tolerate pain. This has been shown in multiple psychological studies and observed by most of us in our clinical population.

More recently, brain imaging studies have documented that subjects with less pain tolerance have greater activation of the cortical areas discussed earlier (ACC, insular cortex, and prefrontal cortex, along with the somatosensory cortex).

Genetic factors undoubtedly play a role in the spectrum of pain tolerance. A study reported in 2005 examined pain tolerance in 202 women and genetic variants for the gene encoding for catecholamine-*O*-methyltransferase (COMT), an enzyme involved in the regulation of catecholamines and enkephalins. After initially measuring pain tolerance with a noxious thermal stimuli, the researchers assessed the genetic makeup of each participant. They found that three genetic variants for COMT accounted for 11% of the variation in pain perception (a large percentage in genetic studies). Figure 11.8 shows how five different combinations of these genetic variants accounted for differing pain responsiveness. Further recent studies by the same research group examined patients in the ER after a motor vehicle accident. They found that those with the pain vulnerable genes were more likely to report neck pain, headaches, and dizziness.

One wonders if subjects who excel at physically demanding professions are more tolerant to pain than those of us with more sedentary jobs. Legend has it that Edward Villella, the famous American dancer, had his feet X-rayed in his thirties

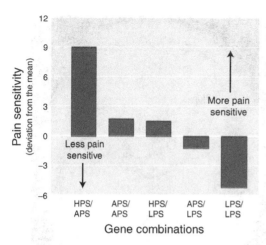

FIGURE 11.8 ● Pain responsiveness categorized by three major combinations of genetic variations for the catecholamine-O-methyltransferase enzyme. LPS, low pain sensitivity; APS, average pain sensitivity; HPS, high pain sensitivity. Subjects with the LPS variation were 2.3 times less likely to develop temporomandibular joint disorder. (Adapted from Diatchenko L, Slade GD, Nackley AG, et al. Genetic basis for individual variations in pain perception and the development of a chronic pain condition. *Hum Mol Genet.* 2005;14(1):135-143.)

and discovered nine old fractures of which he was unaware. Ostensibly what would have crippled us was just an aching foot to Villella. Surprisingly, little has been done to study pain tolerance in professional athletes/performers. One study measured pain tolerance during limb immersion in ice water in ballet dancers. As expected, the dancers endured the ice water longer than nondancers (and men more than women). It is possible that individuals who are successful in physically demanding professions were born with, or developed, better tolerance to pain—along with being stronger and more coordinated and driven to succeed.

DESCENDING PATHWAYS AND OPIOIDS

The discovery of the opioid-mediated pain modulation circuits is one of the great stories in neuroscience. In the late 1960s, it became apparent that the brain exerts a top-down control of pain. A big break came in 1969 with the discovery that electrical stimulation of PAG, the gray matter surrounding the third ventricle and the cerebral aqueduct in the midbrain, induces analgesia. Reynolds implanted electrodes in the PAG of rats and performed abdominal surgery without problems when the electrodes were stimulated. Although the animals did not respond to the pain, they were able to move about the cage (before and after surgery) and displayed a startle response to visual or auditory stimuli even while the electrodes were active.

Subsequent work has led to a detailed knowledge of the descending pain-modulating circuits. Figure 11.9 shows a drawing of the important features of these pathways. Input from the prefrontal areas of the anterior cingulate and insular cortex as well as the hypothalamus and amygdala converges on the PAG. The PAG does not send neurons directly to the dorsal horn, but rather projects by way of intermediary nuclei such as the *rostral ventral medulla* (RVM). Other serotonergic and noradrenergic neurons (not shown) also project down on to the afferent pain neurons. The end result is inhibition and diminution of the pain signal that is sent up the ascending anterolateral tracts to the brain.

Opium

It is likely that opium was used as early as 4000 B.C. by the ancient Sumerians. By the 17th century, the therapeutic value of opium was well known. Morphine was first isolated in 1806 and codeine in 1832. Heroin was introduced to medicine in 1896.

DISORDER SCHIZOPHRENIA

There is a long history of noting increased pain tolerance in patients with schizophrenia, dating back to Kraepelin and Bleuler. More recently, surgeons and internists have written anecdotal reports of patients with schizophrenia who appear to experience little pain despite suffering from extremely painful physical conditions. It is not clear if the pain tolerance is a consequence of the illness, the psychotropic medications, or simply a lack of affect, that is, the patient feels the pain but fails to express it appropriately.

Hooley and Delgado sought to avoid these complicating factors by measuring pain sensitivity in the relatives of patients with schizophrenia. They found that subjects with a family history of schizophrenia showed elevated pain thresholds and tolerance. Of interest, the pain correlated with measures of self-referential thinking, magical ideation, and perceptual disturbances. The pathology of this aberrant pain sensitivity is unknown, but may be part of the genetic makeup of schizophrenia.

Opioid Receptors

The discovery of the opioid receptors was a major breakthrough in understanding the pain modulatory system. Three major classes of opioid receptors have been identified: μ, δ, and κ. However, most of the focus has been on the μ receptor because its activation is required for most analgesics. Indeed the affinity that a medication has for the μ receptor correlates with its potency as an analgesic. *Naloxone* also binds with the μ receptor and acts as the quintessential antagonist for it blocks activation and can precipitate withdrawal.

The opioid receptors are concentrated in the PAG, RVM, and dorsal horn—areas well known for pain modulation. However, the receptor can be found throughout the body, including skin, muscles, and joints, which help explain the benefits as well as typical side effects associated with opioids, for example, constipation and respiratory depression.

Endogenous Opioids

Clearly, animals did not evolve a receptor so that drug abusers could enjoy heroin. In the mid-1970s, the race was on to find the neurotransmitter that the body produces to activate the opioid receptor. The result was the discovery of the β-endorphin, enkephalins, and dynorphins: the three major classes of endogenous opioid peptides. The genes for these peptides are distributed throughout the CNS.

Figure 11.10 gives an example from the dorsal horn of the enkephalins and the μ receptors working together to decrease the pain signal sent to the brain. Note that the μ receptors are on both the presynaptic and the postsynaptic neurons.

Placebo

The use of placebos, substances with no intrinsic therapeutic value, is the oldest treatment known to man. In the modern era of medicine, the placebo response has been equated with the statement

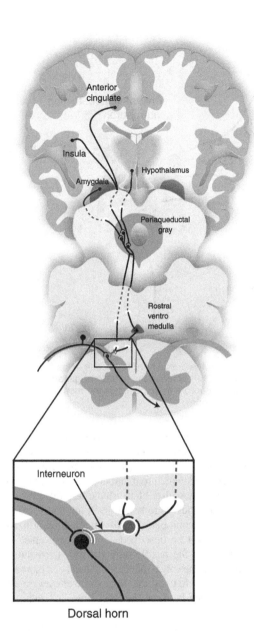

FIGURE 11.9 ● Descending pain-modulating pathways that enable the brain to inhibit the intensity of the ascending pain signals.

The uses and abuses of opium and its analogues have permeated most cultures of the world.

By the mid-1960s, it was known that microinjections of morphine into the PAG or the dorsal horn produced a powerful analgesia and that the opioid antagonist naloxone could block this effect. Furthermore, transection of the axons from the RVM reduces the morphine-induced analgesia. Yet, how does morphine relieve pain?

POINT OF INTEREST

β-endorphin is derived from a larger precursor molecule called *proopiomelanocortin* (POMC), found primarily in the pituitary (see Figure 16.13). POMC contains other biologically active peptides, including adrenocorticotropic hormone (ACTH). Consequently, the stress response—discussed in a previous chapter—includes the release of ACTH as well as β-endorphin into the bloodstream. One wonders about the evolutionary advantage of the simultaneous synthesis and release of these two neuropeptides.

Pain impulse from periphery

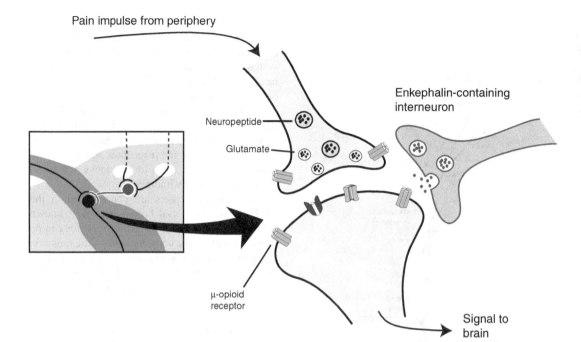

FIGURE 11.10 ● Descending pathways stimulate an interneuron in the dorsal horn to release enkephalins that activate the μ receptors. The effect on the presynaptic neuron is to decrease the release of glutamate and neuropeptides. With the postsynaptic neuron, stimulation of the μ receptors hyperpolarizes the membrane. These two actions result in a smaller signal coming out of the dorsal horn.

"all in your head." Subsequently, it has been recognized that the placebo response is real—and actually in our heads. After the discovery of the endogenous opioid, it was shown that placebo anesthesia could even be reversed with naloxone.

Brain imaging studies of subjects anticipating an effective treatment for pain but given a placebo have shown reduced activity in the pain perception areas and increased activity in the pain modulation areas—those associated with endogenous opioids (Figure 11.11). Thus, placebos work in two ways. First, by decreasing awareness in the pain-sensitive regions and second by increasing activity in regions involved with top-down suppression.

Acupuncture

Acupuncture has been used for thousands of years in China, Korea, and Japan, but only recently introduced to the West. The healing power of acupuncture is believed to work by reestablishing the proper "energy balance" in disordered organs. The treatment is conducted by inserting a needle into specific locations along meridians established through ancient clinical experience. The lack of scientific correlation or good clinical trials can be troubling to those of us who subscribe to a Western orientation of physiology and illness.

One of the difficulties in conducting good clinical trials with acupuncture is separating the specific effect of stimulating the acupoints from the placebo effect. A recent study in London sought to overcome this problem by including two placebo arms along with active acupuncture treatment. The first placebo treatment was with a blunt needle and the patients were aware they were being given an "inert" treatment. The second placebo arm intervention utilized what can best be described as a "stage needle"— when poked, the needle retracted into the handle, giving the appearance that the skin had been pierced. Surprisingly, few of the subjects were aware of the difference between the "stage needle" and real acupuncture.

While these patients—all with osteoarthritis— were being stuck, they were also being scanned with positron emission tomography (PET). The results showed that areas of the brain associated with top-down modulation of pain—dorsolateral prefrontal cortex, ACC, and midbrain—were active with "stage needles" as well as real needles. Only the ipsilateral insula was solely activated by real acupuncture. These results suggest that acupuncture works by way of a large placebo response and also a distinct, but as yet unknown, unique physiological effect.

Stress-Induced Analgesia

Perhaps the most impressive demonstration of top-down modulation of pain is the extreme analgesia

Placebo-induced decrease

Placebo-induced activation

█ Decreased activity in pain-sensitive regions

▒ Increased activity in pain-suppressing regions

FIGURE 11.11 ● The brain imaging studies of the placebo response showing two aspects to the brain's reaction. On the left, control minus placebo shows decreased activity in those areas that perceive pain. On the right, placebo minus control shows increased activity in areas that suppress pain from the top down. PAG, periaqueductal gray. (Adapted from Wager TD, Rilling JK, Smith EE, et al. Placebo-induced changes in FMRI in the anticipation and experience of pain. *Science*. 2004;303(5661):1162-1167.)

shown by individuals at times of stress, for example, the athlete or performing artist who does not appreciate the pain until much later. The classic example was described by Beecher regarding men wounded in battle during the Second World War. He examined 215 men brought to a forward hospital with serious injuries: long bone fractures, penetrating wounds, etc. He found that only 25%, on being directly questioned regarding pain relief, said their pain was severe enough to want morphine. Beecher believed the relief the men experienced, when

taken from the battle and brought to a safe location, blocked the pain.

The modern belief is that stress stimulates opioid-dependent pathways that inhibit the pain signal. However, a group at the University of Georgia has revealed a role for the endocannabinoids in stress-induced analgesia independent of the opioid pathways. Several endocannabinoids rapidly accumulate in the PAG in the midbrain with stress. The group in Georgia demonstrated that stress-induced analgesia in rats could be inhibited with endocannabinoid

In an almost unbelievable brain imaging study, a group in Korea has shown that stimulating a visual-related acupoint—in the foot—activated the visual cortex. The figure shows the cortical activity for visual light stimulation, real acupuncture, and sham acupuncture. These results are difficult to comprehend for those of us who believe in the Western model of medicine and suggest there may be more to this old treatment than we can explain with our current understandings of the brain.

Light and acupuncture (at the visual acupoint 1) stimulate activity in the visual cortex, whereas sham acupuncture does not.

Adapted from Cho ZH, Chung SC, Jones JP, et al. New findings of the correlation between acupoints and corresponding brain cortices using functional MRI. *Proc Natl Acad Sci U S A.* 1998;95(5):2670-2673.

blockers. Their results suggest that higher cortical regions such as the amygdala release endocannabinoids into the PAG during stressful times to suppress pain perception. We appreciate the brain's wisdom in utilizing several mechanisms (endocannabinoids and opioids) to put pain on hold when other events are more important.

CHRONIC PAIN

Until the last half of the past century, pain was thought to be produced by a passive, direct transmission system from peripheral receptors to the cortex. This is called *nociceptive pain* (which we have already discussed earlier) and examples include acute trauma, arthritis, and tumor invasion. There is a veritable medical industry based on locating and correcting the source of the nociceptive pain for patients who are suffering. Unfortunately, most evaluations fail to turn up a cause that explains the pain. One reason is that the traditional model of pain fails to take into account changes in the nerves. Clearly, many patients in pain—particularly chronic, persistent pain—have developed autonomous, maladaptive pain perception independent of tissue damage.

Neuropathic pain is a heterogeneous term used to describe pain that arises from an injured nerve—either centrally or peripherally. Examples of this type of pain are postherpetic neuralgia, diabetic neuropathy, and phantom limb. The distinction between neuropathic and nociceptive pain is important when choosing proper treatment. For instance, neuropathic pain may not respond as well to nonsteroidal anti-inflammatory agents, or opioids, and is better managed with antidepressants and anticonvulsants.

Neuropathic pain is frequently persistent, does not resolve with time, and is resistant to treatment. The pain often disables patients. The pathophysiological mechanisms that underlie these neuropathic pain conditions are beginning to be teased out. One promising area of research is looking at the role of neurotrophic factors in the development of pathologic pain states.

As discussed in previous chapters, tissue injury induces an inflammatory response, which recruits immune cells that release cytokines. The cytokines are literally toxic to the sensory neurons. For example, inflammation interrupts the retrograde transport of neurotrophins from the periphery back to the cell body, where it is needed to maintain normal cell functioning. One neurotrophic factor in particular (glial cell line–derived neurotrophic factor [GDNF]) has been identified as a possible target. Several studies have shown that exogenous GDNF can prevent the development of experimental neuropathic pain.

Pain Memory

A striking example of the brain's elaboration of pain without sensory input can be found in patients after limb amputation. Many will continue to experience pain from lesions that existed on the limb before the surgery—what some call pain memory. For example, a person with an ulcer on the foot at the time of the operation will still feel the presence of the ulcer many months after the limb has been removed.

Several clever clinicians have shown that sufficient local anesthesia of the affected limb several days prior to the amputation significantly reduces the incidence of pain memories. These results suggest that pain has an enduring effect on the brain, which can be attenuated with appropriate treatment.

Gray Matter Loss

A study by a group at Northwestern University further enhances our understanding of the role of the CNS with chronic pain. Apkarian et al. scanned 26 patients with chronic back pain that had persisted for at least 1 year. They compared the results with age-matched controls and found a 5% to 11% loss of gray matter in patients with chronic back pain (Figure 11.12). Further regional analysis showed that the dorsolateral prefrontal cortex was the specific area with greatest decrease in gray matter density. These results suggest that one explanation for chronic pain may be the loss of top-down modulation of pain (e.g., the loss of the placebo response in Figure 11.11).

What causes the gray matter loss with chronic pain? Several explanations are possible. First, the patients could be genetically predisposed to have less gray matter. Small injuries result in persistent pain because the patients lack sufficient CNS modulation of the ascending pain signal. Second, in the next chapter, we will show that medications or abused substances alter the morphology of the cell (see Figure 12.13). Excessive use/abuse may have a toxic effect on neurons in the gray matter. Third, the unremitting pain signal with the associated negative affect and stress may result in an excitotoxic and inflammatory state that essentially wears out the brain circuitry.

Subsequent studies conducted to verify the Apkarian findings have confirmed gray matter loss in patients with migraines, fibromyalgia, and idiopathic facial pain. A group in Oxford demonstrated that thalamic gray matter loss in patients with persistent hip pain was reversed 9 months after successful arthroplasty. These studies demonstrate another example of the remarkable plasticity of the brain.

DEPRESSION AND ANTIDEPRESSANTS

There is a long and well-documented correlation between depression and pain. Patients with chronic pain have a high incidence of depression and patients with depression have an increased expression of painful physical symptoms. Recently, studies have shown that patients with depression and pain are less likely to achieve remission of their depression.

Antidepressants have been shown to be effective in decreasing low back pain and pain in diabetic neuropathy, postherpetic neuralgia, fibromyalgia, and migraines as well as other pains. Traditionally, the tricyclics were used, but with the development of cleaner medications, other agents were tried. Of interest, the selective serotonin reuptake inhibitors (SSRIs) have been disappointing—often not separating from placebo in controlled trials. It appears that only agents

FIGURE 11.12 ● Gray matter loss with chronic back pain. **A.** Decrease in total gray matter volume for patients with chronic back pain compared with controls. **B.** Average for both groups. **C.** The dorsolateral prefrontal cortex is the specific region with decreased gray matter density. (Adapted from Apkarian AV, Sosa Y, Sonty S, et al. Chronic back pain is associated with decreased prefrontal and thalamic gray matter density. *J Neurosci.* 2004;24(46):10410-10415.)

TMS, PFC, AND POSTOPERATIVE PAIN

Transcranial magnetic stimulation (TMS) is a noninvasive procedure that can stimulate the cerebral cortex. The prefrontal cortex (PFC) has been implicated as a region that modulates pain tolerance. A cleaver collaboration between anesthesiology and psychiatry shows that activation of the PFC with TMS can decrease pain perception.

Patients undergoing gastric bypass surgery were randomized to receive 20 minutes of either active or sham TMS immediately after surgery. The total morphine administered by patient-controlled analgesia pumps was tracked as an indirect measurement of pain. The figure shows that patients who received active TMS used approximately 40% less morphine in the 48-hours after the operation.

One 20-minute session of TMS applied to the left PFC postoperatively greatly reduced the total morphine administered to the patients.

Adapted from Borckardt JJ, Weinstein M, Reeves ST, et al. Postoperative left prefrontal repetitive transcranial magnetic stimulation reduces patient-controlled analgesia use. *Anesthesiology*. 2006;105(3):557-562.

that inhibit the reuptake of norepinephrine as well as serotonin are effective for pain reduction. Recently, the newer agents that tout a dual mechanism of action (venlafaxine and duloxetine) have been shown to reduce pain due to diabetic neuropathy. Duloxetine even has an Food and Drug Administration (FDA) indication for peripheral diabetic neuropathy.

How do the antidepressants decrease pain? One possibility could be the beneficial effect of correcting the mood. Yet, SSRIs give disappointing results. Likewise, patients without depression will show some pain reduction. Another possibility is the enhancement of the descending pathways. Some of the fibers projecting from the brain stem

FIGURE 11.13 ● A psychosomatic pain epidemic. The graph shows reports of repetition strain injury at Telecom in Australia by quarter. (Adapted from Hocking B. Epidemiological aspects of "repetition strain injury" in Telecom Australia. *Med J Aust*. 1987;147(5):218-222.)

down onto the dorsal horn of the spinal cord are serotonergic and noradrenergic. More action from these neurons would further dampen the signals from the periphery.

A final possibility for understanding the effectiveness of antidepressants for pain is a cortical mechanism. PET scans of both depressed patients and patients with pain show decreased activity in the prefrontal cortex and increased activity in the insula and ACC. It is possible that antidepressants moderate the pain perception by correcting the cortical imbalance associated with depression and pain.

Epidemic of Unexplained Pain

Let us not forget that pain is highly influenced by one's psychosocial expectations. A good example is the epidemic of vague upper limb pain, from Australia, called *repetitive strain injury* (RSI). This condition was attributed to repetitive keyboard movements by telegraphists, but failed to follow the usual medical model. Reports in the medical literature and sensational media coverage as well as union and legal advocacy produced a dramatic increase in reports of RSI (Figure 11.13). The complaints peaked in 1984 and then declined, as the condition came to be perceived as psychosomatic and the courts went against the litigants. Similar epidemics have occurred in the United Kingdom and Japan.

Another classic study analyzed the development of late whiplash syndrome in Lithuania—a country where few drivers have car insurance or seek legal compensation after an accident. The authors questioned the subjects involved in known rear-end car collisions, 1 to 3 years after the accident, regarding neck pain and headaches, and compared their symptoms with matched control subjects. There was no significant difference between the groups. The authors concluded, "expectation of disability, a family history, and attribution of preexisting symptoms to the trauma may be more important determinants for the evolution of the late whiplash syndrome."

The important point is that the perception of pain is a product of the brain's abstraction and elaboration of sensory input. Many factors affect that process—not just nociceptive signals from the periphery.

QUESTIONS

1. Slow aching pain signals
   a. Aδ fibers.
   b. Aβ fibers.
   c. C fibers.
   d. D fibers.

2. Simultaneous input from these nerve fibers explains the inhibitory effect of the gate theory of pain.
   a. Aδ fibers.
   b. Aβ fibers.
   c. C fibers.
   d. D fibers.

3. Not associated with the affective-motivational pathways of pain
   a. Somatosensory cortex.
   b. "How much does it hurt?"
   c. Medial thalamus.
   d. Anterior cingulate and insular cortex.

4. Condition associated with increased pain tolerance
   a. Depression.
   b. Anxiety.
   c. Fibromyalgia.
   d. Schizophrenia.

5. Not part of the descending pathways of pain
   a. Periaqueductal gray.
   b. Dorsal horn.
   c. Spinothalamic tract.
   d. Rostral ventral medulla.

6. The primary opioid receptor
   a. β receptor.
   b. δ receptor.
   c. κ receptor.
   d. μ receptor.

7. Unlikely explanation for chronic persistent pain
   a. Genetic predisposition.
   b. Diminished placebo response.
   c. Changes in the gray matter.
   d. Damaged nerves.

8. Lacks significant analgesic effects
   a. SSRIs.
   b. Opioids.
   c. Nonsteroidal anti-inflammatory drugs.
   d. Anticonvulsants.

See Answers section at the end of the book.

CHAPTER 12

Pleasure

SEEKING PLEASURE

Voluntary behavior in animals is motivated by the avoidance of pain and the pursuit of pleasure. In this chapter, we will focus on the neuronal mechanisms that guide our choices toward stimuli that give a little reward to the brain.

Our existence—as individuals and as a species—is dependent on using the five senses to recognize and pursue actions necessary for survival. The motivation to pursue a beneficial act is driven in part by giving the brain a brief squirt of euphoria. This reward system has evolved over millions of years to enable an individual to sort through a variety of stimuli and choose the ones that are appropriate.

The orbital aspect of the prefrontal cortex (PFC) is known to play a critical role in goal-directed behavior. Figure 12.1 shows that the relative appeal for an item can be recognized in the brain even down to the level of a single neuron. In this study, electrodes placed in a single neuron in the orbitofrontal cortex registered different levels of activity based on the appeal of the food reward. A raisin generated the largest signal and was the most desired object; cereal was least active and least desired.

Many of our patients, family, and friends struggle with problems that they have created by pursuing the wrong rewards. Clearly, the addicted individual has lost control over his choices (more on this later), but what about the promiscuous

FIGURE 12.1 ● A monkey is taught to view a signal, make a choice, and be rewarded with designated food morsel. **A.** The activity in an individual neuron in the orbitofrontal cortex when the monkey is offered a reward of either a raisin or an apple is shown. **B.** Rewarded with either an apple or cereal. The size of the signal is believed to represent the motivational value, that is, raisin > apple; apple > cereal. (Adapted from Tremblay L, Schultz W. Relative reward preference in primate orbitofrontal cortex. *Nature*. 1999;398(6729):704-708.)

college student, the young adult who accumulates excessive debt on new credit cards, or the child who plays video games instead of doing homework? These people are choosing pleasurable activities that are not to their benefit and even harmful.

The problems are related to how our reward system is designed. We are built for acquiring rewards that were historically in short supply. Now with the extraordinary success of the human race and industrialized civilization, we are exposed to abundance beyond what our wiring has evolved to handle. Junk food, pornography, shopping malls, as well as alcohol, stimulants, and opioids usurp the mechanisms developed to enhance the survival of the hunter–gatherer in all of us.

Happiness

There is clinical evidence to suggest that one's level of happiness remains remarkably fixed. For example, the person winning a lottery or the one suffering the loss of a limb tends to revert to their preexisting level of happiness after a period of euphoria or depression. It seems that happiness is hardwired and closely fluctuates around a genetic "set point" for each person. Unfortunately, there is surprisingly little neuroscience research on this topic.

ANATOMY OF REWARD

Pursuing a reward can be conceptualized as a ball rolling down the hill. Animals will gravitate toward the most enjoyable activity the way a ball rolls to the lowest point. It seemingly happens without effort. However, although we cannot visualize the force of gravity pulling on a moving ball, we continue to tease out the neuroanatomy of the mammalian reward system.

The initial studies came in the mid-fifties when Olds and Milner accidentally discovered that a rat would seek to continue stimulation from a thin electrode implanted in certain parts of his brain. Figure 12.2 shows the relative placement of an electrode in a rat's skull and the apparatus that Olds and Milner used to document the animals' efforts to stimulate themselves. Remarkably, the rats exceeded all expectations in what they were willing to sacrifice to receive stimulation. Depending on

FIGURE 12.2 ● An x-ray showing the placement of an electrode through the skull into the brain of a rat. On the right when the rat presses the level he receives a mild stimulus—and a moment of pleasure. (From Olds J. Pleasure centers in the brain. *Sci Am*. 1956;195:105-112.)

where the electrode was placed, they would press the lever up to 5,000 times in an hour, chose stimulation over food even when starving, and cross an electrified grid for a chance to press the lever.

Fifty years of research has established that the mesolimbic dopamine (DA) systems, including the ventral tegmental area (VTA) and nucleus accumbens (NAc) (also called the *ventral striatum*), are the central structures of reward. These old but effective nuclei lie at the base of the brain (Figure 12.3) and are the structures that were being indirectly stimulated in the Olds and Milner experiments. The NAc and VTA receive signals from a multitude of sources—the most prominent of which are the PFC, amygdala, and hippocampus. It is significant that the input to the NAc and VTA originates from the areas involved in attention, executive decisions, and emotional memories— areas that help the brain negotiate the path to the reward.

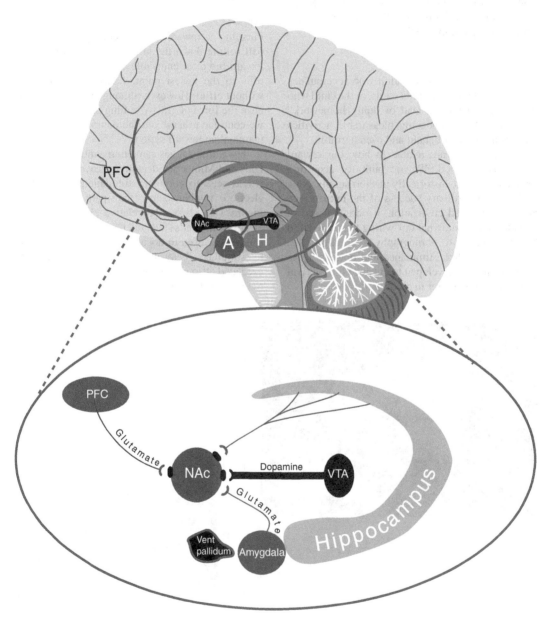

FIGURE 12.3 ● The anatomy of pleasure and reward is mediated in the nucleus accumbens with input from a variety of structures, only a few of which are shown here. NAc, nucleus accumbens; PFC, prefrontal cortex; VTA, ventral tegmental area.

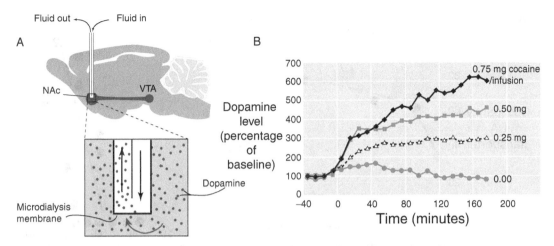

FIGURE 12.4 ● **A.** Microdialysis in a rat brain. **B.** Pettit and Justice found that increasing self-administered doses of cocaine resulted in greater extracellular dopamine at the nucleus accumbens. (Adapted from Pettit HO, Justice JB Jr. Effect of dose on cocaine self-administration behavior and dopamine levels in the nucleus accumbens. *Brain Res.* 1991;539(1):94-102.)

Converging lines of evidence have shown that DA is the primary neurotransmitter that modulates the reward system. Using an implanted microdialysis apparatus, Pettit and Justice were able to regularly sample DA concentration at the NAc. They found a correlation between the amounts of cocaine a rat would self-administer and the extracellular DA at the NAc (Figure 12.4). Alternatively, blocking the effect of cocaine either with a DA antagonist (e.g., haloperidol) or lesioning the dopaminergic cells in the NAc eliminated the self-administration and drug-seeking behavior.

Brain Imaging

More recently, brain imaging studies with human volunteers have further established the link between DA and pleasure. Volkow administered IV methylphenidate (Ritalin) and established a correlation between the dose of the medication and the occupancy of the DA transporter (stimulants work in part by blocking the DA reuptake pump). Additionally by asking the participant how they felt, a correlation between feeling "high" and occupancy of the DA transporter was established (Figure 12.5).

Creative studies with functional imaging scanners have shown that it is not just drugs of abuse (amphetamines, alcohol, nicotine, etc.) that result in enhanced DA at the NAc, but many pleasurable activities. Figure 12.6 gives examples of feelings (looking at beautiful faces, eating chocolate, revenge, etc.) as well as of drugs that have all demonstrated increased DA at the NAc and/or VTA in functional scans in humans.

Figure 12.6 shows only the results with humans. There are additional hedonic experiences that show

similar findings with animals. For example, sexual behavior, violence, opioids, and marijuana all increase DA at the NAc in animals. Furthermore, we can speculate that other pleasurable behaviors—those that would be difficult to investigate in a scanner, such as shopping, gambling, extreme sports, and defeating ones arch enemy—may also deliver a dollop of DA to the NAc. The key point is this: Behaviors that people enjoy seem to precipitate an increase in DA produced at the NAc.

One particularly interesting study conducted at the primate laboratory at Wake Forest University looked at the effect of social rank on DA in monkeys. The monkeys were initially housed individually and scanned for DA D_2 receptors, which were found to be similar for all monkeys. Next, they were housed together in groups of 4. After 3 months, the researchers determined who were the dominant and subordinate monkeys and

DISORDER	COMPLICATED GRIEF

It is not uncommon to see patients who are experiencing prolonged and unabated grief of a loved one. Recent functional brain scans have shown persistent activation of the NAc in patients with such complicated grief: more activity in the NAc correlated with greater yearning when viewing a picture of the deceased. This report suggests that successful adaptation to loss is complicated by the joy of remembering—even when the memory is also painful.

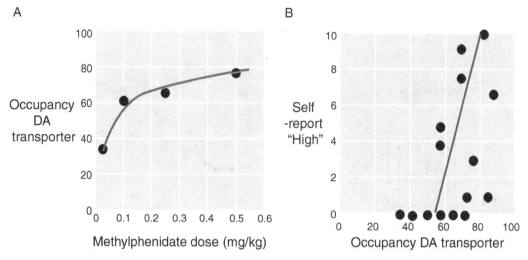

FIGURE 12.5 ● Methylphenidate and occupancy of the dopamine reuptake transporter **(A).** Higher doses of methylphenidate result in increased occupancy of the dopamine transporter, which results in increased dopamine being available to the nucleus accumbens and—at strong enough levels—feeling "high" **(B).** (Adapted from Volkow ND, Fowler JS, Wang GJ, et al. Role of dopamine in the therapeutic and reinforcing effects of methylphenidate in humans: results from imaging studies. *Eur Neuropsychopharmacol.* 2002;12(6):557-566.)

Drugs

1. Cocaine
2. Alcohol
3. Amphetamines
4. Methylphenidate
5. Nicotine

Feelings

6. Romantic love
7. Listening to music
8. Humor
9. Expectation of $$$
10. Inflicting punishment
11. Looking at beautiful faces
12. Social cooperation
13. Eating chocolate
14. Talking about yourself

a. Nucleus accumbens

b. Ventral tegmental area

Drugs

1. Acute Effects of Cocaine on Human Brain Activity and Emotion. *Neuron.* 1997;19:591-611.
2. Alcohol Promotes Dopamine Release in the Human Nucleus Accumbens. *Synapse.* 2003;49:226-231.
3. SPECT Imaging of Srtiatal Dopamine Release After Amphetamine Challenge. *J Nuc Med.* 1995;36:1182-1190.
4. Role of Dopmaine in the Therapeutic and Reinforcing Effects of Methylphenidate in Humans: Results from Imaging Studies. *Eur Neuropsychopharm.* 2002;12:557-566.
5. Nicotine-induce Limbic Cortical Activation in the Human Brain: a Functional MRI Study. *Am J Psych.*1998;155:1009-1015

Feelings

6. Reward, Motivation, and Emotion Systems Associated with Early-Stage Intense Romantic Love. *J Neurophysiol.* 2005;94:327-337.
7. Intensely Pleasurable Responses to Music Correlate with Activity in Brain Regions Implicated in Reward and Emotion. *PNAS.* 2001;98:11818-11823.
8. Humor Modulates the Mesolimbic Reward Centers. *Neuron.* 2003;40:1041-1048.
9. Functional Imaging of Neural Responses to Expectancy and Experience of Monetary Gains and Losses. *Neuron.* 2001;30:619-639.
10. The Neural Basis of Altruistic Punishment. *Science.* 2004;305:1254-1258.
11. Beautiful Faces Have Variable Reward Value: fMRI and Behavioral Evidence. *Neuron.* 2001;32:537-551.
12. A Neural Basis for Social Cooperation. *Neuron.* 2002;35:395-405.
13. Changes in Brain Activity Related to Eating Chocolate. *Brain.* 2001;124:1720-1733.
14. Disclosing Information About the Self is Intrinsically Rewarding. *PNAS.* 2012;109:8038-8043.

FIGURE 12.6 ● Drugs of abuse and pleasant feelings light up the mesolimbic dopamine pathway in functional imaging studies in humans. The studies documenting these findings are listed at the bottom of the figure.

then re-scanned them. The results are shown in Figure 12.7. Note that the dominant monkey now has significantly greater DA D$_2$ receptors in the striatum—an area that includes the NAc.

The researchers also allowed the monkeys to self-administer different doses of cocaine. The graph on the right of Figure 12.7 shows that the dominant monkeys gave themselves less cocaine than the subordinates at different strengths of the drug. This suggests that the "good feelings" that come from being the alpha monkey buffer against seeking external sources of pleasure. This provides some insight into the correlation between increased substance abuse and lower socioeconomic status.

Pleasure versus Novelty

It is overly simplistic to call the NAc the pleasure center. Research with rodents has found that DA will increase at the NAc with adverse stimuli—for example, a foot shock. Likewise, addicts have reported that they have continued to seek their drug, although it is no longer pleasurable.

Some have suggested that the NAc determines the "wanting" and motivation to seek a reward—not the pleasurable experience itself. Volkow, director of the National Institute of Drug Abuse, prefers the term "saliency" to describe the function of DA at the NAc. By salience, she means new and unexpected stimuli that focus attention and motivate to seek more.

Di Chiara has studied the effect of various substances on DA release at the NAc. His group has shown that DA release is strongest for positive, novel reinforcements. Figure 12.8 shows the bump in DA at the NAc when a rat is given chocolate. However, when given the same amount of chocolate on the following day, the bump in DA is no longer significant.

Di Chiara has shown in other studies that habituation does *not* occur with cocaine. Day after day, rats will have a bump in DA at the NAc when given cocaine. Not only is the increase stronger in magnitude (up to 400% over baseline compared with 150% for chocolate) but also does not attenuate like the natural reinforcers. This may in part explain why cocaine is so addictive.

FIGURE 12.7 ● **A.** Drawings of PET scans showing the prevalence of dopamine D$_2$ receptors for monkeys after establishing social hierarchy. **B.** The graph shows that the dominant monkey always self-administered less cocaine at different strengths of the drug compared with the subordinate monkey. (Adapted from Morgan D, Grant KA, Gage HD, et al. Social dominance in monkeys: dopamine D$_2$ receptors and cocaine self-administration. *Nat Neurosci.* 2002;5(2):169-174.)

FIGURE 12.8 ● Habituation. When first given chocolate, a rat shows a significant increase (■) in its dopamine at the nucleus accumbens, which does not occur when given the same food on the following day. (Adapted from Bassareo V, De Luca MA, Di Chiara G. Differential expression of motivational stimulus properties by dopamine in nucleus accumbens shell versus core and prefrontal cortex. *J Neurosci.* 2002;22(11):4709-4719.)

Amygdala

The amygdala along with the frontal cortex influences the mesolimbic DA system. Although better known for its role in fear and avoidance (see Chapter 22), the amygdala plays a role in seeking pleasure. The amygdala is critically involved in the process of acquiring and retaining lasting memories of emotional experiences whether they are pleasurable or traumatic. Studies have shown correlations between the activation of the amygdala during emotionally arousing events and subsequent recall. It is not known if the memories are actually stored in the amygdala or recalled from the cortex by the amygdala.

The process of associating emotional memories with particular events—a special song, helicopters flying overhead, or the smell of a cigarette—is classical conditioning. A demonstration of the role of the amygdala and seeking pleasure can be shown when a rat is conditioned to associate a sound or light with pressing a lever and receiving cocaine. When the cocaine ceases to be delivered, the rat will almost completely stop pressing the lever—extinguishing the behavior. Later, if he hears the conditioned sound or sees the light, he will resume pressing the lever as long as his amygdala is intact. A rat without an amygdala will fail to resume pressing the lever when stimulated with the tone or light. Clearly, the amygdala is essential to remembering the associations.

The Pursuit of Pleasure

People spend time doing what they enjoy. "Time sure flies when you're having fun" is the old saying. The propensity to get "lost" in an activity and lose track of time is a feature of rewarding activities—and something that can be a source of frustration for friends and family who do not enjoy the same activity.

The brain has several internal clocks. The suprachiasmatic nucleus and circadian rhythm is the most renowned internal clock and will be covered in Chapter 16. However, there are lesser known circuits to manage milliseconds, which are essential for sports, dancing, music, and speech. Of relevance to this chapter, these circuits utilize DA and to some extent activate the VTA. Studies with rodents have found that D_2 agonists, such as methamphetamine, accelerate the internal clock whereas D_2 blockers, such as haloperidol, slow down the clock. This may explain why people inaccurately estimate the duration of a pleasurable activity.

People who have the propensity to enjoy work have an adapted advantage over those who do not. We can imagine that nature selects for individuals who possess the traits to enjoy activities that are beneficial, for example, hunting and gathering as well as communicating and planning. Alternatively, some people lose themselves in activities that are not healthy and continue to pursue them in spite of negative outcomes. This behavior and the effects on the brain are the focus of the next section.

POINT OF INTEREST

Albert Einstein is reported to have described his theory of relativity as such: "Put your hand on a hot stove for a minute, and it seems like an hour. Sit with a pretty girl for an hour, and it seems like a minute." Einstein eloquently described how our perception of the passage of time is affected by our feelings of pain and pleasure.

ADDICTIONS CHANGE THE BRAIN

Most of the pleasurable activities that we are wired to pursue occur in nature in limited supply, making it hard to overindulge. Modern life, however, is full of many temptations that activate the mesolimbic pathway. Drugs of abuse, in particular, overwhelm and fundamentally alter the neurons that were never intended to experience such supraphysiologic levels of neurotransmitters. Addictions entail the persistent, destructive, and uncontrollable behaviors that involve obtaining the object of desire.

One simple definition of an addiction is the continued pursuit of a substance or activity in spite of negative consequences. This could apply to gambling, sex, alcohol, smoking, food, and even work. All these activities result in increased DA at the NAc. We focus in this section on drugs of abuse and the changes they cause in the addicted brain. Figure 12.9 shows the location of several commonly abused drugs.

Some drugs have direct effects on the mesolimbic pathway while others work indirectly. The stimulants and nicotine result in increased DA at the NAc. The opioids, alcohol, and phencyclidine (and to some extent nicotine) suppress the inhibitory neurons that modulate the NAc and VTA. With less inhibition, more DA is released to the NAc.

Drug use occurs along a continuum—from casual use to dominating one's life. Addictions result from a combination of genes and environment and develop over time. But once addicted, the drugs alter the architecture of the brain. Tolerance and withdrawal are two clinical manifestations of the changes that occur to the addicted brain. Other clinical examples that show the effects of persistent abuse are as follows:

1. Depression and anhedonia when not using.
2. Less responsive to natural rewards.
3. The capacity to relapse even many years after abstinence.

Global Impairments

One of the most consistently reproducible findings in the addictions field is the reduction in brain volume in chronic alcoholics. Studies have shown decreased total volume and gray matter, particularly in the frontal lobes. These findings co-occur with declines in cognition and memory. Alcoholics evaluated after a period of sobriety show some recovery of tissue volume, whereas those who continue to drink show further reductions.

Recent research has established cigarette smoking as a confounding variable in brain volume reductions and cognitive decline. One study

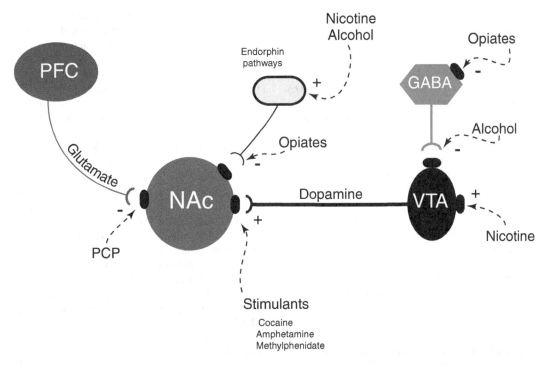

FIGURE 12.9 ● Possible sites of action by drugs of abuse on the mesolimbic pathway. PFC, prefrontal cortex; NAc, nucleus accumbens; VTA, ventral tegmental area; GABA, γ-aminobutyric acid.

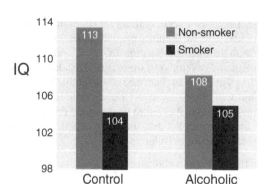

FIGURE 12.10 ● IQ is independently reduced in subjects with heavy alcohol or cigarette use. (Adapted from Glass JM, Adams KM, Nigg JT, et al. Smoking is associated with neurocognitive deficits in alcoholism. *Drug Alcohol Depend.* 2005;82(2):119-126.)

FIGURE 12.11 ● Horizontal PET scans at the level of the striatum. The cocaine abuser has less D_2 receptor binding compared with the control. (Adapted from Volkow ND, Li TK. Drug addiction: The neurobiology of behaviour gone awry. *Nat Rev Neurosci.* 2004;5(12):963-970.)

compared intelligence as measured by IQ in 172 men (Figure 12.10). Alcoholism and smoking were independent risk factors for reductions in IQ. In recent follow-up studies, this same group found alcoholism correlated with a broad range of impairment in executive function, while smoking affected measures that emphasize response speed. It is not known if smoking has a direct neurotoxic effect on cognition or an indirect effect from cardiovascular or pulmonary damage. Interestingly, smokers report that a cigarette enhances their attention and in studies nicotine acutely improves cognitive performance. Yet, the long-term effect on cognition is detrimental.

Dopamine Receptors

The stimulants work by blocking the DA reuptake pump as well as increasing the release of DA, which results in more DA being available to stimulate the NAc. Using positron emission tomography (PET) scans, Volkow has shown decreased D_2 receptors in cocaine addicts during withdrawal (Figure 12.11), which persisted even when tested 3 to 4 months after detoxification. Similar findings have been demonstrated in subjects withdrawn from heroin, methamphetamine, and alcohol. These results show that excessive use of hedonic substances results in a downregulation of the D_2 receptor. This may explain the development of tolerance and need for the addict to take "more." Likewise, this helps us understand why the abstinent user has difficulty experiencing pleasure with the natural joys of life.

Craving and the Frontal Cortex

The addict is someone who has moved from getting high to getting hooked. He is haunted by persistent, intrusive thoughts about his drug, and intensely desires to obtain more. He has lost control. In the literature and on the street, this is called *craving*.

As with obsessions (see Chapter 22), the PFC has been identified as the source of craving. Functional imaging studies have shown enhanced activity in the PFC, particularly the orbital frontal cortex and dorsolateral PFC, when addicts are presented with drug-related cues. For example, cocaine addicts shown pictures of white powder will light up their frontal lobes and will report "drug craving." It is noteworthy that the activity in the PFC correlates with the intensity of self-reported craving.

We discussed in the first section of this chapter the important role the PFC plays in making choices (Figure 12.1). An essential feature of addictions is the inability to make good choices. This problem can be demonstrated in the relative activity of the PFC when addicts are shown various film clips.

In one important study, cocaine users were shown video clips of men smoking crack, sexually explicit scenes, and scenes of nature while in a functional brain scanner. Compared with the controls, the cocaine users showed increased activation in the frontal cortex while viewing videos of men smoking crack but not when shown sexually explicit content. The authors concluded that the drug abusers had developed a heightened response to stimuli associated with drug use, but blunted response to other rewarding stimuli (Table 12.1).

The persistence of cravings and the susceptibility to lose control even after years of abstinence suggest long-term changes in the neurons of the PFC. Several findings with rats suggest that the

TABLE 12.1

Reaction by Cocaine Users to Different Stimuli

Drug-Related Cues	Natural Reinforcing Stimuli
Overrespond	Underrespond
Craving	Lack of interest
Increased activity in prefrontal cortex	Hypometabolism in prefrontal cortex

glutamatergic projections from the PFC to the NAc (Figure 12.3) may be the culprit. The important findings are as follows:

1. Inactivation of the PFC prevents relapse.
2. Glutamate receptor blockade at the NAc prevents relapse.
3. Increased glutamate is released in the NAc during relapse.

These results not only point to the glutamatergic projections as a source of craving but also suggest a possible site to intervene for preventing relapse.

Synaptic Remodeling

The fact that drug-induced adaptations are so permanent suggests that the drugs fundamentally alter the organization of the neuronal circuits and synaptic connectivity. In a series of experiments, Robinson et al. at the University of Michigan have studied the effects of amphetamine, cocaine, and morphine on the structure of pyramidal cells in various parts of the brain. Figure 12.12 shows the neurons from the parietal cortex.

The dendritic spines on the neuron are the postsynaptic receptors for input from other neurons (see Figure 3.4). Presumably, changes in the number of

FIGURE 12.12 ● Photomicrograph of a Golgi-stained pyramidal cell from the parietal cortex. Multiple photographs at different focal planes were merged together to create this composite. The inserts on the right are from the apical (**A**) and basilar (**B**) regions. (From Kolb B, Gorny G, Li Y, et al. Amphetamine or cocaine limits the ability of later experience to promote structural plasticity in the neocortex and nucleus accumbens. *Proc Natl Acad Sci U S A.* 2003;100(18):10523-10528.)

spines reflect changes in the number of synapses on the neuron. In different experiments, Robinson et al. have shown that amphetamine and cocaine will increase the number of spines, whereas morphine results in a decrease. Figure 12.13 shows the drawings of neurons from the NAc in rats exposed to morphine, saline, and amphetamine. One can see that these drugs (and presumably other substances of abuse) induce lasting changes to the brain by altering the morphology of the neural cells.

Molecular Changes

Nestler et al. at the University of Texas Southwestern Medical Center have examined the molecular changes that underlie the long-term plasticity of addiction. As we discussed in Chapter 5, changes in the neuronal architecture are driven by the gene expression. Nestler et al. identified two transcription factors in the NAc that contribute to gene expression and the resulting protein synthesis in the addicted state.

Cyclic adenosine monophosphate response element binding (CREB) is a transcription factor that is activated by increased DA concentrations during drug binges. CREB in turn promotes the production

DISORDER   ANHEDONIA

One of the disturbing effects of a frontal lobotomy was a pervasive lack of motivation. The subjects were left with a general lack of interest in almost everything. While the procedure may have reduced interest in inappropriate activities, it also had a global effect on all interests. This is the challenge for treating the substance abuser: how to selectively eliminate the craving without altering the underlying personality.

Morphine   Saline   Amphetamine

FIGURE 12.13 ● Changes in dendritic spines in the nucleus accumbens from rats exposed to morphine, saline, and amphetamine. Morphine decreases the number of spines, whereas amphetamine induces an increase. (Adapted from Robinson and Kolb, 1997, 2002.)

of proteins that dampen the reward circuitry and induce tolerance. The dampening effects stimulated by CREB are believed to be one of the reasons drug users need to take more of their substance to get the same effect. CREB may also mediate the depression and anhedonia felt by the addicts when unable to get drugs.

However, CREB is only part of the story. It is switched off within days of stopping the drug use, yet the addict remains vulnerable to relapse for a long time. δ-FosB is another transcription factor that may explain the lasting effects of drug abuse. Unlike CREB, δ-FosB accumulates in the cells of the NAc and is remarkably stable. It remains active in the cells for weeks and months after drugs have been stopped. This kind of enduring molecular change may explain why addicts are susceptible to relapse even after years of abstinence.

Relapse

There are three well-known causes for relapsing:

1. Even a minimal use of the drug or a similar drug.
2. Exposure to cues associated with drug use.
3. Stress.

All three causes result in increased release of DA at the NAc, which seems to impair the addict's will to remain abstinent.

The effects of stress on the mesolimbic DA system are mediated in part through the hypothalamic–pituitary–adrenal (HPA) axis. It appears that corticotropin-releasing factor (CRF) and cortisol stimulate the release of DA. Studies with rats have shown that a stressor, such as a foot shock, stimulates the HPA axis as well as reinstates the drug-seeking behavior. Different studies have shown that the reinstatement for heroin, cocaine, and alcohol can be blocked by the administration of a CRF antagonist.

Developmental Disorder?

It is readily apparent that our joys and pleasures change as we age. A latency-age boy is not the least bit interested in sex, but a few years later as an adolescent he is bubbling over with sexual excitement. The old saying, "the difference between men and boys is the price of their toys," describes the development of new sources of pleasure as men age. Changes in the brain most likely accompany the maturing of what we enjoy.

Adolescence is a time characterized by high levels of risk taking and impulsivity. This can be seen as enhanced approach behavior and reduced harm-avoidance behavior—or too much accelerator and not enough brake. In simple terms, the role of the NAc is to enhance the approach behavior, whereas the role of the amygdala is to warn animals to avoid negative situations. A study looking at the activity in these brain areas during reward and loss, with adolescents and adults, sheds some light on this topic.

Ernst et al. examined the activity of the NAc and amygdala in adolescents and adults while they were playing a game with monetary reward. The subjects could win $4 if they made a correct choice. The authors looked at the relative activity of the NAc and amygdala when the subjects won compared with when they lost. Finally, they compared the regional activity for the adults and adolescents. The results (Figure 12.14) show that all subjects had enhanced activity when they won and less when they did not. However, the adolescents showed greater activity in the NAc when winning and less decrease in the amygdala when losing. Specifically, the results show that the adolescent brain is different—more inclined to approach and less inclined to avoid.

The government restricts the use of legally available habit-forming substances and activities to adults, for example, nicotine, alcohol, and gambling. There are many reasons for this policy, but in part it is driven by the belief that early exposure to these hedonic pleasures increases the risk of addiction. With nicotine there is some evidence that early exposure increases the likelihood of developing an addiction as an adult.

Epidemiological studies of adolescents suggest that smoking at a younger age leads to increased addiction to cigarettes. A recent study with rats

FIGURE 12.14 ● Activation in the nucleus accumbens and amygdala is different for adults and adolescents when they win or fail to win during a game with financial reward. (Adapted from Ernst M, Nelson EE, Jazbec S, et al. Amygdala and nucleus accumbens in responses to receipt and omission of gains in adults and adolescents. *Neuroimage.* 2005;25(4):1279-1291.)

has shown that early exposure has lasting effects when compared with later exposure. Exposure to nicotine during the period that corresponds with preadolescence, but not as a postadolescent, increased the self-administration of nicotine as adults. Additionally, the adult rats exposed to nicotine at the younger age had greater expression of the nicotine receptor.

Adolescence is a time of great risk taking and novelty seeking. Unfortunately, many addictions commence during this period. It appears that early use is genetically predetermined and the result of "hanging around with the wrong crowd." Either way, studies suggest that keeping our adolescents involved in wholesome activities—sports, art, camping, and so on—may keep them away from drugs and alcohol until their developing brains are more immune to the damaging effects of hedonic substances.

Treatment

Without a doubt, successful abstinence is most effective when the subject is motivated to stay clean, almost regardless of the treatment approach. A recent analysis of three psychological treatments for substance abuse showed that all were equally effective, and the most important factor was the subject's desire to abstain.

Medications to treat addictions are helpful but not robustly effective. We are still unable to restore the addicted brain to its preexisting condition. Pharmacological treatments generally fall into two categories. The first category is those interventions that interfere with the reinforcing action of the drugs of abuse, for example, naltrexone. The second category is those agents that mimic the action of

the abused substance, for example, methadone. Neither of these treatments cures the underlying central nervous system alterations, but can help in keeping a substance abuser clean.

Most problematic for the recovering addict is the intense craving that leads to relapse. Some addicts even report craving dreams during withdrawal. Efforts are underway to find medications that will decrease the thoughts and desires stimulated by memories of drug use. Much of the focus has been on agents that affect glutamate and γ-aminobutyric acid, but as yet no substantial interventions have been discovered. The challenge is to selectively eliminate the craving for drugs without affecting the interest in the natural reinforcing stimuli.

Are Stimulant Medications Neurotoxic?

The diagnosis and treatment of attention-deficit/hyperactivity disorder (ADHD) has increased dramatically over the past decade. Psychostimulants such as methylphenidate and amphetamine remain the most effective and widespread pharmacological interventions for ADHD. These medications are potent inhibitors for the DA reuptake transporter and result in increased DA stimulation of postsynaptic neurons.

Although effective in improving attention and decreasing impulsivity, the long-term effects of these agents are not well studied. A meta-analysis of stimulant therapy and substance abuse shows that the medications did not promote substance abuse later and may even decrease the potential. However, we have seen in this review that other substances that increase DA at the NAc result in changes to the molecular and structural character of neurons. It is unknown if such changes occur with sustained use of the psychostimulants.

Two studies with methylphenidate in rats found enduring behavioral effects after treatment during early development. As adults, these rats showed signs of reduced responsiveness to normal stimuli and increased reactions to aversive situations. These findings are similar to what we see with addicts when they are not using their drug of abuse. A compelling study by Kolb et al. found that exposure to amphetamine has enduring impairments on the development of dendritic branching and spine formation 3 months after stopping the medication. However, these studies have been criticized for using rodents, high doses of the medications, and administering the medication by injection.

A recent study by a group at Johns Hopkins Medical Institute examined the neural effects of amphetamine administered orally to nonhuman primates in equivalent doses comparable to that used on patients with ADHD. The researchers taught a small group of baboons and squirrel monkeys to orally ingest a racemic mixture of dextro- and levo-amphetamine (similar to what is found in Adderall) twice a day. The plasma amphetamine levels were measured and corresponded to doses reported in humans. Treatment continued for 4 weeks. Two weeks after stopping medication, the animals were sacrificed and their brains were analyzed.

The baboons that had self-administered amphetamine showed significant reductions in striatal DA. Likewise, the DA transporter protein (the protein blocked by the amphetamine) was significantly reduced in the striatum (Figure 12.15). Similar results were found in the squirrel monkeys, a different primate species. For comparison, the serotonin levels were concomitantly measured, and they remained equal in the amphetamine and control groups.

While we must be cautious when we extrapolate from animal studies to humans, we must also be vigilant about avoiding harmful treatments. The history of medicine is replete with interventions that initially seemed safe, only to show problems later. Our understanding of DA receptor antagonism shows that supraphysiologic doses, as one gets with cocaine, can result in detrimental changes to the neurons. The long-term effects of smaller, controlled doses with stimulant medications, especially after years of continuous use, remain unknown.

CONCLUSION

The good news—we are designed to experience pleasure. The bad news—pleasure is supposed to wane. We are only meant to feel satisfied for a short period. We are built to "lead lives of quiet desperation." People satisfied with their accomplishments fall behind. Some of the patients we see, particularly the chronic schizophrenic and seriously depressed, are cursed with a lack of motivation and joy. They are unable to work toward a goal that will be rewarding and bring them pleasure.

Likewise, we frequently deal with patients who create havoc in their lives through their excessive pursuit of pleasurable substances and activities. An understanding of the neuroscience of pleasure helps us conceptualize that patients, such as this, fail to find joy in alternative, natural reinforcers. Our task with these patients is to assist them in developing healthy activities that will stimulate the mesolimbic cortical pathway, but not alter the chemical or cellular substrate.

FIGURE 12.15 ● **A.** Significant reduction in dopamine transporter after 4 weeks of oral amphetamine treatment in nonhuman primate. **B.** Drawing of cross section of the basal ganglia stained for dopamine transporter. Darker *brown = more dopamine* transporter. (Adapted from Ricaurte GA, Mechan AO, Yuan J, et al. Amphetamine treatment similar to that used in the treatment of adult atte0ntion deficit/hyperactivity disorder damages dopaminergic nerve endings in the striatum of adult nonhuman primates. *J Pharmacol Exp Ther.* 2005;315(1):91-98.)

QUESTIONS

1. Cocaine induces euphoria by
   a. Inhibiting GABA.
   b. Stimulating GABA.
   c. Inhibiting DA reuptake.
   d. Stimulating DA reuptake.

2. Heroin induces euphoria by
   a. Inhibiting GABA.
   b. Stimulating GABA.
   c. Inhibiting DA reuptake.
   d. Stimulating DA reuptake.

3. Microdialysis allows
   a. Pharmacologic stimulation at precise locations.
   b. The development of conditioned behaviors.
   c. Biopsy of cellular tissue.
   d. Continuous sampling of extracellular fluid.

4. Pleasurable feelings include all of the following, except
   a. Increased DA at the NAc.
   b. DA receptor antagonism.
   c. Increased activity of the VTA.
   d. Receptor stimulation.

5. All of the following are involved with the development of tolerance, except
   a. Activation of the PFC.
   b. Habituation.
   c. Downregulation of DA receptors.
   d. Accumulation of inhibitor transcription factors.

6. All of the following are involved with craving, except
   a. Hypometabolism of the PFC to natural stimuli.
   b. Hypermetabolism of the PFC with drug cues.
   c. Enhanced GABA activation.
   d. Glutamatergic activation of the NAc.

7. The Alpha monkey has
   a. Increased glutamatergic activation of the NAc.
   b. Increased frontal lobe metabolism.
   c. Greater propensity to self-administer stimulants.
   d. Increased DA receptors.

8. Enhanced transmission of all of the following can result in relapse, except
   a. GABA.
   b. Glutamate.
   c. DA.
   d. CRH.

9. All of the following result in increased spine formation in rats, except
   a. D-Amphetamine.
   b. Heroin.
   c. Methylphenidate.
   d. Cocaine.

See Answers section at the end of the book.

CHAPTER 13

Appetite

SET POINT

In spite of great fluctuation in the quantity and frequency of eating, we all maintain remarkable precision between energy expenditure and energy intake. Social factors, emotions, and time of day, as well as taste, satiety, and personal habits, influence our eating patterns, yet we maintain a reasonably stable body weight month after month. This is referred to as *energy homeostasis* or simply a metabolic "set point."

Evidence of a set point comes from a variety of sources. If a rat is deprived of food, then, when offered a normal diet, it will overeat for a short period and return its body weight to its preexisting level. Likewise, after being force-fed to increase body weight, it will limit its food intake to return to normal weight (Figure 13.1). The brain and body work in harmony to keep the body weight at a specific point.

The human corollary to this is the disturbingly low success rates that people have with most diets. In a review of long-term efficacy of dietary treatment interventions for obesity, Ayyad and Anderson found that only 15% of the patients fulfilled at least one of the criteria for success 5 years after the study. Unfortunately, most people who diet will slowly return to their preexisting weight within 1 year.

Several lines of research suggest that the set point is genetically controlled. Adoption studies provide a unique way to separate the effects of genetics from environment on body weight by comparing children with their biologic parents and with the parents from the house in which they were raised. In an analysis of Danish adoptees, Stunkard et al. found a strong relation between weight class of the adoptees and the body mass of the biologic parents. However, there was no correlation between the weight class of the adoptees and their adopted parents, suggesting that genetic makeup, not environment, is a major determining factor in one's body weight.

Yet, obesity was a rare condition 50 years ago. Clearly, our genes have not evolved in half a century. There must be other explanations for the significant change in body weight that is occurring in first-world nations. The Pima Indians of Mexico and Arizona can provide some insight on this issue.

The Pima Indians separated into two tribes approximately 700 to 1,000 years ago—one tribe remained in Mexico and the other settled in what is now known as Arizona. In spite of their similar genetic makeup, they have remarkably different average body weights. The Arizona Indians have a high prevalence of obesity and non-insulin-dependent diabetes mellitus, whereas their Mexican relatives are not overweight and have little diabetes. The difference can be best explained by understanding the divergent lifestyles these two populations developed.

The Mexican Pima Indians have remained in the mountains, continuing a traditional rural lifestyle. They exert considerable physical energy working the farms and eat a diet high in starch and fiber. The Arizona Indians, on the other hand, were forced to move onto reservations and abandon their former way of life. There they lead more leisurely lives and eat a diet high in fat and sugar.

The obesity problem that the Pima Indians suffer from has been attributed to a "thrifty gene"—a gene that promotes saving and storing calories. Two thousand years ago, such a genetic predisposition would enhance the survival for those struggling with the fluctuations of prosperity and famine. However, with plentiful high caloric, highly palatable food, the "thrifty gene" promotes accumulation and storage beyond what is healthy. So the weight problem is genetic, but influenced by what is available in the environment.

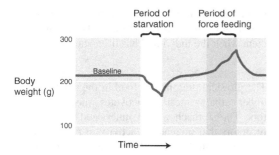

FIGURE 13.1 ● A rat will return its body weight to its preintervention weight when allowed to eat a regular diet. (Adapted from Keesey RE, Boyle PC. Effects of quinine adulteration upon body weight of LH-lesioned and intact male rats. *J Comp Physiol Psychol*. 1973;84(1):38-46.)

The concept of a set point helps us understand the difficulties encountered by anyone trying to diet. One of the mechanisms the brain uses to return the body weight to its baseline set point became apparent in the Minnesota Starvation Experiment. This was an experiment conducted with conscientious objectors in Minnesota toward the end of the Second World War to help the military understand the condition of the starving civilians in Europe.

Participants were subjected to a semistarvation diet for 6 months with the goal of losing approximately 25% of their weight. From our perspective, one of the more interesting symptoms these men experienced during the experiment was obsessive thought about food. Not unlike the cravings discussed in the previous chapter, food became the principal topic of their thoughts, conversation, and daydreams. Reading cookbooks and collecting recipes became an intensely interesting pastime for many men. Eating, either mentioned in a book or shown in a movie, was a cue that put the men at heightened risk for breaking their diet. The urge to eat was so powerful that the researchers established a buddy system so that participants would not be tempted to cheat when away from the dorm. Clearly, their brains were focusing on what the body needed.

The brain can also adjust the energy expenditure as another way to maintain a stable body weight. Figure 13.2 shows a thermodynamic perspective of energy expenditure. Energy enters an organism as food and exits as heat or work. Energy is stored as fat or glycogen and mobilized when needed. Total energy expenditure can be subdivided into three components: obligatory energy expenditure, physical activity, and adaptive thermogenesis.

Adaptive thermogenesis is the other major obstacle the brain uses to thwart weight loss. Changes in sympathetic tone alter energy expenditure. For example, activation of the sympathetic nervous system results in catabolic breakdown of adipose tissue and produces energy. Figure 13.3 shows the changes in energy expenditure in healthy subjects after a 10% alteration in body weight. Not only does the brain increase adaptive thermogenesis when the body gains weight but also turns it down in response to weight loss—a frustration many dieters have experienced.

HOMEOSTATIC MECHANISMS

The key point is that despite large day-to-day fluctuations in food intake and energy expenditure, our weight remains within a relatively narrow range.

FIGURE 13.2 ● Energy accumulation and expenditure must be in balance for an organism to maintain a stable body weight. Adaptive thermogenesis is regulated by the brain and can vary in response to changes in diet or temperature. (Adapted from Lowell BB, Spiegelman BM. Towards a molecular understanding of adaptive thermogenesis. *Nature*. 2000;404(6778):652-660.)

FIGURE 13.3 ● Total energy expenditure is increased in response to weight gain and decreased when weight is lost. (Adapted from Leibel RL, Rosenbaum M, Hirsch J. Changes in energy expenditure resulting from altered body weight. *N Engl J Med.* 1995;332(10):621-628.)

This is accomplished through feedback loops between the brain and the body. Brain lesion and stimulation studies in the 1940s identified the hypothalamus as a major center controlling food intake. Although the initial studies turned out to be overly simplified, the hypothalamus remains an important command center for weight maintenance.

But what are the signals the brain receives and sends? Interrupting or enhancing these signals may provide opportunities for interventions to stem the obesity epidemic. The best way to understand the current conceptualization of the central nervous system (CNS) homeostatic mechanisms is to separate the short-term signals from the long-term ones.

Short-Term Signals

The short-term signals tend to affect meal size rather than the overall energy storage. The signals comprise nutrients and gut hormones in the circulation as well as afferent signals sent up the vagus nerve. These signals to the brain result in the sensation of satiety but do not produce sustained alteration in body adiposity.

Nutrients

Glucose is the primary nutrient that mediates satiety. Hypoglycemia increases hunger sensations and stimulates eating. Glucose infusions will decrease the food intake. Other nutrients in the systemic circulation, such as fats and amino acids, play a real but limited role in signaling to the brain the effects of a recent meal. High levels of these nutrients tell the brain to stop eating, but the brakes are insufficient when the individual has been starving.

Mechanoreceptors

The physical presence of food in the stomach and upper small intestine activates mechanoreceptors. The stomach wall is innervated with stretch receptors that increase in activity in proportion to the volume in the stomach. We usually think of the vagus as a conduit from the brain to the gut, but as much as 80% of the neural traffic is flowing in the opposite direction (see Figure 2.9). The vagus nerve transmits signals about gastric distension to the hindbrain. This may be the reason some patients with vagus nerve stimulators report weight loss.

Gut Hormones

Numerous gut hormones are involved in food intake regulation. The most widely studied hormone is *cholecystokinin* (CCK). CCK is released from endocrine cells in the mucosal layer of the small intestine in response to fats and proteins. CCK inhibits further food intake through several mechanisms, such as stimulating the vagal nerve and inhibiting gastric emptying. Additionally, there are CCK receptors in the brain. The injection of CCK directly into the ventricles will inhibit eating. CCK appears to have central and peripheral mechanisms to put the brake on a meal.

Although CCK will limit food intake, its long-term administration does not induce significant weight loss. In studies with rats, the repeated administration of CCK resulted in smaller but more frequent meals. Thus, the overall energy balance was not altered. Figure 13.4 summarizes the short-term signals regulating food intake.

There are many other gut hormones that also inhibit eating, for example, glucagon-like peptide-1 (GLP-1) and peptide tyrosine–tyrosine. *Ghrelin* is of most interest as it is the only gut hormone that stimulates hunger. Produced in the stomach, fasting increases the levels of ghrelin, which then fall after a meal. Peripheral and central administration of ghrelin increases the food intake. In contrast to CCK, there is some evidence that ghrelin has long-term effects on weight and may be a potential culprit in obesity. Some studies suggest that reduced ghrelin production is one of the reasons gastric bypass surgery is so effective (see Figure 13.10).

The Joy of Eating

Eating is more than just sustenance; it is one of the great pleasures of life. The perception of pleasure that we get from some foods is most likely an adaptation that enhanced the survival of our ancestors

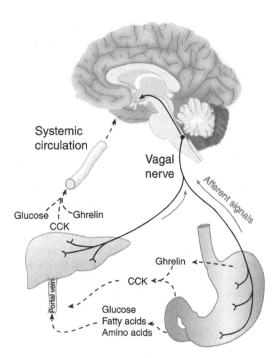

Systemic circulation

Vagal nerve

Afferent signals

Glucose
Ghrelin
CCK

Ghrelin

CCK

Glucose
Fatty acids
Amino acids

Portal vein

FIGURE 13.4 ● Short-term signals from the intestines (hormones in the circulation and stimulation of the vagus nerve) signal to the brain that the body is full. CCK, cholecystokinin. (Adapted from Havel PJ. Peripheral signals conveying metabolic information to the brain: short-term and long-term regulation of food intake and energy homeostasis. *Exp Biol Med*. 2001;226(11):963-977.)

| DISORDERS | YOUR GRANDFATHER'S DIET |

A remarkable study from an isolated community in Sweden has shown that a man's risk of death from cardiovascular disease and diabetes is affected by his grandfather's diet during his grandfather's slow growth period—ages 9 to 12 for boys. Using records of harvest success or failure during the 19th century, the researchers found increased risk of heart disease and diabetes if the grandfather lived through bountiful harvests during his slow growth period. Alternatively, grandfathers who grew up during times of famine sired grandchildren who lived longer. The mechanism, derived in part from rodent studies, is believed to be transgenerational epigenetic inheritance (see Figure 6.12).

---

during lean times. However, with the abundance of inexpensive highly palatable refined foods, genes that favored sweet foods cause us to overeat.

Certain foods increase dopamine at the nucleus accumbens (see Figure 12.6). Additionally, the endogenous opioids appear to be more active during a good meal. Other evidence suggests that eating is a highly valued pleasure that can resemble an addiction. For example, obese individuals have reduced D_2 receptors in the striatum and activation of the orbitofrontal cortex when craving food. Clearly, dopamine and the endogenous opioids are signals that influence energy consumption.

Long-Term Signals

Long-term signals tell the brain about the overall energy storage, not just the caloric content of the recent meal. In the 1950s, it was suggested that adipose tissue releases a hormone that signals the hypothalamus about the current state of energy storage.

Termed an *adiposity signal*, the elusive hormone must have the following three traits:

– Circulate in the blood in proportion to the amount of stored fat
– Cross the blood–brain barrier and stimulate specific receptors in the brain
– Produce changes in caloric intake and energy expenditure when levels of the hormone fluctuate

Leptin

It was not until the discovery of *leptin* in 1994 that the first adiposity signal was identified. The mutant ob/ob mice (ob = obese) have an alternation in one gene, which results in hyperphagia and weight gain of three to five times the normal. Identifying the locus of the genetic defect allowed the cloning of the protein that the ob/ob mice were missing: leptin.

Leptin is primarily produced in white fat cells and circulates in direct proportion to the total fat load. The largest concentration of leptin receptors is found in the arcuate nucleus of the hypothalamus. Mice that lack leptin are obese. When given exogenous leptin, they reduce the food intake and lose weight (Figure 13.5).

Other hormones have been proposed as adiposity signals, the most prominent of which is *insulin*. The role of insulin is complicated because its primary function is to enhance the glucose intake into the muscle and adipose tissues. Yet, insulin secretion is influenced by total body fat, and in turn it can elicit a reduction in body weight. Insulin appears to

FIGURE 13.5 ● Two ob/ob mice, both of which are missing the gene to produce leptin. The mouse on the right has received daily leptin injections for 4.5 weeks and weighs about half as much as the mouse on the left. (From Amgen Inc., Thousand Oaks, California.) Photo by John Sholtis.

work in parallel with leptin. Figure 13.6 shows a schematic representation of these adiposity signals.

Arcuate Nucleus

The hypothalamus is at the heart of the regulation of the body's energy metabolism. So it is no wonder that the largest concentration of leptin receptors is found in the arcuate nucleus of the hypothalamus. The arcuate nucleus is located at the base of the hypothalamus next to the third ventricle (Figure 13.7). Two groups of neurons have been identified within the arcuate nucleus that mediate the leptin signal: proopiomelanocortin (POMC) and neuropeptide Y (NPY).

Proopiomelanocortin

The POMC neurons put the brakes on eating. The POMC neuropeptide is cleaved to produce α-melanocyte–stimulating hormone (α-MSH), which is a potent suppressor of food intake. The effects of α-MSH are mediated through the melanocortin (MC) receptors, particularly MC3R and MC4R, which are strongly expressed in the hypothalamus.

High levels of leptin as well as other circulating hormones will stimulate the POMC neurons. Conversely, low levels of leptin inhibit the POMC neurons. Thus, POMC neurons and α-MSH are directly responsive to circulating hormones that signal an excess of adipose tissue.

Neuropeptide Y

The NPY neurons work to increase the food intake and decrease the energy expenditure. The NPY

FIGURE 13.6 ● Adipose tissue secretes hormones in proportion to the total fat stored. The hormones in turn affect the energy expenditure and food intake in relation to their levels in the circulation.

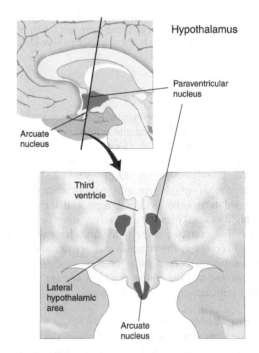

FIGURE 13.7 ● Two sections of the brain showing the location of the arcuate nucleus within the hypothalamus along with two other important nuclei for the control of energy balance.

neurons express a peptide called *agouti-related peptide* (AGRP), which is an antagonist at the MC4 receptor. Consequently, activation of the NPY neurons blocks the effects of α-MSH and the POMC neurons. The role of NPY neurons and AGRP in the accumulation of calories has been demonstrated in many experimental conditions (see Figure 6.11):

1. Stimulation of the NPY neurons increases food intake.
2. Increased expression of AGRP results in increased food intake.
3. During starvation, there is increased activation of the NPY neurons and increased expression of AGRP.
4. Leptin inhibits the NPY neurons and AGRP expression.

Thus, there is an accelerator and brake relationship between the NPY neurons and the POMC neurons that responds to signals from the body about the long-term status of energy storage (Figure 13.8). Of particular relevance to the current epidemic of obesity is the unequal relationship between each set of neurons. While they provide equal stimulation of the downstream effort neurons, only the NPY neurons directly inhibit the POMC neurons. The POMC neurons do not inhibit the NPY neurons. Consequently, there appears to be a slightly greater emphasis on the accumulation of calories. In other words, the accelerator is stronger than the brake, which, from an evolutionary perspective, would seem to enhance the survival in times of low food supply or famine.

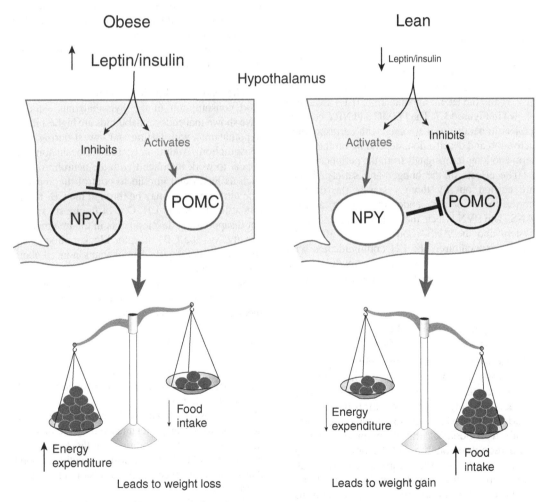

FIGURE 13.8 ● The presence or absence of adiposity signals, such as leptin and insulin, has opposite effects on the NPY and POMC neurons. In turn, the activation of the NPY and POMC neurons has different effects on energy balance and body weight. NPY, neuropeptide Y; POMC, proopiomelanocortin.

STRESS

Many patients will report that food is a source of comfort when they are "stressed out." Several lines of evidence suggest there may be a correlation between the hypothalamic–pituitary–adrenal axis and the ability to resist the pleasures of food:

1. Childhood stress is associated with increased weight problems in adolescence and adulthood.
2. Corticotropin-releasing hormone and cortisol stimulate the release of dopamine at the nucleus accumbens, which makes it harder to resist temptations.
3. Glucocorticoids increase fat deposits.
4. Stressed rats given access to sweet water have lower glucocorticoid levels.

Downstream Targets

The downstream effects of the arcuate neurons are numerous and largely remain mysterious. Two important sites are the paraventricular nucleus (PVN) and the lateral hypothalamic (LH) area, also shown in Figure 13.7. The POMC and NPY neurons project in parallel to these sites with corresponding activation and deactivation, depending on the short-term and long-term signals from the periphery.

The effects of the hunger and satiety signals are carried out by three systems: the cerebral cortex (behavior), the endocrine system, and the ANS. The PVN affects the output of the endocrine system and the ANS—both of which affect the energy expenditure. The LH communicates with the cerebral cortex, which in turn modulates the food-seeking behavior. This simplified analysis of

POINT OF INTEREST

Smoking has one legitimate virtue: appetite suppression. Smokers are generally thinner and typically gain about 10 lb when they cease smoking. Recent research has identified the anorexic mechanism. Nicotine binds with a subunit of the nicotine acetylcholine receptors on the POMC neurons. This activates the POMC neurons, which leads to reduced food intake and weight loss. This receptor subunit may be accessible to pharmacologic manipulation turning on one benefit of smoking without the toxic effects.

the downstream effects of signals from the body is shown in Figure 13.9.

Endocannabinoids

It has been known for a long time that marijuana stimulates the appetite. The naughty boys at our colleges called it *the munchies*. Stimulation of the cannabinoid (CB_1) receptor by the main active component of marijuana, Δ^9-tetrahydrocannabinol, is believed to induce this behavior. Clinicians have successfully utilized this effect when treating anorexic conditions such as AIDS (acquired immunodeficiency syndrome)-related wasting syndrome. With animals, it has been found that the endocannabinoid system is activated with short-term fasting or the presentation of palatable food, thereby inducing appetite.

The CB_1 receptor is involved with the regulation of food intake at several levels. First, it enhances the motivation to seek and consume palatable food, possibly by interactions with the mesolimbic pathways. Studies with rodents show that endocannabinoids enhance the release of dopamine at the nucleus accumbens and may synergize the effects of the opioids.

The endocannabinoid system also stimulates food consumption in the hypothalamus. Studies have shown that endocannabinoids are highest in the hypothalamus with fasting and lowest during food consumption. Additionally, the endocannabinoids appear to work in concert with the neurohormones such as leptin and ghrelin to control the appetite. The ultimate effect may be through the CB_1 receptors at the PVN and LH. One of the most exciting but disappointing developments in the treatment of obesity was the CB_1 receptor blocker rimonabant (the anti-munchie pill). Rimonabant induced about a 10-lb weight loss, but it also led to the emergence of anxiety, depression, and suicidal thinking. The Food and Drug Administration (FDA) rejected the medication and it was withdrawn in Europe.

EATING DISORDERS
Obesity

Fifty years ago, obesity was a rare disease. Readily available palatable food accompanied by a sedentary lifestyle has now resulted in an epidemic of obesity. Most disturbing is the rapid rise in childhood obesity. Clearly, diet and exercise are first-line interventions for this condition, but these efforts are a constant uphill battle against a genetic set point that favors rich, sweet food that historically was in short supply.

After the discovery of leptin, there was great excitement about the prospect of a treatment for obesity. Leptin was shown to reduce obesity in

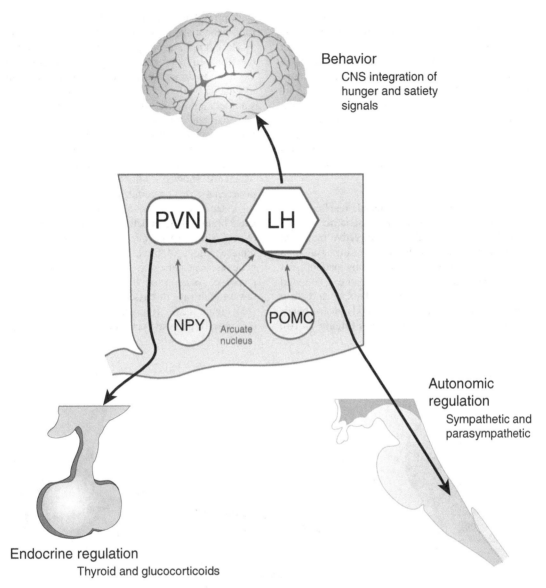

Behavior
CNS integration of hunger and satiety signals

PVN   LH

NPY   Arcuate nucleus   POMC

Autonomic regulation
Sympathetic and parasympathetic

Endocrine regulation
Thyroid and glucocorticoids

FIGURE 13.9 ● The PVN and lateral hypothalamus (along with others) influence the three major effort pathways so that the body can maintain a stable energy balance. CNS, central nervous system; PVN, paraventricular nucleus; LH, lateral hypothalamic; NPY, neuropeptide Y; POMC, proopiomelanocortin.

genetically leptin-deficient humans and rodents (Figure 13.5). Unfortunately, the magnitude of weight loss in most obese humans who received exogenous leptin in studies has been modest. In actuality, most obese people have high levels of circulating leptin, but for some reason fail to respond to the signal. This has generated speculation that obesity may be associated with, or even caused by, a resistance to leptin, as is seen with insulin resistance in type 2 diabetes.

Why cannot we find a pill that tells the brain, "I'm full"? It is not for lack of trying. The fen–phen debacle (fenfluramine/phentermine)—with its modest weight loss and potential for pulmonary hypertension or valvular disease—has spooked the field. Likewise, a recent follow-up of patients who took benzedrine or dexedrine for weight loss in the sixties showed a 60% greater chance of developing Parkinson's disease. There are a number of stimulant medications such as phentermine and benzphetamine that suppress appetite, but they are used only for short-term weight loss—say 8 to 12 weeks.

The dilemma is to find a medication that is effective and safe for long-term use. We know of four medications that were rejected (or not accepted) by the FDA and one that was voluntarily withdrawn from the market in this short period of time. Recently, the FDA reconsidered and accepted Belviq (lorcaserin), a serotonin 2C receptor agonist that is believed to activate POMC. The benefits are mild—roughly 13-lb weight loss compared with 5 to 6 lb for patients on the placebo. Unfortunately, when it comes to medications that control weight, it is difficult to deceive the brain without unintended damages—or at least that is the case so far.

Gastric Bypass Surgery

One success during the past decade has been gastric bypass surgery. Also called bariatric surgery, it is clearly not only the most effective treatment for morbid obesity but also the most invasive—and not without significant risks. Many patients not only lose substantial weight but also can be cured of secondary problems such as diabetes and sleep apnea. There are two primary methods: gastric banding and Roux-en-Y gastric bypass (Figure 13.10).

Both procedures mechanically limit the amount of food in the stomach, which reduces the caloric intake.

Recent research suggests that one of the reasons the Roux-en-Y procedure may be more effective has more to do with changes in gut hormones than mechanical effects. In a small non-randomized study comparing the two procedures, the patients who had the Roux-en-Y showed greater weight loss along with greater changes in gut hormones (Figure 13.10). Not shown in the figure are the other hormones such as GLP-1 and peptide YY, which also showed significant differences at 1 year between the two procedures.

A separate study by a different group investigated brain activation before and after a Roux-en-Y bypass. Subjects were cued with auditory and visual representations of food, while a functional magnetic resonance imaging (MRI) followed their brain response. As expected, the food cues activated the reward pathways discussed in the previous chapter (see Figure 12.6). Remarkably, after the surgery, the reward pathway activation was significantly

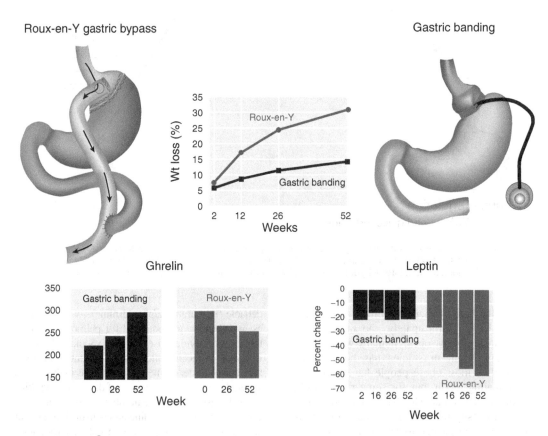

FIGURE 13.10 ● The superiority of Roux-en-Y gastric bypass surgery to produce substantial weight loss which may be due to changes in hormones that regulate appetite. (Adapted from Korner j, Inabnet W, Febres G, et al. Prospective study of gut hormone and metabolic changes after adjustable gastric banding and Roux-en-Y gastric bypass. *Int J Obesity.* 2009;33:786-795.)

reduced in response to food cues. In other words, the subjects did not have as much food cravings after the bypass surgery.

Taken together, these studies suggest that Rouxen-Y procedure dampens numerous hormones and neurotransmitters that mediate the neural response to food. Maybe one reason it is so hard to find a pill that reduces appetite is because one molecule cannot replicate the panoply of hormones released by the gastrointestinal tract that regulate the body's energy balance.

Purging

It is tempting to speculate that patients with anorexia and bulimia have set points that favor lean body mass, in other words, some pathology in their hypothalamus. However, most of the studies point to the involvement of other areas of the brain. Specifically, the symptoms of anxiety, perfectionism, and obsessions about body image are more consistent with disorders in the prefrontal cortex and amygdala. Likewise, eating disorder patients who have lost significant weight experience food cravings similar to what the men in the Minnesota Starvation Experiment experienced. Finally, the neuropeptide and neuroendocrine alterations present when patients are restricting intake return to normal levels when the patients recover. Eating disorder patients struggle with a drive to be thin, but this is not likely to be caused by pathological appetite signals.

PSYCHIATRIC MEDICATIONS

Weight gain is one of the most difficult side effects associated with psychiatric treatment and is often a reason patients stop effective treatments. Surprisingly, little is known about the mechanism of this problem. The new antipsychotic agents have been of particular concern. The FDA has required all manufacturers to include black box warnings documenting concerns about weight gain as well as the development of diabetes and hypercholesterolemia.

The mechanism of the weight gain remains a mystery. One compelling study examined the affinity for various receptors (serotoninergic, adrenergic, dopaminergic, histaminergic, and muscarinic) compared with reports of short-term weight gain. They determined that the strongest correlation for gaining weight is with H_1 histamine receptor activity ($r = -0.72$). Table 13.1 shows the relative risk of weight gain from the second-generation antipsychotic agents, as determined by a consensus group that included the American Diabetes Association and the American Psychiatric Association (as well as others), compared with the H_1 affinity.

The histamine neurons are known to be involved with energy homeostasis—an effect enhanced by modafinil. Additionally, centrally administered histamine increases the activity of leptin in rodents. Inversely, the blocking effect of the antihistamines may result in weight gain through decreased energy metabolism as well as increased appetite. However, diphenhydramine (Benadryl) is

---

TREATMENT **LONGEVITY**

Caloric restriction (CR) is the most reproducible intervention to extend life. Rhesus monkeys whose caloric intake is restricted by 30% live longer. The figures (A) show the survival curves for age-related mortality and overall mortality for the monkeys with CR compared to controls. The CR monkeys have less diabetes, cancer, and cardiovascular disease. Furthermore, MRIs show that CR monkeys have more brain volume and less CNS fluid (B). CR appears to prevent cell loss and brain atrophy associated with aging. While beneficial, it is unlikely that humans can muster the self-control to use CR to prevent age-related CNS decline.

Adapted from Colman RJ, Anderson RM, Johnson SC, et al. Caloric restriction delays disease onset and mortality in rhesus monkeys. *Science*. 2009;325:201-204. Brain scans courtesy of Ricki Colman and the University of Wisconsin-Madison.

TABLE 13.1

The Relation between the Risk of Weight Gain with Second-Generation Antipsychotic Agents and Affinity for the H_1 Histamine Receptor

	Weight Gain	Amount of Drug Needed to Block H_1 Histamine
Clozapine	+++	1.2
Olanzapine	+++	2
Quetiapine	++	11
Risperidone	++	15
Aripiprazole	+/–	29.7
Ziprasidone	+/–	43

considered weight neutral, so there must be more than just H_1 affinity causing the weight problems associated with antipsychotic medications.

Patients on antidepressants or mood stabilizers are also often caught between maintaining an ideal body size and the negative consequences of effective treatment. Long-term studies find weight gain and increased risk of diabetes mellitus DM in patients treated with these medications. What could be causing this? One theory is that patients are regaining the weight they lost prior to starting treatment. More likely explanations are that psychiatric mediations increase the food craving or reduce the resting metabolic rate. Unfortunately, there is scant evidence to identify a specific mechanism.

Few psychiatric medications induce weight loss. Bupropion and topiramate have demonstrated beneficial effects on weight, but results are modest and few studies exist. Amphetamines were the original "diet pills" and were freely prescribed in the fifties and sixties. In the early seventies, due to problems with addiction and occasional psychosis, the government deemed this class of medications Schedule II and required new studies to establish effectiveness. These steps, for all intents and purposes, stopped the use of stimulants as diet pills. More recently, the quick removal of dexfenfluramine (Redux) in the 1990s and the massive lawsuits that followed portend further research with stimulants for weight control.

The mechanism by which stimulants induce weight loss is not as straightforward as one would expect. These medications—affectionately called "speed" and "uppers" on the street—actually reduce motor activity: *the paradoxical effect*. Figure 13.11 documents this effect in a group of boys with no behavioral or learning difficulties and an average IQ of 130. Motor activity was measured by a little

sensor the children wore around their ankles during a 2-hour test period. The graph shows that, with few exceptions, the boys reduced the motor activity while on amphetamine. (Some clinicians incorrectly interpret this normal response to stimulants as an indication that the subject has ADHD.)

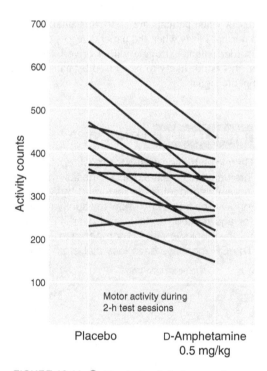

FIGURE 13.11 ● Physical activity in normal prepubertal boys decreased when they were on amphetamine compared with placebo. (Adapted from Rapoport JL, Buchsbaum MS, Zahn TP, et al. Dextroamphetamine: cognitive and behavioral effects in normal prepubertal boys. *Science.* 1978;199(4328):560-563.

| TREATMENT | NUTRITION AND MENTAL HEALTH |

There is a growing body of evidence correlating nutrition and mental health. Separate studies in the UK, Spain, and Australia have shown that increased consumption of a Western diet (processed food, refined grains, and sugary products) is associated with more depressive symptoms. Although unproven as a therapeutic intervention, maybe a healthy diet rich in fruits and vegetables should be a prescription we give to every patient.

A more recent study analyzed resting energy expenditure (see Figure 13.3) in 14 normal men and women given methylphenidate. Subjects received 0.5 mg/kg of methylphenidate or placebo in a blinded, crossover study. While on methylphenidate the resting energy of the subjects increased by 7%. Other studies with humans have consistently shown decreased caloric intake while on stimulants. Subjects will consume a normal quantity when eating, but eat less frequently.

The stimulants appear to increase energy expenditure and reduce energy intake—which on the surface is exactly what we want. Unfortunately, the stimulants also have a host of adverse CNS effects. Of interest, some of the recently rejected appetite suppressants also had psychiatric adverse effects such as depression, anxiety, and suicidal ideation—a prime reason the FDA turned down these medications. There is an interesting, and as yet poorly understood, association between medications that reduce appetite and mental health—further evidence that obesity is more than just energy consumption.

QUESTIONS

1. All of the following support the concept of a metabolic "set point," except
   a. Most diets fail.
   b. Forced feeding leads to increased energy expenditure.
   c. The "thrifty gene" promotes weight gain when high caloric food is readily available.
   d. Adaptive thermogenesis is unchanged by caloric intake.

2. Patients with anorexia nervosa and participants in the Minnesota Starvation Experiment share which of the following symptoms?
   a. Perfectionistic personality traits.
   b. Obsessive thoughts about food.
   c. Altered metabolic "set point."
   d. Increased energy expenditure.

3. Short-term signals about hunger and satiety include all of the following, except
   a. Leptin.
   b. CCK.
   c. Glucose.
   d. Ghrelin.

4. Adiposity signals must be able to do all of the following, except
   a. Cross the blood–brain barrier.
   b. Change in relation to the amount of stored fat.
   c. Alter afferent signals from the vagus nerve.
   d. Inhibit or enhance caloric intake.

5. The largest concentration of leptin receptors are in the
   a. Amygdala.
   b. Arcuate nucleus.
   c. Adrenal cortex.
   d. Anterior corticospinal tract.

6. The AGRP does which of the following?
   a. Antagonist at the MC4 receptor and stimulates eating.
   b. Antagonist at the MC4 receptor and inhibits intake.
   c. Agonist at the MC4 receptor and stimulates eating.
   d. Agonist at the MC4 receptor and inhibits intake.

7. The Melanocortin system
   a. Has been implicated as a cause of AN.
   b. Stimulates foraging for food.
   c. Potentiates the endocannabinoid receptor.
   d. Suppresses the food intake.

8. The effects of the brain's assessment of caloric needs are carried out by all of the following, except
   a. Endocrine hormones.
   b. Changes in behavior.
   c. Modulation of the "set point."
   d. Alterations in the ANS.

See Answers section at the end of the book.

CHAPTER **14**

Anger and Aggression

DIAGNOSIS

Anger and aggression are fundamental reactions throughout the animal kingdom. Defending against intruders and hunting for the next meal are traits that were essential for the survival of our ancestors. However, some individuals are too aggressive. We all know a few dogs (and relatives for that matter) that are easily agitated and quick to bite. Animals and people with this tendency are a significant social problem.

Terms such as *road rage*, *spouse abuse*, and *school violence* are all too common in our daily papers. Yet, the *Diagnostic and Statistical Manual* (DSM) does not include a category for inappropriate anger. It has been suggested this is because men created DSM and they do not see anger as a problem. (PMS, on the other hand, is now a disorder!)

The absence of a diagnostic category is clinically relevant. For example, a small Danish pharmaceutical company in the 1970s was pursuing a treatment for aggression, called *serenics*. In spite of promising results, the company shelved the medication when it became clear the US Food and Drug Administration would not approve the medication because aggression is not a specific disorder. Consequently, although psychologists and other counselors provide treatment for "anger management," there is no sanctioned pharmacologic intervention for excessive anger and irritability.

Aggression is clearly influenced by one's culture and upbringing. Violence on TV and early physical abuse increase the likelihood a person will be aggressive. Alternatively, the context in which an assault occurs determines the appropriateness of the aggression. For example, fighting on the ice at hockey games is accepted, but fighting in the stands is not. These are issues beyond the scope of this text. We are interested in the processes in the brain that generate or fail to impede violence toward another.

Two Kinds of Aggression

Working with cats, Flynn at Yale, and Siegel at the University of Medicine and Dentistry of New Jersey, identified two types of aggressive behavior. One is more predatory—similar to hunting—the cat quietly and calmly stalks his prey. The other type of aggression is defensive. Here the cat is agitated and makes a big display of his feelings, in part to avoid a fight, but is also ready to respond if provoked. In the cat, these different responses can be elicited by electrical stimulation of different regions of the hypothalamus.

MECHANISMS IN THE BRAIN
Hypothalamus

In a series of experiments over many years, Flynn and Siegel placed electrodes into the hypothalamus of cats and searched for the regions that would, with stimulation, elicit aggression. Remarkably, they found separate regions that elicited the two kinds of aggressive behaviors observed in cats. Figure 14.1 shows the location of the hypothalamus and the two general areas (lateral and medial) on either side of the third ventricle that correspond with predatory and defensive aggression.

Figure 14.2 shows an example of predatory aggression elicited in a cat by stimulation of the *lateral hypothalamus*. The bite to the back of the neck is preceded by quiet, stealthy circling of the rodent. It is worth noting that the researchers used cats in these experiments that would not bite the rat before the hypothalamic stimulation.

Figure 14.3 shows the defensive type of aggressive behavior induced by stimulating the *medial hypothalamus*. In this case, the cat becomes aroused (high sympathetic tone, increased heart rate, dilated pupils, etc.) and displays hostile behavior (hissing, growling, arching back, piloerection, etc.). The different features of each kind of aggression are summarized in Table 14.1.

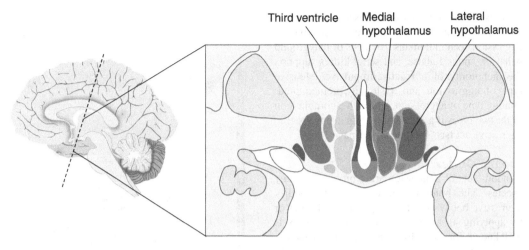

FIGURE 14.1 ● The medial and lateral regions of the hypothalamus.

FIGURE 14.2 ● Predatory attack (quiet bite) against a rat induced by stimulating the lateral hypothalamus. (From Flynn JP. The neural basis of aggression in cats. In: Glass DC, ed. *Neurophysicology and Emotion*. New York: Rockefeller University Press; 1967:40–60.)

FIGURE 14.3 ● Defensive attack elicited by stimulating the medial hypothalamus. (From Flynn JP. The neural basis of aggression in cats. In: Glass DC, ed. *Neurophysicology and Emotion*. New York: Rockefeller University Press; 1967:40–60.)

TABLE 14.1

The Different Features of Predatory and Defensive Aggression

	Predatory Aggression	Defensive Aggression
CNS location	Lateral hypothalamus	Medial hypothalamus
Sympathetic tone	Calm	Autonomic arousal
Behavior	Stealthy movement, bite to back of rat's neck	Hissing, arching back, paw swipe, piloerection
Evolutionary function	Hunting	Protection
Quality	Hidden, premeditated	Overt, reactive

CNS, central nervous system

These two pathways and subsequent behavior elicited in the cat also describe the two basic kinds of aggression seen in humans. Analysis of playground behavior, spousal abuse, and serial killers supports the dichotomy of a reactive/impulsive/defensive type of aggression and a stealthy/premeditated/hunting type of aggression, although a combination of the two types is a common finding in any specific aggressive act (see Treatment box, page 166).

Frontal Cortex

Random acts of aggression are a problem for any species. The brain has mechanisms to modify aggressive behavior either by putting on brakes or by applying an accelerator. The frontal cortex is well known for controlling the impulsive behavior. Impairment of the frontal cortex is the equivalent of taking off the brakes on aggressive impulses. The most famous example of this is Phineas Gage. Gage was a foreman at a railroad construction company in Vermont in 1848. A tamping iron was blown through his left frontal skull when a spark inadvertently ignited the explosive powder.

Gage's skull has been preserved, and Figure 14.4 shows a reconstruction of the path the tamping iron took through his skull. Remarkably, he recovered, was out of bed within a month, and lived another 12 years. However, his personality had drastically changed. While before the accident he had been efficient, balanced, and responsible, now he was fitful, impulsive, unfocused, and easily agitated.

If we imagine that the frontal cortex applies the brakes to the array of primitive impulses that arise from the subcortical brain, then we can see how taking the brakes off (due to a poorly functioning frontal cortex) allows the expression of feelings that would normally be subdued. Specifically, a poorly functioning frontal cortex allows more aggressive impulses to be expressed. Alternatively, a healthy, active frontal cortex puts the "brakes" on inappropriate aggressive behavior.

Experiments out of Siegel's lab provide alternative evidence of the important role the frontal cortex plays in restraining aggression. In this study, a cat has one electrode in his lateral hypothalamus and one in the lateral aspect of his frontal cortex. What is being measured is the time until the cat attacks the rat after stimulation of the electrodes. With just hypothalamic stimulation, the cat only waits approximately 12 seconds before attacking. However, with stimulation of both the hypothalamus and the frontal cortex, the time to attack is doubled (Figure 14.5).

This study was repeated with many cats with electrodes in different locations of the frontal cortex. Similar results were found. Clearly, the frontal cortex

A   B

FIGURE 14.4 ● **A.** The skull of Phineas Gage and the tampering iron that exploded through his head in 1848. **B.** Drawing of a computerized reconstruction of the path the rod took through his skull and brain. The damage involved both left and right prefrontal cortices. (Adapted from Damasio H, Grabowski T, Frank R, et al. The return of Phineas Gage: clues about the brain from the skull of a famous patient. *Science*. 1994;264:1102-1105.)

FIGURE 14.5 ● The time it takes a cat to attack a rat after the hypothalamus is stimulated is greatly increased when the frontal cortex is simultaneously stimulated. (Adapted from Siegel A, Edinger H, Dotto M. Effects of electrical stimulation of the lateral aspect of the prefrontal cortex upon attack behavior in cats. *Brain Res*. 1975;93:473-484.)

TREATMENT PSYCHOSURGERY

There are few studies in the medical literature involving the hypothalamus and aggression in humans, with the exception of a few reports of psychosurgery. For example, in Japan, Sano and Mayanagi performed 60 posteromedial hypothalamotomies in the 1960s for aggressive behavior. Most patients also had a history of seizures and mental retardation. In a follow-up report conducted in 1987, Sano and Mayanagi reported the absence of violence and aggression in 78%, with apparently normal endocrine function. Although a drastic procedure, it accentuates the central role of the hypothalamus with aggressive behavior.

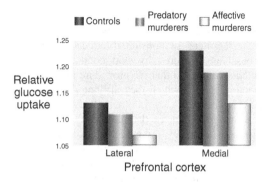

FIGURE 14.6 ● The relative activity in the lateral and medial aspect of the prefrontal cortex of predatory and affective murderers compared with normal controls. (Adapted from Raine A, Meloy JR, Bihrle S, et al. Reduced prefrontal and increased subcortical brain functioning assessed using positron emission tomography in predatory and affective murderers. *Behav Sci Law*. 1998;16(3):319-332.)

has an inhibitory effect on aggressive expressions. It is unfortunate that we have not found a way to "beef up" a wimpy frontal cortex.

One of the most consistent findings with humans and violence is frontal lobe dysfunction. With the advent of neuroimaging capabilities, many researchers have looked at the activity in the prefrontal cortex (PFC) in men with violent histories. In a review of the literature on the topic, Brower and Price concluded that significant frontal lobe dysfunction is associated with aggressive dyscontrol—in particular, impulsive aggressive behavior.

A study of convicted murderers by Raine et al. provides further insight on this topic. Raine separated a group of murderers into those who committed planned, predatory violence and those who perpetrated affective, impulsive violence. Positron emission tomography scans were conducted on these subjects along with normal controls, examining the activity in the frontal cortex. The results are shown in Figure 14.6. Both groups of murderers had less activity in the PFC compared with controls, but the impulsive, affective group had the least. One wishes there was a way for men in prison to exercise and strengthen their frontal cortex as much as they exercise their biceps.

Amygdala

There is conflicting information about the role of the amygdala and aggressive behavior. Although better known for being activated during fearful situations, the amygdala may have a broader function in processing emotional stimuli. Early studies with monkeys showed that the bilateral removal of the amygdala produced an animal that was placid—neither frightened nor aggressive. This is called the *Klüver-Bucy syndrome*, after the two researchers

who performed the experiments. This and other research suggest that the amygdala is instrumental in recognizing whether a stimulus is threatening and that an overactive amygdala can lead to excessive defensive aggression.

There are reports in the literature of bilateral amygdalotomies for untreatable aggression in humans. Some of the reports are disturbingly optimistic. A group from India reported on 481 cases, stating that 70% showed excellent or moderate improvement after 5 years (see Prefrontal Lobotomy box, page 18 for another example of psychosurgery hyperbole). A report about two cases in Georgia provides a more balanced assessment of the procedure.

Two individuals who were essentially institutionalized because of aggressive behavior received amygdalotomies after years of failed medical therapies.

DISORDER VIOLENCE AND AGE

Age has a profound effect on the likelihood of being violent. The incidence of violent crime rises rapidly until the ages of 18 to 22 and then gradually declines over the next three decades. The very young and very old are the least violent. There are many sociocultural variables that contribute to this trend. However, the delay in the maturing of the brain compared with the fully developed physical body provides one explanation (see Figure 8.7). The young adult does not have enough containment by the frontal cortex of his aggressive impulses.

The procedures resulted in reductions but not elimination of the assaultive behavior. Pre- and postassessments demonstrated reduced autonomic arousal as measured by skin conductance. The authors concluded that the procedure resulted in a "taming effect," which they attributed to reduced perceptions of threats. In other words, an overactive amygdala causes the individual to perceive threats where they do not exist. Removing the amygdala decreases the false perceptions.

Other research suggests that the amygdala is *underactive* in those with aggressive problems (see section "The Psychopath" in the subsequent text). Recent imaging studies have found that amygdala dysfunction is associated with criminal psychopaths. One study in Finland showed decreased volume of the amygdala in a group of psychopaths. Another study used functional magnetic resonance imaging to examine the activity of the amygdala during memory tasks involving negatively charged words. The psychopaths showed less amygdaloid activity compared with controls (Figure 14.7). These studies suggest that an underactive amygdala may facilitate aggression.

The work by Siegel with his cats may shed light on the conflicting data about the role of the amygdala in aggressive behavior. We must remember that the amygdala is not just one organ but is made up of multiple nuclei (see Figure 2.7). Siegel found with cats that stimulating the lateral and central groups facilitates predatory attacks and suppressed defensive rage. Conversely, stimulation of the medial aspect of the basal complex has just the opposite effect. This subtle difference within the amygdala would be hard to identify in humans with current imaging technology. The amygdala may be overactive with different subtypes of aggression and underactive with others. Alternatively, it could be that different nuclei are activated for the different types of aggression.

An old case recently came to our attention that emphasizes the points of this section. Charles Whitman was described as an intelligent, loyal young man who was leading an uneventful life until he started to struggle with episodes of anger in his early twenties. In March 1966, he sought psychiatric help at the University of Texas Medical Center, but failed to return after the initial, psychoanalytic evaluation. In August, after killing his mother and wife—whom he professed to love—he climbed the tower at the University of Texas and shot 48 people, killing 16. At autopsy, a walnut-sized glioblastoma was discovered beneath the thalamus pressing on the hypothalamus. The tumor also extended into the temporal lobe and was compressing the amygdala.

It is impossible to identify what caused the emergence of Whitman's unimaginable violence. He was abusing amphetamines (Dexedrine) at the time of shooting and was raised in a dysfunctional family with an abusive father. However, it is likely that some of the murderous rage resulted from the tumor's compression of the hypothalamus and amygdala.

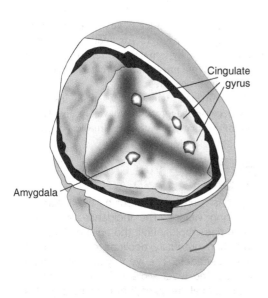

FIGURE 14.7 ● Criminal psychopaths showed less activity in the amygdala along with parts of the cingulate gyrus when recalling negative affective words compared with controls. (Adapted from Kiehl KA, Smith AM, Hare RD, et al. Limbic abnormalities in affective processing by criminal psychopaths as revealed by functional magnetic resonance imaging. *Biol Psychiatry*. 2001;50:677-684.)

HORMONES AND NEUROPEPTIDES
Testosterone
Everyone "knows" that testosterone stimulates aggression. Males fight more than females. It seems like a "no-brainer." Fortunately, the role of testosterone and aggression is not as simple as it first seems.

In 1849, Arnold Adolph Berthold, a German physician, conducted an experiment that is considered the first formal study of endocrinology (Figure 14.8). With this elegant little study, he demonstrated the importance of a substance from the testes (later discovered to be testosterone) and aggressive behavior.

Berthold knew that male chicks grow into roosters with typical secondary sexual characteristics, displaying sexual and aggressive behavior. In the experiment, Berthold removed the testes from chicks, which curtailed their normal development

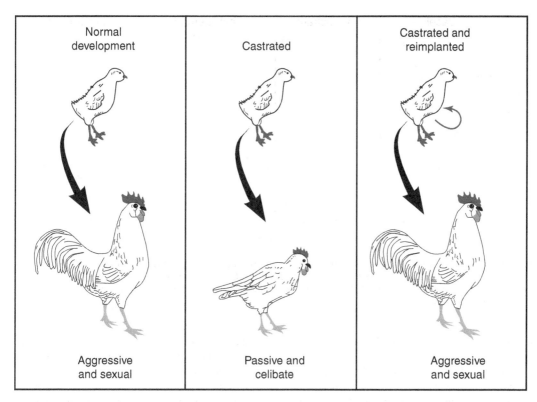

FIGURE 14.8 ● Berthold established in 1849 that a substance in the testes was necessary for the development of male behavior and body structure. (Adapted from Rosenzweig MR, Breedlove SM, Watson NV. *Biol Psychol*. 4th ed. Sunderland, MA: Sinauer; 2005.)

and eliminated the sexual and aggressive behavior. In a second group, he reimplanted the testes into the abdominal cavity. If the testes could establish a blood supply, the chick would develop into a normal rooster with the usual sexual and aggressive tendencies. Berthold concluded that the testes release a substance that affected the male body structures and behaviors.

Research with laboratory animals in the years since Berthold have consistently demonstrated similar correlations between testosterone and aggressive behavior. A good example by Wagner et al. shows the effect of castration on bite attacks on an inanimate target for adult male mice (Figure 14.9). Before castration and with testosterone replacement, the male mice will frequently bite the target. However, in the absence of the hormone, bite attacks drop close to the frequency seen with females.

For humans, it is not so easy to establish a direct link between plasma testosterone and magnitude of hostility. Conflicting results are found throughout the literature. In particular, it is hard to establish the cause and effect. For example, a popular study is to compare testosterone levels in male prisoners with their crimes. As expected, the more aggressive

prisoners have higher levels of testosterone, but so do the socially dominant, non-aggressive inmates. A recent study with baboons sheds light on this issue. The researchers followed the changing social rank for 125 adult males from five social groups over 9 years. Simultaneously, they collected fecal samples to measure testosterone as well as glucocorticoid (stress hormone). Their results are shown in Figure 14.10. It appears that plasma testosterone rises as one ascends the social ladder. The inverse is true for the glucocorticoids except for the highest ranking male. (Sapolsky, in an editorial on this article, expressed sympathy for the poor CEO [alpha male] who, although at the top of the pyramid, is more stressed than his immediate subordinate.)

Another popular belief is that exogenous steroids that some athletes take to enhance performance increases aggression in most men: "roid rage." This too is murky. In the best study of the effects of supraphysiologic doses of testosterone on normal men, Tricker et al. found no difference in anger for those on either testosterone or placebo, as noted by the spouse or by self-report after 10 weeks. Likewise, studies of sexual predators treated with antiandrogens have demonstrated

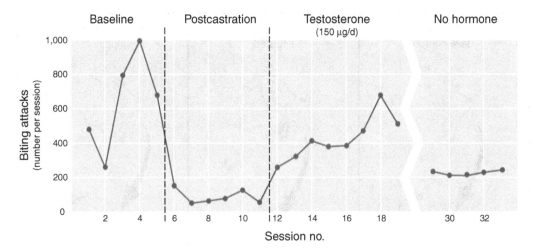

FIGURE 14.9 ● Baseline bite attacks for male mice are markedly diminished with castration. This effect can be reversed temporally with testosterone replacement. (Adapted from Wagner GC, Beuving LJ, Hutchinson RR. The effects of gonadal hormone manipulations on aggressive target-biting in mice. *Aggress Behav.* 1980;6:1-7.)

remarkable decreases in libido but with little change in aggression.

It appears that testosterone, besides its physical affects on sexual characteristics, has behavioral affects that might best be described under the umbrella of dominance behavior, that is, a display of behaviors to achieve and maintain a higher social status. There are a host of behaviors such as staring, tone of voice, cajoling, projecting confidence, and monopolizing the conversation that can advance one's social position. These behaviors, what we sometimes call "mojo," might be enhanced by testosterone. This is in stark contract to the traditional view of testosterone as a hormone that incites antisocial, egotistical, and even aggressive behaviors.

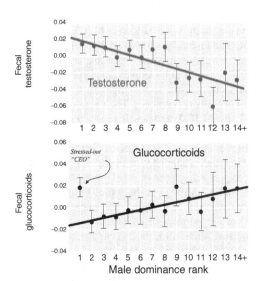

FIGURE 14.10 ● Testosterone levels rise as baboons ascend in social rank. Glucocorticoids, with the exception of the alpha man, descend with rank. (Adapted from Gesquiere LR, Learn NH, Simao CM, et al. Life at the top: rank and stress in wild male baboons. *Science.* 2011;333:357-360.)

Vasopressin

Vasopressin, better known for its role as an *antidiuretic hormone* and its physiologic effect on water retention and bedwetting, is increasingly recognized as playing an important in social attachment. Many neuropeptides have multiple functions in the brain: both physical and behavioral. We are only beginning to understand the role of vasopression in the aggressive behaviors. When given to hamsters, rats, and voles, for example, vasopressin will increase their aggressive display. Alternatively, vasopressin receptor blockers will decrease aggression.

A remarkable study by Coccaro et al. has looked at cerebrospinal fluid (CSF) vasopressin and aggression in 26 subjects with personality disorders. Figure 14.11 shows the correlation between CSF vasopressin and a life history of aggression against other people. The importance of vasopressin in social interactions goes beyond aggression. We also see this peptide involved with bonding and will discuss it further in Chapter 17. In the future, this may be a neuropeptide with great interest for the mental health community.

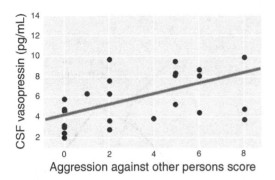

FIGURE 14.11 ● Cerebrospinal fluid vasopressin levels correlate with aggression in subjects with personality disorders. (Adapted from Coccaro EF, Kavoussi RJ, Hauger RL, et al. Cerebrospinal fluid vasopressin levels: correlates with aggression and serotonin function in personality-disordered subjects. *Arch Gen Psychiatry*. 1998;55:708-714.)

Nerve Growth Factors

It is interesting to ask whether fighting changes the brain. That is, does winning or losing alter the structure of the brain in a manner that develops aggressive or submissive personalities? We know there is a strong relationship between experience and neurobiology, for example, enriched environments

cause enhanced nerve cell growth (see Figure 8.5). Likewise, we know that the growth and development of neurons are enhanced by nerve growth factors (NGFs). Finally, we know that animals that are repeatedly on the losing side of fights will develop a syndrome called *conditioned defeat*.

A group in Italy has examined the effect of winning and losing on growth factors in mice. Figure 14.12A shows the rapid and sustained release of NGF into the bloodstream immediately after a fighting episode. Further studies looked at growth factors in areas that are known for the proliferation of new nerve cells, for example, the subventricular zone (SVZ) (see Figure 8.3). The researchers found enhanced levels of NGF as well as brain-derived neurotropic factor (BDNF). However, the levels depended on who won the fight.

Figure 11.12B shows the results of NGFs in the SVZ after three consecutive days of fighting episodes. It was only the subordinate mouse that had increases in NGF. The dominant mouse had increased levels of BDNF. These results suggest that winning or losing turns on different genes which may affect which growth hormones are released and which nerves are "fertilized." If this is true, it may explain why winners and losers behave differently.

FIGURE 14.12 ● **A.** Fighting results in an increase in nerve growth factor (NGF). **B.** In the subventricular zone, NGF only increases for the subordinate mouse, whereas brain-derived neurotropic factor (BDNF) increases for the dominant mouse. (Adapted from Fiore M, Amendola T, Triaca V, et al. Fighting in the aged male mouse increases the expression of TrkA and TrkB in the subventricular zone and in the hippocampus. *Behav Brain Res*. 2005;157(2):351-362 and Branchi I, Francia N, Alleva E. Epigenetic control of neurobehavioural plasticity: the role of neurotrophins. *Behav Pharmacol*. 2004;15(5-6):353-362.)

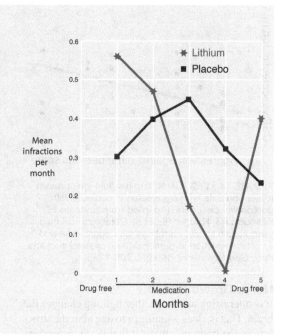

TREATMENT LITHIUM

One of the most unique treatment studies for aggressive behavior was conducted in a prison in Connecticut in the 1970s. Volunteers with a history of violence were randomly assigned to receive lithium or placebo. The exclusion of inmates with psychosis was the only psychiatric criterion applied to this study. The number of infractions reported by the institutional staff that was blind to the treatment administered served as the measure of response. The following figure shows the results.

Although the study has methodological problems (small *n*, high dropout rate for those on lithium), it nonetheless demonstrates the powerful effect that lithium has on violent behavior. This is consistent with lithium's well-documented capacity to decrease suicide—which can be considered violence against oneself. What lithium does in the brain to reduce violence remains a mystery.

SEROTONIN

There is actually a more robust association between low serotonin and aggression than between low serotonin and depression. Because there is no feasible way to directly measure serotonin in humans or animals, most studies examine the correlation between violence and CSF 5-hydroxyindoleacetic acid (5-HIAA), a metabolite of serotonin.

Studies with monkeys have found high rates of wounding, violence, and inappropriate aggression in subjects with low CSF 5-HIAA. Analysis of these monkeys has shown that they are not necessarily uniformly more aggressive. However, they are more likely to engage in rough interactions that escalate into unrestrained aggression with a high probability of injury. This behavioral trait can be viewed as poor impulse control, which could underlie the aggressive tendency.

A group has studied the relationship between 5-HIAA and violence in a longitudinal study of free-ranging rhesus monkeys secluded on a small island on the coast of South Carolina. The researchers captured 49 two-year-old males and measured their CSF 5-HIAA. Two years is the age for a monkey that corresponds to middle to late childhood in humans and is a particularly dangerous age for male monkeys. This is a phase of life when males move from their group of origin to a new social group. The monkeys were followed for up to 4 years.

By the time most of the subjects had reached young adulthood, 11 had died. Figure 14.13 shows the percentage of subjects that died and the percentage that had survived, separated by their CSF 5-HIAA concentrations at the start. Note that all those in the high concentration group were still alive. The researchers observed that those monkeys with the lowest levels of 5-HIAA were much more

FIGURE 14.13 ● The percentage of 2-year-old monkeys who are still alive after 4 years, separated by the metabolite of serotonin (5-HIAA) in the CSF. (Adapted from Higley JD, Mehlman PT, Higley SB, et al. Excessive mortality in young free-ranging male nonhuman primates with low CSF 5-hydroxyindoleacetic acid concentrations. *Arch Gen Psychiatry*. 1996;53(6):537-543.)

likely to engage in risky behavior, including aggressive acts directed at older, larger males. They would pick fights they could not win. They were not only aggressive but also impulsive.

Studies with humans are equally impressive. A variety of researchers from many different sites have shown the following results:

1. Lower 5-HIAA correlates with greater suicide intent and higher lethality in those who have attempted suicide.
2. 5-HIAA levels show an inverse correlation with lifetime histories of aggression.
3. Low 5-HIAA levels predict recidivism for violent offenders.
4. Acute tryptophan depletion, which causes a transient decline in brain serotonin, will result in increased irritability and aggression.

Most relevant for the practicing clinician are the studies with selective serotonin reuptake inhibitor (SSRIs) and aggression. Several double-blind, placebo-controlled studies have found reduced aggression with SSRIs in patients with personality disorders, autism, schizophrenia, and dementia. While there are no medications with FDA approval for treating aggression, a serotonin reuptake inhibitor might not be a bad place to start.

THE PSYCHOPATH

Being violent is not the same as being cruel or mean. Violence in defense of oneself or one's family is not even considered a crime. Alternatively, there are many examples of violence that seems to have no purpose other than being mean and inflicting emotional or physical pain.

Psychopathy is the closest definition we have in psychiatry to describing cruel or mean behavior. It is not included in the DSM. The Psychopathy Checklist-Revised created by Robert Hare defines psychopathy and is made up of two factors. The first factor includes impulsive aggression and a wide variety of offenses, which correlates closely with antisocial personality disorder in the DSM.

The other factor defines the emotional shallowness of the psychopath: superficial, egotistical, lack of remorse, lack of empathy, and manipulative. This factor has a smaller correlation with antisocial personality disorder and more closely resembles what we would consider cruel and mean. It tends to persist as the subject ages, although the impulsive, aggressive factor decreases with maturity. The older psychopath is no more empathetic or remorseful, but less likely to be violent.

Hare has suggested that the psychopath lacks some internal control. We know very little about this which is unfortunate because psychopaths are a huge drain on society and there remains no effective treatment. However, the advent of functional imaging studies brings some insight to the neural workings of the average psychopath.

Raine has shown that men with antisocial personality disorders have decreased prefrontal gray matter when compared with normal controls or substance abusers. This suggests a lack of containment from the frontal cortex, similar to what has been discussed earlier. Unique to the psychopath are findings showing low autonomic arousal and less activity in the amygdala.

Resting Heart Rate

One of the most consistent physiologic findings in psychiatry is the correlation between low resting heart rate and aggressive behavior in children. Furthermore, a low heart rate in a child is predictive of future criminal behavior independent of all other psychological variables. Some people speculate that the low heart rate reflects a fearless, stimulus-seeking temperament. A fascinating study from Europe supports this conclusion.

The study is based on Pavlovian (classical) conditioning. When presented repeatedly with a neutral stimulus followed by an aversive stimulus, most people will show some anxiety when seeing the neutral stimulus in anticipation of what will follow. Birbaumer et al. scanned 10 criminal psychopaths out on bail and 10 healthy controls repeatedly presented with neutral pictures followed by painful stimuli. The controls showed increased activity in areas underlying conditioned fear response: amygdala, orbitofrontal cortex, insula, and anterior cingulate (Figure 14.14). Remarkably, the psychopaths showed almost no activity in these areas. This disconnect between emotion and cognition may be the neural basis for the cold, detached demeanor of psychopaths. It is also one more reason your authors will never be successful criminals.

The Pleasure of Violence

The lack of fear alone does not seem sufficient for some of the cruel actions perpetrated by psychopaths. Many people can utilize their fearless temperament to help others. For example, decorated bomb-disposal operators have been shown to have unusually low heart rates during experimental simulations. We can imagine that other high-stress professions are overly represented with individuals who are innately calm: firefighters, air-traffic controllers, trauma surgeons, etc. Something else is needed to understand the behavior of the psychopath. A study with rats suggests a possible neurologic mechanism to explain what else may be aberrant with psychopaths.

Healthy controls   Psychopaths

FIGURE 14.14 ● Healthy controls show a robust fear response in anticipation of an adverse stimulus. Psychopaths fail to develop a similar fear. (Adapted from Birbaumer N, Veit R, Lotze M, et al. Deficient fear conditioning in psychopathy: a functional magnetic resonance imaging study. *Arch Gen Psychiatry.* 2005;62(7):799-805.)

First, we must acknowledge that many people enjoy violence. One has to only look at what is popular at the movies, in video games, and on the news to recognize that blood sells. Second, as we described in Chapter 12, the nucleus accumbens lights up with dopamine during pleasurable activities: cocaine, sex, gambling, and so on. It seems logical that violence induces a squirt of dopamine at the nucleus accumbens.

The missing study is shown in Figure 14.15. In this experiment, male rats were implanted with

FIGURE 14.15 ● Increase in dopamine at the nucleus accumbens following an aggressive encounter with another rat. (Adapted from van Erp AM, Miczek KA. Aggressive behavior, increased accumbal dopamine, and decreased cortical serotonin in rats. *J Neurosci.* 2000;20:9320-9325.)

micropipettes that sampled the extracellular concentration of dopamine at the nucleus accumbens every 10 minutes. The sampling was done during an aggressive encounter with a naive male intruder in which two to six bites and at least 140 seconds of aggressive behavior were displayed by the rat under study. The graph shows that dopamine significantly rose above baseline for up to 60 minutes after the encounter. The thrill of victory?

Imaging studies of humans suggest similar neural mechanisms. Researchers in Switzerland set up an elaborate study to examine the activity in the brain when a subject is playing a game with an untrustworthy partner. In instances when the subject wants to retaliate after the partner keeps all the money, there was increased activity in the dorsal striatum—an area that contains the nucleus accumbens. Furthermore, the stronger the activity in the striatum the more willing the subject was to incur a deficit to make the other person suffer.

Using these data, we can conceptualize in an overly simplified manner that violence and aggression give a squirt of pleasure to the aggressor. This could explain why some people seem to enjoy watching or inflicting acts of aggression. Furthermore, the psychopath may experience the most joy of all.

In summary, the neurobiology of the psychopath may be a constellation of problems: inadequate constraint from the frontal cortex, insufficient fear of consequences, and too much activation of the nucleus accumbens. It could be that psychopathy, like alcoholism or cocaine dependence, is an addiction—although in this case the addiction is to violence. This could explain why psychopathy, like other addictions, is so difficult to treat and does not respond well to traditional interventions.

DISORDER   TEMPORAL LOBE EPILEPSY

There is a subgroup of patients with temporal lobe epilepsy who have aggressive outbursts between seizures. Some have attributed this to an interictal syndrome often called *episodic dyscontrol*. However, many of these patients have alternative explanations for their aggression, for example, low IQ and antisocial personality disorder. The concept remains controversial but may apply to a few patients with seizure disorder.

More appealing is the prospect that patients with aggressive outbursts may be having unrecognized subclinical temporal lobe seizures. Unfortunately, this has been difficult to substantiate. However, the anticonvulsants do show some positive effects as treatment for aggression, although the benefits are primarily limited to those with impulsive aggressive acts rather than premeditated acts.

QUESTIONS

1. When dealing with a patient with an anger problem and trying to make the right diagnosis, which of the following do you not do?
   a. Refuse to treat him because there is no DSM diagnosis for anger.
   b. Call it a variation of bipolar disorder.
   c. Call it a wastebasket term, such as depression not otherwise specified (NOS) or anxiety NOS.
   d. Call it intermittent explosive disorder because it sounds good, even although you know it does not actually apply.

2. Which of the following is not associated with predatory aggression?
   a. Activation of the lateral hypothalamus.
   b. Stealthy movement.
   c. Autonomic arousal.
   d. Premeditated.

3. In simple terms, the frontal cortex plays what role with anger?
   a. Activates the autonomic neuron system.
   b. Applies the brakes on the impulses.
   c. Modulates the nucleus accumbens.
   d. Activates the lateral hypothalamus.

4. All of the following apply to the amygdala and aggression, except
   a. Klüver-Bucy syndrome.
   b. Shows less activity with criminal psychopaths.
   c. Different nuclei could be activated with different subtypes of aggression.
   d. Facilitates the expression of the serotonin receptor.

5. Testosterone
   a. Is the primary cause of fighting.
   b. Increases plasma levels for the loser.
   c. May show a better correlation with social dominance.
   d. Stimulates overt hostility in weight lifters.

6. After a fight, the dominant mouse has which of the following?
   a. Decreased testosterone and decreased NGF.
   b. Decreased testosterone and increased BDNF.
   c. Increased testosterone and decreased NGF.
   d. Increased testosterone and increased BDNF.

7. All of the following statements about low CSF concentration of the serotonin metabolite 5-HIAA are true, except
   a. Common with major depression.
   b. Correlates with greater lifetime history of aggression.
   c. Predicts relapse for criminal offenders.
   d. Associated with greater suicide intent.

8. The psychopath can be conceptualized as having all of the following, except
   a. Low resting heart rate.
   b. Activated frontal cortex.
   c. Hypofunctioning amygdala.
   d. Increased activity at the nucleus accumbens.

See Answers section at the end of the book.

CHAPTER 15

Sleep and Circadian Rhythms

NORMAL SLEEP

Sleep remains a mystery. We spend roughly a third of our lives in this suspended state. All mammals sleep, as does most of the animal kingdom. Even the fruit fly sleeps—although not enough. Most people look forward to sleeping, especially if they have been deprived of sleep. Without enough sleep, people function as poorly as if they are drunk. Significant sleep deprivation will cause psychosis and physical problems. What is it that happens to us when we sleep?

The average length of sleep is approximately 7.5-hours per night (Figure 15.1). Remarkably, some people, called *nonsomniacs*, require much less. Meddis studied a retired nurse who was happily functioning on an hour of sleep a night. She reported she had needed little sleep all her life.

FIGURE 15.1 ● The duration of sleep for adults is normally distributed around a mean of 7.5-hours per night. (Adapted from Hobson JA. *Sleep*. New York, NY: Scientific American Library; 1989.)

When studied in Meddis's sleep laboratory, she did not sleep the first night and then slept, on average, only 67 minutes for each of the remaining four nights. She did not complain of being tired or wanting more sleep. (As an aside, some in the psychiatric community might diagnose this woman with a bipolar spectrum disorder, although her condition may simply be a variant of sleep need.)

Most people show deterioration in performance when deprived of sleep. Figure 15.2 shows the results of neurobehavioral tasks for subjects deprived of differing amounts of sleep. One group was totally sleep deprived for 3 days, two other groups were restricted to 6 or 4-hours of sleep per night for 14 days, and the control group got 8-hours of sleep per night. Figure 15.2A shows the effects of sleep restriction on a sustained attention task, whereas Figure 15.2B shows the effects on a test of memory. Note how chronic sleep deprivation takes a toll on the subjects' performance as the study progresses. Of interest, the subjects were largely unaware of their impairments—a finding that is not uncommon when cognition declines.

A recent intervention with medical interns working in an intensive care unit in a Boston hospital demonstrated a practical application of this knowledge. Interns who had their workday limited to 16-hours (compared with the traditional 24+ hours) got more sleep each week and made half the attentional errors during on-call nights compared with the interns following the traditional schedule.

Stages of Sleep

For centuries, sleep had been considered a passive, uniform process that simply restored the body. That changed in 1953 when Nathaniel Kleitman and Eugene Aserinksy examined electroencephalographic (EEG) recordings from sleeping healthy subjects. They discovered that sleep comprises

◆ 8 h sleep/night
✲ 6 h sleep/night
● 4 h sleep/night
■ Total sleep deprivation

A

Better

Behavioral
alterness

Worse

B

Better

Working
memory

Worse

0   2   4   6   8   10 12 14
Day of sleep restriction

FIGURE 15.2 ● The effects of total sleep deprivation for 3 days and chronic sleep restriction for 14 days are measured with neurobehavioral tasks. The Psychomotor Vigilance Task (**A**) measures alertness and attention. The Digit Symbol Substitution Task (**B**) measures working memory. (Adapted from Van Dongen HP, Maislin G, Mullington JM, et al. The cumulative cost of additional wakefulness: dose-response effects on neurobehavioral functions and sleep physiology from chronic sleep restriction and total sleep deprivation. *Sleep*. 2003;26(2):117-126.)

Awake

Alpha activity   Beta activity

Stage 1   Drowsy period

Theta activity

Stage 2   Light sleep

Sleep
spindle

Stage 3   Moderate sleep

Slow wave sleep

Stage 4   Deep sleep

Delta activity

REM

FIGURE 15.3 ● Characteristic electroencephalographic rhythms during the stages of consciousness. REM, rapid eye movement. (Adapted from Horne JA. *Why We Sleep: The Functions of Sleep in Humans and Other Mammals*. Oxford: Oxford University Press; 1988.)

different stages that repeat in characteristic patterns throughout the night. They identified the three states of consciousness as awake, non-rapid eye movement (non-REM) sleep, and rapid eye movement (REM) sleep. Non-REM sleep has been further subdivided into four stages.

Electroencephalographic Patterns

Figure 15.3 shows the characteristic EEG patterns during the different stages of sleep. From an awake state to the deepest sleep of stage 4, there is a progression of decreasing frequency and increasing amplitude of the EEG activity. Stage 1 sleep, also

called the *drowsy period*, is so light that most people when awoken from this stage will say that they were not asleep. Stage 2 sleep shows the development of sleep spindles, which are periodic bursts of activity resulting from interactions between the thalamus and the cortex. Stage 3 and 4 sleep, also called *slow wave sleep* (SWS), are the deepest stages of sleep characterized by the development of delta waves. REM sleep is the most unusual finding that Kleitman and Aserinksy discovered. In REM sleep, the EEG activity is remarkably similar to the awake state, but the body, or at least major muscles, is paralyzed.

In a typical night, a person cycles through five episodes of non-REM/REM activity (Figure 15.4A). The first REM episode occurs after approximately 90 minutes of sleep. The time to the first REM occurrence is called *REM latency* and is usually reduced in patients who are exhausted as well as those with depression, narcolepsy, and sleep apnea. The deepest stage of sleep occurs only in the early phases of the night. The REM episodes increase in length as the night unfolds.

All mammals sleep. Mammals living in the water are able to sleep, but still they must regularly surface for air. Additionally, from the day they are born until they die, dolphins are continuously moving and avoiding obstacles. They do not have a period of immobility that in terrestrial mammals marks the state of sleep. How do they do all this and still sleep?

Studies of EEG tracings of the bottlenose dolphin show that they rest one hemisphere at

a time (see figure). Note how the large amplitude waves of SWS are only present in one hemisphere at a time. The eye contralateral to the brain hemisphere showing slow waves is usually closed while the other eye is almost always open. Lastly, these dolphins do not display REM activity, which may be an adaptation so they can keep moving.

Electroencephalographic tracings from bottlenose dolphins. (Adapted from Mujhametov LM. Sleep in marine mammals. In: Borbely AA, Valatx JL, ed. *Sleep Mechanisms*. Munich: Springer; 1984 and Purves D, Augustine GJ, Fitzpatrick D, et al. *Neuroscience*. 3rd ed. Sunderland, MA: Sinauer; 2004.)

Figure 15.4B shows some of the other physiologic changes that take place during the stages of sleep. The most remarkable findings are the differences in physiologic activity between non-REM and REM sleep. Non-REM sleep is characterized by limited eye movement and a decrease in muscle tone, heart rate, and respirations. Metabolic rate and body temperature are also decreased in these stages. They reach their lowest levels during stage 4 sleep. REM sleep, as the name implies, is characterized by rapid, darting movements of the eyes along with paralysis of most major muscle groups. Heart rate and respirations increase almost to the level found when awake. Penile/clitoral erections also occur during REM sleep—a finding that helps rule out physiologic impotence.

Muscle Tone

Muscle activity varies depending on the phase of sleep. During non-REM sleep, the muscles are capable of movement, but they rarely do so. On the other hand, REM sleep is characterized by a loss of skeletal muscle tone. Respiratory muscles along with the muscles of the eyes and the tiny muscles of the ear remain active in REM sleep.

Brain Imaging

Brain imaging studies during sleep reveal a pattern that is consistent with EEG findings. During non-REM sleep, positron emission tomography (PET) studies show decreased cerebral blood flow and energy metabolism. The greatest decreases correlate with greater depth of sleep. Alternatively, REM sleep shows a cerebral energy metabolism, which is equal to that occurring during awakening.

William Dement, a prominent sleep researcher from Stanford, has eloquently summarized the difference between the phases of sleep. He has characterized non-REM sleep as an idling brain in a movable body. In contrast, REM sleep is an active, hallucinating brain in a paralyzed body.

Changes with Aging

Total sleep duration and the proportions of time spent in various stages change as people age. Figure 15.5 shows the duration of sleep across the life span. Neonates (on the left of the figure) spend most of their time sleeping, with a large percentage of that time in REM sleep. Some have suggested that REM serves a developmental purpose and this is why neonates and young children require so much time in this phase.

FIGURE 15.4 ● Physiologic changes in a healthy volunteer during 8 hours of sleep. REM, rapid eye movement. (Adapted from Purves D, Augustine GJ, Fitzpatrick D, et al. *Neuroscience.* 5th ed. Sunderland, MA: Sinauer; 2011.)

DISORDERS   SLEEPWALKING AND NIGHT TERRORS

Approximately 40% of people are *sleepwalkers* as children, although few are sleepwalkers as adults. This behavior usually occurs in the first stage 4 non-REM period of the night. In a typical episode, the child's eyes will be open and the child will avoid obstacles when moving about the room or house. The cognition is clouded and the child will usually have no memory of the event. The best intervention is to gently guide the sleepwalker back to bed.

Night terrors are characterized by extreme terror and an inability to be awakened. Typically occurring in children between the ages of 4 and 7, this condition affects only approximately 3% of the population. As with sleep walking, it develops in the deep stages of non-REM sleep. Night terrors are not to be confused with nightmares, which are vivid dreams during REM sleep.

The child appears in a state of panic, and may even scream and cry. Fortunately, it usually returns to sleep in 10 to 20 minutes and little is remembered the next day. The greatest toll may be on the parents who have to comfort the frightened child. The best intervention is support.

On the right side of Figure 15.5 is a meta-analysis of sleep duration from childhood to old age. Note the gradual reduction in the deepest stages of sleep and the increase in awakening after sleep onset as people age. Dissatisfaction with sleep is a common complaint in the elderly, and the origins of those complaints can be seen in this figure.

Dreaming

Historically, it has been believed that dreaming is limited to REM sleep. A thorough analysis of what people are experiencing at different stages of consciousness reveals that dreams occur in all stages of sleep, but the content varies. Researchers gave college students a pager and instructed them to

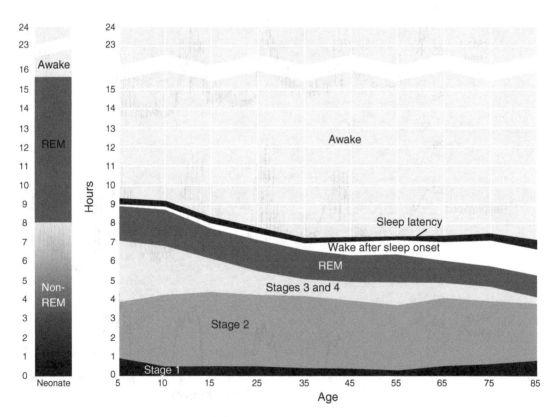

FIGURE 15.5 ● Sleep duration across the life span. Neonates are shown on the left and on the right is a meta-analysis of sleep parameters in healthy individuals across the life span. REM, rapid eye movement. (Adapted from Ohayon MM, Carskadon MA, Guilleminault C, et al. Meta-analysis of quantitative sleep parameters from childhood to old age in healthy individuals: developing normative sleep values across the human lifespan. *Sleep.* 2004;27(7):1255-1273.)

FIGURE 15.6 ● A special home-based sleep-monitoring system (**A**) allows researchers to correlate dream content with the stage of consciousness (**B**). REM, rapid eye movement. (Adapted from Fosse R, Stickgold R, Hobson JA. Brain-mind states: reciprocal variation in thoughts and hallucinations. *Psychol Sci.* 2001;12(1):30-36.)

sleep with a special nightcap that recorded eye and head movement (see Figure 15.6A). The students were considered to be in non-REM sleep when there was an absence of eye movement. REM sleep was defined as rapid eye movements without head movement. The students dictated what they were doing, thinking, and feeling when they were paged or spontaneously awoke.

The results showed that the subjects had dreams at all stages of sleep; however, the nature of dreams was different. In non-REM sleep, the dreams are more thoughts—as though the person is solving a problem. In REM sleep, the dreams are illogical, bizarre, and even hallucinatory. Figure 15.6B shows the decrease in thoughts as the subject goes from an awake state to REM sleep and the corresponding marked increase in hallucinations.

NEURONAL CIRCUITS

Until the 1940s, sleep was generally conceptualized as the body's reaction to the lack of stimulation, that is, the brain passively turns "off" when there is no input. We now know that sleep is an active process initiated and terminated by different regions of the brain.

Suprachiasmatic Nucleus

The master clock of the brain is the suprachiasmatic nucleus (SCN) located in the anterior hypothalamus

(Figure 15.7). The SCN orchestrates circadian rhythms throughout the brain and body. The SCN is synchronized (entrained) by signals from the retina, which are activated by inputs from the sun. When humans are prevented from receiving cues about the solar day (such as living in a cave for weeks), the 24-hour sleep–wake cycle will gradually increase to approximately 26-hours—a condition that is called *free-running*.

The SCN is made up of some of the smallest neurons in the brain and has a volume that is approximately 0.3 mm³. Output from the SCN synchronizes other cellular oscillators throughout the brain and body. Studies with hamsters have established the

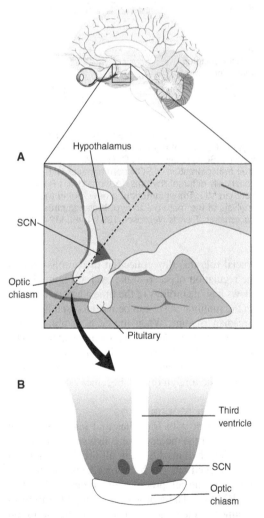

FIGURE 15.7 ● A sagittal view (**A**) and frontal view (**B**) of the human suprachiasmatic nucleus (SCN). (Adapted from Bear MF, Connors BW, Paradiso MA, eds. *Neuroscience: Exploring the Brain.* 3rd ed. Baltimore, MD: Lippincott Williams & Wilkins; 2007.)

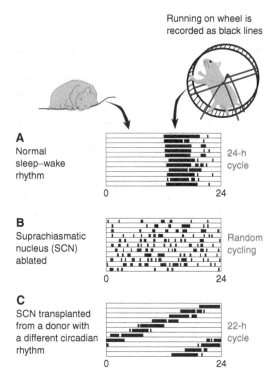

Running on wheel is recorded as black lines

A
Normal sleep–wake rhythm

24-h cycle

0   24

B
Suprachiasmatic nucleus (SCN) ablated

Random cycling

0   24

C
SCN transplanted from a donor with a different circadian rhythm

22-h cycle

0   24

FIGURE 15.8 ● **A.** An usual 24-hour circadian rhythm. **B.** Lack of rhythm after the suprachiasmatic nucleus (SCN) is destroyed. **C.** New 22-hour rhythm after transplantation of SCN from hamster with genetically different rhythms. (Adapted from Ralph MR, Lehman MN. Transplantation: a new tool in the analysis of the mammalian hypothalamic circadian pacemaker. *Trends Neurosci.* 1991;14(8):362-366.)

TREATMENT **MELATONIN**

Under normal circumstances, the SCN is reset each day by signals of light from the retina. However, melatonin secreted during the dark cycle from the pineal gland can also entrain the SCN. This justifies the use of melatonin to promote sleep in those with delayed sleep onset or to reset the internal clock that is disrupted with jet lag. Studies with melatonin agents have been effective although less robust than we might hope. Success with melatonin requires proper timing of administration. Taking a dose at the wrong time will not only be ineffective but can make things worse!

The buildup and breakdown of these proteins takes 24-hours. Figure 15.9 shows the daily fluctuation in the proteins PER and CRY from a mouse SCN. Note the 6-hour lag between the buildup of the messenger RNA (gene expression) and the production of the proteins. Although the functions of PER and CRY remain to be elucidated, this molecular mechanism is believed to drive the 24-hour cycling of the SCN.

An area of great interest involves the genes that control these proteins in humans and their role with sleep disorders. For example, mutations of CLOCK and PER have been found in some individuals with delayed or advanced sleep phase syndromes.

---

crucial role this tiny collection of neurons play in the regulation of sleep–wake cycles. Figure 15.8A shows how recordings of the time a hamster spends on the running wheel can be used to establish their circadian rhythm. When the SCN is ablated, the 24-hour rhythm is lost and no regular pattern can be identified. If the hamster receives a transplant from a strain of mutant hamsters with a 22-hour circadian rhythm, the foreign rhythm becomes established.

Molecular Mechanisms

Recent work with fruit flies and mice has begun to tease out the molecular mechanisms that control circadian rhythm. Although all the details remain to be worked out, the basic mechanism is becoming clear. The cell produces two proteins: CLOCK and BMAL1. These proteins bind together to form a dimer, which then activates the transcription of other proteins, called *PER (Period)* and *CRY (Cryptochrome)*. PER and CRY form a dimer that inhibits the transcription of CLOCK and BMAL1, providing a negative feedback loop.

FIGURE 15.9 ● Fluctuations of gene expression and protein levels in the mouse suprachiasmatic nucleus (SCN). These proteins are believed to be the molecular signal of circadian rhythm. (Adapted from Pace-Schott EF, Hobson JA. The neurobiology of sleep: genetics, cellular physiology and subcortical networks. *Nat Rev Neurosci.* 2002;3(8):591-605.)

Additionally, of great interest to us is the question of damaged *clock* genes and psychiatric disorders. Clearly, sleep impairments have a strong correlation with psychiatric disorders, but as yet there is only limited evidence implicating *clock* genes as the culprits.

Ascending Arousal Systems

In 1949, the Italian neurophysiologists Horace Magoun and Giuseppe Moruzzi discovered the first circuits governing sleep and wakefulness. They found that stimulating a group of neurons in the midline of the brain stem aroused a sleeping animal. Likewise, lesions of this region resulted in persistent sleep. They called this region the *reticular activating system.*

It is likely that Magoun and Moruzzi were stimulating many different sets of ascending arousal neurons during their experiments. Further study in the intervening years has identified several of the important nuclei and neurotransmitters. One group is the cholinergic neurons with cell bodies located near the pons–midbrain junction. These neurons project to the thalamus and activate the thalamic relay neurons that are crucial for the transmission of information to the cerebral cortex. Stimulation of these nuclei causes high-frequency, low-amplitude EEG activity.

The second group comprises four neuronal systems: the noradrenergic neurons of the locus coeruleus, the serotoninergic neurons of the raphe nuclei, the dopaminergic neurons from the periaqueductal gray matter, and the histaminergic neurons in the tuberomammillary nucleus (see Chapter 4, for further details). These neurons project to the hypothalamus and throughout the cerebral cortex.

All five neuronal systems are active during arousal and quiescent during non-REM sleep. However, the cholinergic neurons resume their activity during REM sleep while the monoaminergic neurons slow down even further. This is another example of how wakefulness and REM sleep (conditions that seem so similar) are different. A summary of these arousal networks is given in Table 15.1.

The Sleep Switch

In general, most people experience a relatively rapid transition from arousal to asleep or vice versa. This transition can be conceptualized as the flipping of a switch. The closest approximation to a "sleep switch" in the brain is the ventrolateral preoptic nuclei (VLPO). The VLPO has projections to the main components of the ascending arousal system shown in Table 15.1. The VLPO is inhibitory and primarily active during sleep. In other words, an active VLPO induces sleep by putting the brakes on the arousal nuclei. People with damage to their VLPO experience chronic insomnia.

Conversely, the VLPO must be inhibited so that people can wake up. Indeed, the VLPO receives inputs from the monoaminergic neurons—the very neurons that it inhibits. So the "sleep switch" has mutually inhibitory elements in which activity from one side shuts down the other side and disinhibits its own actions. This helps explain the relatively abrupt change from awake to asleep that occurs in most mammals (Figure 15.10).

Narcolepsy

A problem with such a switch is that rapid, unwanted transitions from one state to another can occur when it is unstable. Presumably, this is the mechanism of narcolepsy. Attacks of irresistible sleepiness as well as episodes of physical collapse and loss of muscle tone during emotional situations

TABLE 15.1

A Summary of the Major Neuronal Systems That Mediate Arousal and Comprise the Ascending Reticular Activating System

Neurotransmitter	Cell Bodies	Projections	Active During
Cholinergic	Nuclei of pons–midbrain junction	Thalamus	Awake and rapid eye movement
Noradrenergic	Locus coeruleus		
Dopaminergic	Periaqueductal gray matter	Hypothalamus and cerebral cortex	Awake
Serotoninergic	Raphe nuclei		
Histaminergic	Tuberomammillary nucleus		

A

FIGURE 15.10 ● A schematic diagram of the "sleep switch." (**A**) Locus coeruleus (LC), tuberomammillary nucleus (TMN), and raphe nuclei in the awake state are stabilized by the orexin neurons. They also inhibit the VLPO. (**B**) In the sleep state, the VLPO inhibits the orexin neurons as well as the LC, TMN, and raphe nuclei. VLPO, ventrolateral preoptic nuclei. (Adapted from Saper CB, Scammell TE, Lu J. Hypothalamic regulation of sleep and circadian rhythms. *Nature.* 2005;437(7063):1257-1263.)

FIGURE 15.11 ● Neuronal degeneration of orexin neurons in lateral hypothalamus of a patient with narcolepsy compared with a control. (Courtesy of Jerome Siegel.)

(*cataplexy*) characterize narcolepsy. In 2000, it was discovered that patients with narcolepsy have few orexin neurons in the hypothalamus (Figure 15.11). Orexin neurons (also called *hypocretin*) are mainly active during wakefulness and reinforce the arousal system.

It appears that patients with narcolepsy have lost the stabilizing influence of the orexin neurons and can abruptly switch from one state of consciousness to another. In other words, they have a floppy "sleep switch." Patients with narcolepsy do not sleep more than normal individuals, but they just take more naps during the day and awaken more frequently during the night.

The link between SCN and the "sleep switch" is more confusing than one might expect. SCN actually has few direct projections to the VLPO and orexin neurons. There appears to be a third system: the dorsomedial nucleus of the hypothalamus (DMH). Why might the brain have evolved a three-stage pathway for control of sleep? Well, the SCN is always active during the light cycle and the VLPO is always active during sleep. Without an intermediate step, nocturnal animals could not sleep during the day.

The DMH receives projections from the SCN and sends projections to the VLPO. However, the DMH appears to do more than just relay signals from one nucleus to another. There are many factors that influence the sleep–wake cycle: hunger, stress, and sleep debt—not just the cycle of the sun. In turn, many physiologic functions are affected by the DMH: eating, temperature, and corticosteroid cycles, as well as sleep and arousal. The three-stage pathway allows greater integration of multiple factors and greater flexibility in behavioral response.

WHY DO WE SLEEP?

Life is competitive. However, when we sleep, we can neither advance our position nor protect ourselves or our families. From this perspective, sleep is a costly process. So it must be important for us to pay such a high price. As one researcher puts it, "If sleep doesn't serve an absolutely vital function, it is the biggest mistake evolution ever made."

TREATMENT NARCOLEPSY

Amphetamines were first used in 1937 as a treatment for narcolepsy and remain popular. More recently, modafinil, an agent with minimal potential for abuse and a different mechanism of action, has become the first-line treatment for patients with the disorder. Modafinil works by indirectly activating the histamine network—the opposite effect of an antihistamine. Although effective for excessive daytime sleepiness, modafinil has limited benefits for cataplexy. Some clinicians add a tricyclic antidepressant or a newer antidepressant with dual action to decrease cataplectic attacks. Such a combination will affect histamine, serotonin, and norepinephrine—all components of the "sleep switch."

OBESITY

A recent analysis of more than a thousand volunteers found a U-shaped curvilinear association between sleep duration and body mass. Subjects who slept, on average, 7.7-hours per night had the lowest weight, whereas those sleeping for more or less time were heavier. The authors suggest that the cause may be due to changes in the hormones regulating appetite, such as leptin and ghrelin.

A rat deprived of sleep will die faster than when it is deprived of food. Humans with fatal familial insomnia, an inherited disease that develops in the middle age and results in degeneration of the thalamus, usually die within 24 months (although there may be other reasons for death). Humans forced to remain awake will pursue sleep with a vigor that rivals sex and food. When allowed to sleep, they will make up for the loss by sleeping deeper and longer—called *sleep rebound*. Clearly, something essential happens when we sleep, and most of us suffer when we are short changed. But what is it?

It has been proposed that mammals have a *homeostatic sleep drive*—as though there is some "vital energy" that needs to be restored each day or, inversely, some "toxin" that needs to be cleared while we sleep in order for us to function effectively when awake. However, no one has identified a neural mechanism to explain the sleep drive—no neuropeptide that needs to be restored or no annoying enzyme that needs to be removed. As yet, we can only postulate as to why bats, dolphins, cats, and humans need sleep.

Development

Some have speculated that sleep serves to establish brain connections during the critical periods of development. For example, all the twitching that infants exhibit during sleep may serve to help babies get control of their muscles. If this theory is true, then it would explain why we sleep most when young and less as we age. Additionally, species that are more mature at birth (e.g., those that can thermoregulate and ambulate) have sleep durations close to adult levels.

Frank and his group have conducted studies that suggest sleep enhances the plasticity of the developing cortex. We discussed the devastating effects that occluding an eye at critical periods has on normal development in Chapter 8. Frank and his group took this research one step further. They occluded an eye of 1-month-old cats for 6-hours. Then one group was allowed to sleep for 6-hours and the other group

was kept awake in darkness for an equal amount of time. Both groups were anesthetized and their visual cortex was probed. Electrodes inserted almost parallel to the visual cortex recorded activity from different locations while a light shone in the cat's eyes.

The results are shown in Figure 15.12. Compare these results with the study results shown in Figure 8.12. Note that the cats that were allowed to sleep developed the typical pattern of unilateral ocular dominance. That is, the opened eye dominates the neurons in the visual cortex. The cats that did not sleep maintained a more even distribution of ocular dominance. This research suggests that the effects of occluding an eye are not fully processed until the animal is asleep; to put this in another way, the changes in the brain that develop with experience are imprinted during sleep.

Taken together, these observations suggest that sleep is instrumental to normal development. However, Siegel has noted an almost complete absence of sleep for dolphin mothers and their newborns after birth. The calf will gradually increase its sleep to adult amounts over a period of months. This is the opposite of what is seen with terrestrial mammals, which suggests that sleep is either not essential for normal development or dolphins have adapted alternative mechanisms.

Neurogenesis

A group at the University of California, Los Angeles examined the effects of sleep deprivation

DREAM ENACTMENT

In the REM state the mind is active, but the body is virtually paralyzed. We dream but we only move our eyes. Unfortunately, some people lose the ability to induce muscle paralysis—a condition called *REM sleep behavior disorder*. Often this condition precedes by many years the emergence of a neurodegenerative disorder such as Parkinson's disease.

Patients who fail to suppress the muscle tone during REM sleep are condemned to act out their dreams. Such patients thrash about in bed and frequently hurt themselves or their partners. In some cases, it even gets violent. In cats, a similar condition has been elicited with small lesions of the pons just above the locus coeruleus. In humans, it has been harder to find a specific lesion. It is presumed that some subtle disruption of the balance between atonic and motor generation may be occurring in the spinal cord, brain stem, or even higher cortical areas.

FIGURE 15.12 ● The effects of sleep and sleep deprivation on ocular dominance plasticity during the critical period of visual development in 1-month-old cats. (Adapted from Frank MG, Issa NP, Stryker MP. Sleep enhances plasticity in the developing visual cortex. *Neuron*. 2001;30(1):275-287.)

on neurogenesis. Adult rats were deprived of sleep for 4 days and then examined for new cells in the dentate gyrus of the hippocampus. There was a 68% reduction in new cells in the sleep-deprived group compared with the controls. Stress hormones did not mediate the change, as the serum corticosterone levels were not significantly different in the two groups.

Energy Conservation
Sleep may be a form of energy conservation across the 24-hour day, the way hibernation conserves energy through a winter. An animal that is protected in a warm location minimizes the energy expenditure that will later need to be replaced. However, conserving energy does not explain the drive to sleep or sleep rebound.

Restoration
Comparing sleep amounts across species sheds some light on the function of sleep. One established relationship in biology is the inverse correlation between body mass and metabolic rate, that is,

smaller animals have higher metabolic rates and a higher metabolic rate means greater metabolic activity in the brain. Greater activity in the brain means greater metabolic by-products. Small animals with higher metabolic rates tend to sleep longer. For example, bats and opossums sleep approximately 18 to 20-hours per day, whereas elephants and giraffes sleep as little as 3 to 4-hours a day.

A high metabolic rate results in increased oxidative stress produced from the mitochondria. Higher rates of oxidative stress have been linked to aging, arthritis, and dementia in the mouse. Sleep may be the time that the brain "cleans up" and repairs the damage that accumulated during the day.

Siegel et al. have shown that sleep deprivation in the rat results in increased oxidative stress, which can be reversed with sleep. Additionally, they have shown that tissue damage occurs in the brain stem, hippocampus, and hypothalamus with sleep deprivation. Siegel believes that wakefulness produces a gradual toxic state that is corrected with sufficient sleep. Animals with a higher metabolic rate require greater sleep amounts to repair the more extensive wear and tear on their neurons during arousal.

Memory Consolidation
The idea that sleep improves the consolidation of memories has been debated and studied for more than 80 years. There is still no consensus. The underlying hypothesis proposes that information acquired during the day is reviewed and strengthened during sleep. Many different experimental designs have shown that memory for procedures or the ability to recognize patterns improves after sleeping—or even just napping during the day. However, memories for facts (declarative memory) do not seem to improve with sleep. So, the relationship between sleep and memory depends on the material learned.

It was discovered in the 1970s that some neurons in the rat hippocampus fire when the animal is in a specific location or moving toward that location. These cells were called *place cells*. It was subsequently shown that specific patterns of activity by the place cells during the day were reactivated during non-REM sleep that night. That is, the synchronicity established between hippocampal cells and cortical neurons when the rat is running from place to place is repeated again when the animal sleeps. This suggests that the hippocampus revisits the events of the day "off-line" and possibly orchestrates the consolidation of memories to long-term cortical stores.

Pierre Maquet et al. in Belgium have taken this one step further and used functional imaging studies to look at the activity in the human hippocampus

A

B

C

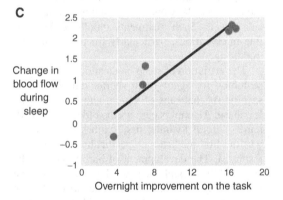

FIGURE 15.13 ● Hippocampal reactivation during non-REM sleep and memory consolidation. The sagittal (**A**) and horizontal (**B**) sections show the areas of the right hippocampus that were reactivated during sleep and correlated with improved scores on the task. (Adapted from Peigneux P, Laureys S, Fuchs S, et al. Are spatial memories strengthened in the human hippocampus during slow wave sleep? *Neuron*. 2004;44(3):535-545.)

the night after learning a new task. Participants were instructed to memorize the route through a complicated virtual town. It was observed that regions of the hippocampus that were active during the task were reactivated during subsequent non-REM sleep. Of particular interest, everyone improved on the task the following day. However, those with the greatest activity expressed during SWS also showed

the greatest improvement navigating the virtual town the following day (Figure 15.13).

In conclusion, sleep appears to serve a number of functions none of which explain a homeostatic drive to sleep. A universal function, across species, that can explain the irresistible urge to lie down on a couch after a heinous night on call has yet to be discovered.

MOOD DISORDERS

There is a long-standing suspicion that mood disorders are initiated or at least maintained by circadian dysfunction. Several lines of evidence suggest this to be true for depression. For example:

1. Depression has a diurnal variation—worse in the morning.
2. Insomnia is one of the most common complaints.
3. Insomnia resolves with effective treatment.
4. Sleep deprivation is an effective, although short-lived, antidepressant.

Seasonal Affective Disorder

Seasonal affective disorder (SAD), also called *winter depression*, is most suggestive of circadian changes affecting mood. Many mammals display seasonal fluctuations in behavior that is regulated by the change in day length. Hibernation may be the extreme form of this seasonal change. Humans with SAD develop symptoms of depression in the winter, along with weight gain, increased sleep, and decreased activity. This array of symptoms resembles changes seen in animals preparing to hibernate.

The changes in daylight hours are transmitted from the retina to the SCN. The SCN activates the paraventricular nucleus of the hypothalamus, which indirectly (by way of the sympathetic nervous system) inhibits the pineal gland. When the SCN is inactive during darkness, the inhibition is reduced, and the pineal gland secretes melatonin. In other words, melatonin is secreted during the night when the "brakes" are off. The duration of elevated nightly melatonin provides every tissue with information about the time of day and the time of year. Some have called the pineal gland both a *clock* and a *calendar*. For example, animals that hibernate, such as the Syrian hamster, produce more melatonin in winter and less in summer.

Recent research has examined melatonin secretion in 55 patients with SAD in summer and winter. They found that for patients with SAD the nocturnal duration of melatonin secretion was longer in winter than in summer, but there was no change in duration for the healthy volunteers. Other research has found that early morning light therapy for patients with SAD improved their mood and produced phase advances of the melatonin rhythm. In total, these results suggest that the neural circuits that mediate season change in mammals may be impaired in patients with SAD.

Bipolar Disorder

Bipolar disorder is another condition associated with circadian dysfunction. The delay in sleep onset and reduction in sleep duration accompanying a manic episode are clear examples of disrupted circadian rhythm. Additionally, the mood stabilizer lithium is known to lengthen the circadian period, which may be one of its mechanisms of action.

Of particular interest is the predictive value of sleep disruption and mania. It is well known that a decreasing need to sleep can precede a manic episode. There is some evidence that the prevalence of bipolar disorder, particularly the rapid cycling subgroup, is increasing. Although the increased use of antidepressants and/or illicit drugs is a possible cause, another explanation may be sleep disruption due to the modern lifestyle.

Wehr et al. believe that individuals with bipolar disorder are predisposed to exacerbations of the illness when sleep deprived. Because manic behavior interferes with sleep and sleep deprivation makes mania worse, a vicious downward cycle can be established. They describe a highly educated, successful individual who developed bipolar disorder

in his mid-forties. Despite aggressive pharmacologic management, he cycled between depression and mania every 6 to 8 weeks. He also showed great fluctuations in his sleep–wake phases across these cycles.

The group intervened by encouraging the subject to remain in bed rest in a dark room for 14-hours each night. This was later tapered to 10-hours per night. Remarkably, his mood and sleep stabilized. Periods of hyperactivity and hypoactivity were greatly reduced. The effects were still present after 1 year. It is worth noting that he remained on divalproex sodium and sertraline. The authors believe that enforced bed rest synchronized and stabilized the circadian rhythms, which were so easily disrupted by his modern lifestyle. If nothing else, this case highlights the importance of good sleep hygiene for any patient.

Treating Insomnia

Insomnia is generally a long-term problem. Hypnotic medications are not without risk. Nonpharmacologic interventions, such as cognitive behavior therapy and stimulus control, are as effective as medications, show enduring benefits, and have no side effects. Such treatments should be the first-line interventions, particularly for the young and middle aged.

The evolution of sleep medications is a story of searching for agents with shorter duration, more specific mechanisms of action, and less potential for abuse. Alcohol is perhaps the oldest sleep medicine. Chloral hydrate, first synthesized in 1832, was the first medication specifically indicated for insomnia. The development of barbiturates in the early 1900s brought a new class of agents that were widely used for 50 years. The introduction of benzodiazepines in the 1960s provided a treatment that was effective and safer.

As shown in Figure 5.3, benzodiazepines work by sensitizing the γ-aminobutyric acid (GABA) receptor, which in turn increases the movement of negatively charged chloride ions into the cell and ultimately enhances the activity of the GABA neurons. More GABA activity means more inhibition of the central nervous system.

There are two benzodiazepine receptor subtypes on the GABA receptor. The traditional benzodiazepines bind to both, but the newer agents (zolpidem, zaleplon, and eszopiclone) bind to just one subunit. This subunit mediates the sedating and amnesic effects, but not the anxiolytic, or myorelaxation. Whether this selective binding translates into fewer side effects remains to be determined.

The chronic use of sleep aids for insomnia remains controversial. Some epidemiological data

DISORDER HYPERAROUSAL

Trouble in sleeping is a common complaint. Some patients cannot turn off the arousal networks at bedtime. Patients with anxiety disorders, attention-deficit/hyperactivity disorder, and hyperthymic temperament will often complain that they cannot stop thinking when trying to sleep. Patients who abuse alcohol, opioids, and marijuana often use the substance as a hypnotic and frequently show rebound insomnia when substance free. Furthermore, insomnia is a risk factor for relapse with recovered alcoholics.

A recent neuroimaging study of patients with insomnia showed that these patients had a greater global cerebral metabolism while awake and asleep compared with controls. Additionally, the patients showed a smaller decline in relative metabolism from waking to sleep states in some of the structures discussed earlier, for example, ascending reticular activating system and hypothalamus.

have documented increased mortality with chronic hypnotic use, presumably due to residual cognitive impairment the following day. Fortunately, a recent placebo-controlled study with eszopiclone demonstrated enduring benefits for sleep and improved

functional status during the day for the 6 months of the trial. However, many patients, once started on a sleeping pill, will take something for years. We still do not know if such a treatment is beneficial in the long run.

QUESTIONS

1. Which do you typically see in stage 2 of sleep?
   a. Sleep spindles.
   b. α-Waves.
   c. δ-Activity.
   d. SWS.

2. REM latency is decreased in all of the following, except
   a. Depression.
   b. Generalized anxiety.
   c. Narcolepsy.
   d. Sleep apnea.

3. Which of the following is true?
   a. The average length of sleep is 8-hours per night.
   b. The deepest sleep occurs in the latter third of the night.
   c. Muscle tone increases during REM sleep.
   d. PET scans show decreased cerebral blood flow during SWS.

4. Which of the following is true about dolphin sleep?
   a. They never show REM sleep.
   b. Newborn calves sleep the most during the neonatal period.
   c. They close their eyes and navigate by echolocation.
   d. They sleep on the surface so they can breathe.

5. All of the following are true regarding sleep and aging, except
   a. We sleep less as we age.
   b. Arousal after sleep onset increases with age.
   c. REM sleep increases in the latter part of life.
   d. SWS decreases with aging.

6. Which of the following is active during the night in humans?
   a. The SCN.
   b. Orexin neurons.
   c. The ventrolateral preoptic nucleus.
   d. Tuberomammillary nucleus.

7. Which of the following systems is active during arousal and REM sleep?
   a. Noradrenergic.
   b. Dopaminergic.
   c. Histaminergic.
   d. Cholinergic.

8. Possible functions for sleep include all of the following, expect
   a. Memory consolidation.
   b. Energy conversation.
   c. Neurotransmitter reaccumulation.
   d. Metabolic restoration.

See Answers section at the end of the book.

CHAPTER 16

Sex and the Brain

SEXUAL DIMORPHISM

Humans are sexually dimorphic (*di*, "two"; *morph*, "type"). That is, we come in two styles. How one conceptualizes these differences depends on one's perspective. Table 16.1 summarizes the major categories of sexual dimorphism. In this chapter, we focus on how the hormones change the morphology of the brain and how this affects the behavior and sexuality.

Pink and Blue

In general, men and women behave differently and enjoy different activities. The etiology of this difference remains a hotly debated topic. Is it nature or nurture—genetic or environmental? With humans, it is almost impossible to tease out these opposing causes. The signals a baby receives about its sexual identity start early—in the nursery. Typically, boys favor construction and transportation toys. Girls show less rough physical play and prefer toys such as dolls. Is this a product of learned gender social roles or something more innately wired in the brain?

A study with vervet monkeys suggests that the choices of toys children make to play with are more ingrained than some might think. Monkeys in large cages at the University of California, Los Angeles Primate Laboratory were allowed 5 minutes of exposure to individual toys classified as "masculine" (police car and ball) or "feminine" (doll and pot). The amount of time they were in direct contact with each of the toys was recorded. Figure 16.1 shows a male and female monkey playing with the toys and the percent time that each gender spent in contact with the toys. These results show that even nonhuman primates who are not exposed to social pressure regarding toy preference will choose gender-specific toys.

If we remember the important role of pleasure in determining behavioral preferences, we can speculate that the monkeys spend more time with the toys they enjoy. Likewise, we can speculate that the association between an object and the pleasure is hardwired in the brain. Furthermore, some of this "wiring" must have arisen early in human evolution before the emergence of our hominid ancestors.

The Boy Who Was Raised as a Girl

One of the more remarkable stories of sexually dimorphic behavior involves a tragic story of a boy raised as a girl. David was 8 months old in 1966 when his entire penis was accidentally burned beyond repair during a routine circumcision. Dr. John Money, a psychologist at Johns Hopkins Hospital with expertise in sexual reassignment, convinced the family to proceed with surgical sex change and raise the boy as a girl. Dr. Money believed that sexual identity/orientation developed

---

TABLE 16.1

Different Ways of Conceptualizing Sexual Dimorphism

Perspective	Example
Chromosomal	XX, XY
Gonadal	Ovaries, testes
Hormonal	Estrogen, androgens
Morphological	Genitalia, body size, body shape
Behavioral	Nurturing, aggressive, hunter, gatherer, etc.
Sexual	Identity, orientation, preference

Female with doll

A "Feminine" toys

■ Males
■ Females

B "Masculine" toys

Male with truck

FIGURE 16.1 ● Male vervet monkeys spent more time in contact with "masculine" toys while females spent more time with "feminine" toys. (From Alexander GM, Hines M. Sex differences in response to children's toys in nonhuman primates (*Cercopithecus aethiops sabaeus*). *Evol Hum Behav.* 2002;23:467-479.)

after 18 months of age and children could adapt to a new sexual identity if the procedure was started early enough. David provided an ideal case study as he had an identical twin brother with a normal penis.

Amazingly, Dr. Money reported in the medical literature that the reassignment was a success, but it was in actuality a disaster. David, whose name was changed to Brenda, did not want to wear dresses, or play with dolls. She preferred to play with guns and cars. She could beat up her brother and threw a ball like a boy. Worst of all, this unusual behavior was not well received at school. She was relentlessly teased for her masculine traits. Brenda was shunned by the girls and not accepted by the boys.

By the time Brenda was 14 years old she was still unaware of the sexual reassignment and remained distressed. A local psychiatrist who was treating Brenda convinced the parents to reveal the truth. Brenda recalls her reaction, "Suddenly it all made sense why I felt the way I did. I wasn't some sort of weirdo."

David immediately decided to revert to his genetic sex. Within several months, he began going

out in public as a boy. He stopped estrogen and started testosterone. He had bilateral mastectomies and several operations to rebuild male genitalia. He eventually married in his twenties although he could not have children. However, he battled with depression and the demons from this childhood experience. In May 2005, at the age of 38, he killed himself.

The significant point about this case is that in spite of being raised as a girl and in spite of the presence of estrogen hormones and the absence of testosterone, David continued to have male pattern psychosocial and psychosexual development. Larger case studies are consistent with David's experience. One analysis of XY individuals assigned female roles at birth due to a severe pelvic defect (cloacal exstrophy) found that all showed masculine tendencies. Slightly more than half chose to declare themselves male when older. These studies suggest that something permanent happens in utero that determines sexual identity/orientation.

Environment

It would be naive to dismiss the significance of environment on sexually stereotypical behaviors. History is replete with examples of men and women showing varying amounts of masculine and feminine behavior that are clearly molded by shifts in social norms. Kim Wallen reviewed 30 years of research with rhesus monkeys and attempted to separate hormonal and social influences. For example, rough and tumble play is one of the most robust sexually dimorphic behaviors. Juvenile males wrestle more frequently than females in almost every rearing condition. However, if reared in a group with only males, they (males or females?) actually engage in less rough play. Likewise, mounting behavior is seen more with males than females. However, when reared in isolated, same-sex environments, males display less mounting while females display more such behavior.

Rust et al. looked at gender development in preschool children and the effect of an older sibling. They discovered that having an older brother was associated with greater masculine and less feminine behavior in boys and girls. However, boys with older sisters were more feminine but not less masculine, whereas girls with older sisters were less masculine but not more feminine.

Together, these studies suggest interplay between hormones and environment. That is, biologic factors predispose individuals to engage in specific behaviors, which can be modified by social experience.

GONADS

The gonads (ovaries and testes) serve two major functions. First, they produce eggs or sperm to pass on DNA to the next generation. Second, they produce the sex hormones that not only promote the development of secondary sexual characteristics but also drive the behavior that increases the chances of an egg and sperm meeting.

HORMONES

Figure 14.8 shows the classic experiment by Berthold who was the first to establish that the testes contain a substance that controls the development of male secondary sexual characteristics. In Chapter 7, we discussed the relationship between the cortex, hypothalamus, pituitary gland, and end organ. Briefly, with input from the cortex, the hypothalamus produces gonadotropin-releasing hormone (GnRH), which in turn stimulates the anterior pituitary gland to produce luteinizing hormone (LH) and follicle-stimulating hormone (FSH). LH and FSH stimulate the gonads to produce the sex hormones.

Cholesterol is the precursor of all steroid hormones. Figure 7.7 shows the three major steroids synthesized from cholesterol: glucocorticoids, mineralocorticoids, and the sex steroids. The sex steroids are synthesized in the adrenals or gonads. Because the steroid hormones are lipid soluble and easily pass through the cell walls, they are released as they are synthesized.

Testosterone, as shown in Figure 16.2, is converted into 17-β-estradiol (E2) and an androgen, 5-α-dihydrotestosterone (DHT). (An androgen is a generic term for a hormone that stimulates or maintains male characteristics.) Amazingly, much of the androgen effects in the brain are actually implemented by 17-β-estradiol. For example, an injection of estrogen to a newborn rat is more masculinizing than an injection of testosterone.

Why do the maternal estrogens not masculinize all fetuses? One of the functions of α-fetoprotein during pregnancy is to bind with maternal estrogens, which are then cleared through the placenta. This protein, which does not bind testosterone effectively, prevents estrogens from reaching the brain.

We have discussed in other chapters how the sex steroids can work directly on synaptic receptors or indirectly through gene transcription (see Figures 5.3, 7.1, and 7.3). These different effects are summarized in Figure 16.3. The direct effects are fast, while the indirect effects take longer to

FIGURE 16.2 ● The sex hormones are synthesized from cholesterol. Testosterone serves as a prohormone for 17-β-estradiol.

transpire. Because the sex hormones can influence neural function, they are sometimes called *neurosteroids* in neuroscience literature.

Differentiation and Activation

The development of sexual dimorphism is dependent on the sex hormones. The presence of testosterone at critical periods of time both masculinizes and defeminizes the brain. Likewise, the absence of testosterone feminizes and demasculinizes the brain. In 1959 William C. Young et al. published a classic paper that rivals Berthold's work with roosters in helping us to understand the fundamental principles of hormones and behavior.

To understand Young's study it is important to be aware of the different sexual postures males and females display at appropriate times.

FIGURE 16.3 ● Steroids can directly affect the transmitter synthesis/release or postsynaptic transmitter receptors. They can also indirectly influence gene transcription. (Adapted from Bear MF, Connors BW, Paradiso MA, eds. *Neuroscience: Exploring the Brain.* 3rd ed. Baltimore, MD: Lippincott Williams & Wilkins; 2007.)

Female rodents will stand immobile and arch their backs: *lordosis*. Males will *mount* such a receptive female. Females and males rarely (although not completely) exhibit the opposite behavior. Researchers use the presence or absence of lordosis and mounting as expressions of sexual behavior. For example, castration of a male stops his mounting behavior. But this can be reinstated with injections of testosterone.

Young's group sought to understand the effects of early and late exposure to sex hormones on sexual behavior. Their experiment, which is shown in Figure 16.4, started with injecting testosterone in a pregnant female guinea pig. Their first observation (not shown in the figure) was that female pups exposed to high doses of androgens in utero were born with masculinized external genitalia.

The rest of the study focused on the female pups, which were allowed to mature and were then spayed. Later, they were all given estrogen and progesterone to stimulate female sexual behavior. Each was paired with a normal male guinea pig. Sometime later, the procedure was reversed. All were injected with testosterone and paired with a receptive female. The results were striking. The females exposed to testosterone in utero failed to display lordosis when given estrogen and progesterone. However, they would mount other females when given testosterone. The control group displayed the opposite behavior.

This elegant experiment established a clear distinction between the differentiating effects of sex hormones during development and the activating effects during adulthood. The females exposed to testosterone in utero had alterations in the organization of their brains that prevented the normal activation by female sex hormones as an adult.

Human Congenital Anomalies

Occasionally, people are born with genetic alterations that give us insight into the differentiation and activation of human sexual dimorphism. One such condition is *congenital adrenal hyperplasia*. Children with this condition are exposed to excessive androgens due to overactive fetal adrenal glands. Paradoxically, the condition is caused by an impaired ability of the fetal adrenal gland to produce cortisol. Because the pituitary fails to receive the appropriate negative feedback, it continues to secrete adrenocorticotropic hormone (ACTH), which in turn induces hyperplasia of the androgen-producing cells of the adrenal cortex.

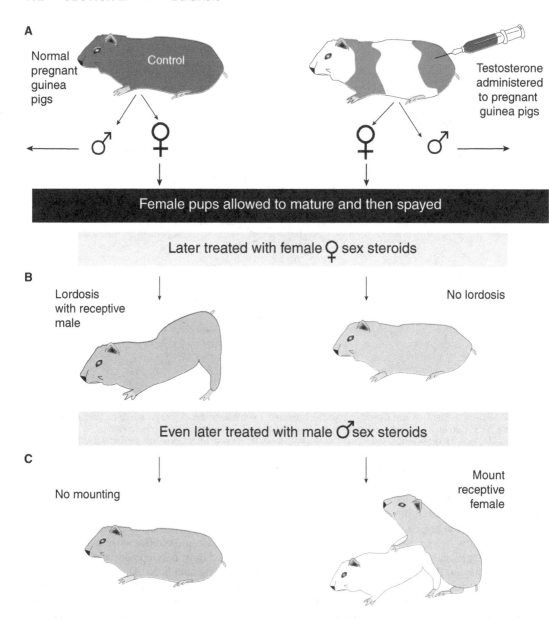

FIGURE 16.4 ● Guinea pigs exposed to testosterone in utero (**A**) fail to show feminine sexual behavior (**B**) when given female sex hormones and instead act like males (**C**) when given testosterone.

As we might predict from Young's studies with guinea pigs, human males are unaffected by the exposure to excess adrenal androgens in utero. Females, on the other hand, are born with masculinized external genitalia. Additionally, the females tend to exhibit more rough and tumble play as children. As adults, they have an increased tendency to prefer other females as partners.

An extraordinary condition in men provides a different example of anomalous sexual development. *Androgen insensitivity syndrome* (AIS) is a condition in which XY (male) individuals are born as normal appearing females. The problem is caused by a mutation in the androgen receptor. These individuals produce testosterone, but the cells are unable to recognize it. Consequently, there is no activation of the genes necessary for male characteristics.

These individuals are born looking like normal little girls and are raised as such (Figure 16.5). Typically, the problem is only recognized when they fail to menstruate in adolescence. Unfortunately, they are unable to conceive as they have failed to develop uteri, fallopian tubes, and ovaries.

FIGURE 16.5 ● This person with complete androgen insensitivity syndrome has an XY genotype, but has developed unambiguous feminine characteristics. (Courtesy of John Money.)

However, their behavior is unequivocally feminine. Hines et al. examined the psychological development of 22 XY individuals with complete AIS compared with 22 XX normal controls and found no differences on any measure of psychological outcome. They concluded that these results argue against the need for ovaries and two X chromosomes in the development of traditional feminine behavior. Likewise, it reinforces the importance of the androgen receptor in masculine development. It is an interesting thought that all humans (both men and women) would develop into women unless other hormones intervene. The default model for mankind is a woman!

NEURONAL CIRCUITRY
Nerve Growth
Gonadal steroids grow more than just testes and breasts—they also cause selective neuronal growth. As shown in Figure 16.3, gonadal steroids stimulate gene expression through the androgen and estrogen receptors. These receptors, once bound with the hormone, also function as transcription factors, which, in turn, stimulate gene transcription and protein synthesis. Ultimately, the gonadal steroids can affect the nerve volume, dendritic length, spine density, and synaptic connectivity.

Woolley et al. demonstrated this effect by administering estradiol or placebo to ovariectomized rats and examining the structure and function of the hippocampal cells. Figure 16.6 shows two CA1 pyramidal cells and a closer examination of their dendritic spines. The estradiol-exposed neurons had 22% more spines and 30% more *N*-methyl-D-aspartate glutamate receptors than the controls. Furthermore, the treated neurons exhibited

Control   Estradiol

CA1 pyramidal cell   CA1 pyramidal cell

FIGURE 16.6 ● Ovariectomized rats treated with estradiol display greater spine formation on CA1 pyramidal cells from the hippocampus. (Adapted from Woolley CS, Weiland NG, McEwen BS, et al. Estradiol increases the sensitivity of hippocampal CA1 pyramidal cells to NMDA receptor-mediated synaptic input: correlation with dendritic spine density. *J Neurosci.* 1997;17(5):1848-1859.)

less electrical resistance to cellular input. So not only did the estrogen change the structure of the neuron but also the function.

Growth Factor Proteins

The astute reader might wonder about the role of growth factor proteins with sex hormones and nerve plasticity. Indeed, there is considerable evidence linking gonadal steroids with growth factors such as brain-derived neurotrophic factor (BDNF). However, it is unclear if the sex hormones stimulate the production of the growth factor protein, or work synergistically with them, or both. A study looking at the rat motor neuron sheds some light on this question.

The motor neurons projecting from the spinal cord to the skeletal muscles in rodents are generally similar for males and females. However, the male requires the additional innervation of the *bulbocavernosus* muscles around the penis, which are necessary for erections and copulation (Figure 16.7). Consequently, the motor neurons in the lumbar region of the spinal cord of the male rat (collectively called the *spinal nucleus of the bulbocavernosus* [SNB]) are approximately four times larger than in the female. These motor neurons regress in the female shortly after birth. Similar regression occurs with castrated males, although androgen treatment will preserve the motor neurons.

The dendrites of the motor neurons have extensive branchings that make connections spanning several spinal segments. Cutting the SNB motor neurons results in regression of the dendrites. Previous research has shown that testosterone or BDNF can limit the dendritic regression.

Yang et al. took this a step further. They cut the SNB motor neurons in castrated males. Then they put BDNF over the cut axons or administered testosterone, or both, in different groups of rats. A month later, the motor neurons were injected with a marker that allows visualization of the dendrites and axons after the animal is sacrificed. Figure 16.8 represents a computer-generated composite section marking the presence of the SNB motor neurons for the three groups of rats. The BDNF plus testosterone group preserved substantially more dendritic branching than seen with either alone (similar to what would be seen in a normal control). This suggests that BDNF and testosterone act synergistically to maintain the SNB motor neuron morphology.

Songbirds

The study of the sexually dimorphic brain structures of the songbirds is one of the great stories of neuroscience—one that transformed our recognition of

A

B   Cross section of lumbar spinal cord

Female   Male

SNB

FIGURE 16.7 • **A.** The male rat has bulbocavernosus muscles that are needed to control the penis for copulation. **B.** Cross sections of the female and male lumbar spinal cord show the presence of the spinal nucleus of the bulbocavernosus for the male, but not the female (**A.** Adapted from Breedlove SM, Arnold AP. Hormonal control of a developing neuromuscular system. II. Sensitive periods for the androgen-induced masculinization of the rat SNB. *J Neurosci.* 1983;3(2):424-432.)

the dynamic quality of the brain. The leader in this research is Fernando Nottebohm at the Rockefeller University in New York. He and others wanted to understand why male songbirds sing and females seldom do.

They initially looked at the syrinx (vocal cords) trying to find out the differences, but without success. Later, they focused on the neuronal mechanisms that control singing: the high vocal center (HVC), robust nucleus (RA), and area X. These nuclei send projections to the XII cranial nerve which controls the syrinx. Lesions of the HVC bilaterally will silence a bird.

The big discovery came when they realized that the song nuclei are approximately three times larger in males (Figure 16.9). This was the first discovery of sexual dimorphism in the brain.

Testosterone

BDNF

Testosterone
and BDNF

FIGURE 16.8 ● Composite lumbar cross sections showing the extent of spinal nucleus of the bulbocavernosus motor neurons that remain 1 month after surgical excision. Testosterone plus brain-derived neurotrophic factor preserved more of the motor neurons than either alone. (Adapted from Yang LY, Verhovshek T, Sengelaub DR. BDNF and androgen interact in the maintenance of dendritic morphology in a sexually dimorphic rat spinal nucleus. *Endocrinology*. 2004;145(1):161-168.)

Furthermore, they showed that the size of the HVC correlates with the number of song syllables a male canary sings.

Their next discovery has fundamentally altered the way we think about the brain. Adult canaries change their songs every year, which is accomplished by adding new syllable types and discarding others. Remarkably, this occurs through the birth and death of neurons in the song nuclei. Nottebohm et al. were the first to show that working neurons develop in adult warm-blooded vertebrates—an idea that received a cool reception when first presented in 1984.

The reason for discussing this topic in this chapter is the fact that much of the differences in the male canaries' nuclei and song production are controlled by the testosterone. Evidence to support this include the following:

1. The nuclei of the adult song system have high concentrations of testosterone.
2. Adult males with higher testosterone sing more than the adults with less testosterone.
3. Females given testosterone will sing more and show increased volume of their HVC and RA.
4. Drops in testosterone levels at the end of the breeding season correspond with the death of HVC neurons.

Hypothalamus

The hypothalamus is instrumental in regulating gonadotropin secretion. Specifically, the anterior aspect of the hypothalamus is known to control a wide variety of mating behaviors: desire, sexual behavior, and parenting. Lesions in this area can lead to alterations in sexual behavior. The *preoptic area* (POA) in the rat is an area where significant differences between the sexes are found (see Figure 2.8). In the male rat, the POA is five to seven times larger than in the female. The difference is so prominent that it can be accurately identified with the naked eye. This region of the POA is called the *sexually dimorphic nucleus of the preoptic area* (SDN-POA). Female rats given androgens will develop an SDN-POA approximately the size of that of a male. As with the SNB motor neurons, it appears that the androgens preserve the nerve cells, which otherwise waste away.

Humans

Allen et al. examined the anterior aspect of the hypothalamus in a postmortem analysis of 22 human brains: half of each sex. They focused their attention on an area that is the human equivalent of the rat SDN-POA. They identified four cell groupings within the anterior hypothalamus, which they called the *interstitial nuclei of the anterior hypothalamus* (INAH). They numbered the INAH from 1 to 4 and reported that INAH-2 and INAH-3 are approximately twice as large in males compared with females. Figure 16.10 shows the actual comparative micrographs through the INAH of males and females.

Sexual Orientation

Simon LeVay took this work one step further and compared the INAH for females, heterosexual males, and homosexual males. He confirmed the work by Allen et al., that is, two of the four interstitial nuclei are sexually dimorphic. However, even more interesting, he found that INAH-3 was twice as large in heterosexual men as it was in homosexual men. Although this provides compelling evidence that

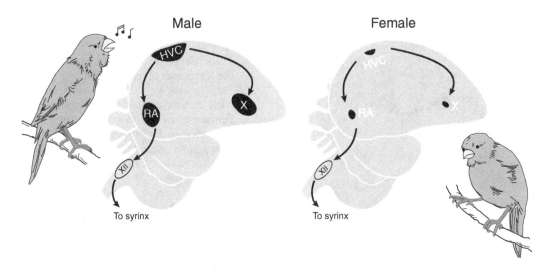

FIGURE 16.9 ● The difference in the song nuclei in canaries explains why males sing but females rarely do. HVC, high vocal center; RA, robust nucleus. (Adapted from Nottebohm F. The road we travelled: discovery, choreography, and significance of brain replaceable neurons. *Ann N Y Acad Sci*. 2004;1016:628-658.)

FIGURE 16.10 ● Representative micrographs showing the interstitial nuclei of the anterior hypothalamus for women (top) and men (bottom). Note that INAH numbers 2 and 3 are less distinct in women. (From Allen LS, Hines M, Shryne JE, et al. Two sexually dimorphic cell groups in the human brain. *J Neurosci*. 1989;9(2):497-506.)

sexual orientation is "hardwired," we must be cautious for there could be other explanations. For example, almost all of the homosexual men died of acquired immunodeficiency syndrome (AIDS), whereas only approximately one-third of the heterosexual men died of AIDS. Likewise, there was considerable overlap in the size of the nuclei between groups, implying that it is impossible to predict the sexual orientation of any individual based on the measurement of his INAH-3.

Other researchers have addressed this topic in different species. Approximately 8% of the domestic male sheep display sexual preference for other males. A group in Oregon identified a cluster of cells within the POA of the anterior hypothalamus (analogues to the INAH) that is significantly larger in rams than in ewes. They compared these nuclei for rams with different sexual preferences and found it was twice as large in heterosexual rams as it was in homosexual rams. Hence, an animal model that is consistent with the work by LeVay.

More recently, a group in Amsterdam (the capital of the sex trade industry) examined the INAH-3 nucleus from the brains of individuals with and without gonadotropin hormones compared with male-to-female transsexual individuals with completed sex reassignment surgery. The volume of the INAH-3 nucleus was larger in the males compared with females and transsexual subjects. Furthermore, they counted the neurons in the nucleus for each group and found a similar relationship as shown in Figure 16.11.

Taken together, the above studies suggest a possible explanation for the continuum of human sexual behavior. Small differences in nuclei in the anterior hypothalamus produce significant differences in sexual identity and behavior. Early exposure to sexual hormones during critical periods or other environmental factors or genetics may alter the development of nuclei that steer one's sexual orientation and preferences.

PSYCHIATRIC DISORDERS
Cognitive Decline

There is considerable evidence that estrogens (and presumably testosterone) are neuroprotective. Figure 16.6 shows the robust increase in spine formation that can be induced by estrogen in hippocampal neurons. Presumably, such an arborization of the neurons enhances neural connections. Research with rodents and nonhuman primates demonstrates beneficial effects of estrogen on cognition. Multiple observational studies in humans have found that hormone replacement protects against the development of Alzheimer's disease, although there are other risks of continued hormone replacement.

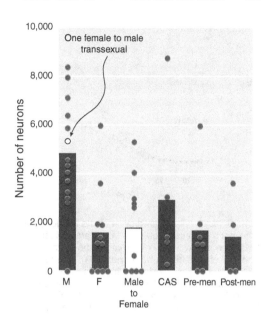

FIGURE 16.11 ● Postmortem analysis of the number of neurons in the INAH-3 nucleus for males (M), females (F), male-to-female transsexual, and castrated males due to prostate cancer (CAS). All the women are separated by menopausal status in the last two bars. One female to male transsexual is included with the males. (Adapted from Garcia-Falgueras A, Swaab DF. A sex difference in the hypothalamic uncinate nucleus: relationship to gender identity. *Brain*. 2008;131:3132-3146.)

Figure 16.12 is an example of one such observational study with humans. This was a study of more than 3,000 elderly people from one county in Utah. The objective was to test for the development of Alzheimer's disease and see if a history of hormone

TREATMENT HOMOSEXUALITY

A few mental health professionals across the country offer treatment for individuals who want to be heterosexual rather than homosexual. Hardly any studies exist that establish the effectiveness of such treatment. In 2003 Robert Spitzer published a survey of 200 individuals who reported changing their sexual orientation after therapy. Many reported changing from predominantly or exclusively homosexual to predominantly heterosexual. Few reported complete changes. The report drew heated criticism. In 2012 Spitzer apologized to the gay community and acknowledged the study was flawed. That is, the study did not assess the credibility of the subject's reports of change in sexual orientation.

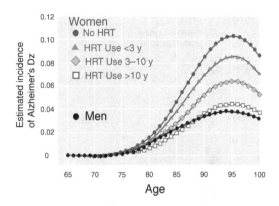

FIGURE 16.12 ● A prediction of the incidence of Alzheimer's disease calculated from data collected about men and women over 3 years shows the beneficial effects of sex hormones. HRT, hormone replacement therapy. (Adapted from Zandi PP, Carlson MC, Plassman BL, et al. HRT and incidence of Alzheimer's disease in older women: the Cache County Study. *JAMA.* 2002;288(17):2123-2129.)

replacement therapy (HRT) was protective. Note that the men (who presumably maintain adequate levels of sex hormones) fare better than the women in terms of developing Alzheimer's disease. Likewise, the women who took HRT displayed a dose–response effect. That is, the longer a woman took HRT the less likely she was to develop Alzheimer's disease.

Clinical trials of HRT and cognition have not been as uniformly positive as we would hope. A review of the studies suggests that unopposed estrogen improves the verbal memory in women younger than 65 years. For older women, the results are neutral. Janicki and Schupf, in a recent review of hormonal influences on cognition and Alzheimer's progression, concluded that "overall data from epidemiologic studies, observational studies and clinical trials of HRT, studies of endogenous hormones, and evaluation of genetic variants involved in estrogen biosynthesis and receptor activity indicate that estrogen plays an important role in the pathogenesis of cognitive decline and risk for Alzheimer's Disease in both men and women." So while estrogen may not be the panacea for preventing Alzheimer's disease, it does appear to have some neuroprotective benefits.

Sexual Dysfunction

A survey of adults between the ages of 18 and 59 in the United States found a high prevalence of sexual dysfunction: 31% for men and 43% for women. The most common complaint for men was premature ejaculation, whereas for women it was lack of interest. There are pharmacologic interventions

available for premature ejaculation. For example, the selective serotonin reuptake inhibitors make it harder to have an orgasm, although they are not U.S. Food and Drug Administration (FDA) approved for this indication.

Lack of interest in sex, on the other hand, is difficult to treat. Certainly, the qualities of the relationship, secondary medical conditions, and the presence of other psychiatric disorders have strong influences on the joy of sex. However, some women find sex lacking. As many as one in three women never or infrequently achieve orgasm during intercourse—the number is still only one in five with masturbation. Studies with twins show a genetic component to orgasmic ability. Estimated heritability for difficulty achieving orgasm during intercourse is 34%—on par with anxiety and depressive disorders (see Table 6.1).

Dopaminergic mechanisms may play a large role in modulating sexual drive and orgasmic quality. As discussed in Chapter 12, the dopamine pathways to the nucleus accumbens are active in motivated behavior. Dopamine agonists such as the stimulant medications and cocaine are anecdotally reported to enhance human sexual behavior. More recently, genetic studies have shown that different genotypes of the dopamine D4 receptor correlate more or less closely with sexual desire and arousal. This suggests that biology as well as environmental signals (in close proximity to Mr or Miss Right) interact to determine the sexual experience.

The prospect of giving women an approved medication to enhance sexual desire, although of interest to the pharmaceutical industry and feared by domineering fathers everywhere, is currently not an option. The phosphodiesterase-5 inhibitors (e.g., Viagra) have been tested in large trials for female sexual dysfunction and failed to enhance the interest any more than placebo. The testosterone patch, although effective for some patients, failed to win the FDA approval owing to safety concerns.

Recent research suggests that α-melanocyte–stimulating hormone (α-MSH) may be, what some call, a genuine aphrodisiac. We mentioned in Chapter 11 that a large precursor neuropeptide in the pituitary gland, proopiomelanocortin (POMC), is cleaved to form active neuropeptides, which include ACTH, β-endorphin, and α-MSH (see Figure 16.13). α-MSH is the peptide that also causes the skin to darken in patients with Addison's disease and also suppresses appetite (see Chapter 13). The story is told that a company was testing a melanocortin product as a possible tanning agent that did not require sun exposure. During early testing the medication triggered erections in most of the men. *Eureka!* Subsequently, a peptide analog of α-MSH called *bremelanotide* (a melanocortin receptor agonist) was developed for further study.

Research with animals has shown that bremelanotide enhances female sexual solicitation in rats. The female rats became overtly flirtatious in a rodent sort of way—even climbing through little holes in the walls to get to the males. A study with married women in Iran (of all places) using an intranasal spray to administer the medication reported greater intercourse satisfaction in those receiving the active medication. Unfortunately, testing has been halted due to increased blood pressure in a few subjects. The company is considering subcutaneous administration as a means to eliminate the hypertensive adverse effect.

It is not clear why the pituitary neuropeptide α-MSH enhances sexual interest. Studies in which the medication was injected directly into a female rat's lateral ventricles found increased solicitations, establishing that its effects are mediated centrally. Additionally, α-MSH activated the Fos proteins (markers of gene expression) in the POA of the hypothalamus as well as the nucleus accumbens—areas that would be consistent with sexual pleasure.

Mood Disorders

The lifetime prevalence of mood disorders in women is approximately twice that of men. Although the cause of this difference remains undetermined, one possible explanation is the sex hormones—or more specifically, the fluctuation in sex hormones. Figure 16.14 shows the alterations in estrogen levels for a hypothetical woman across her life span. The times of greatest risk for mood disturbances are during times of fluctuating estrogen levels: menarche, premenstrual syndrome (PMS), postpartum, and perimenopausal.

The correlation between dropping sex hormones and depressive symptoms is not limited to women. The difference is the fluctuations. Men typically have stable testosterone levels. However, when testosterone drops, psychiatric symptoms become more prevalent. In one veterans administration (VA) study, the researchers followed up the testosterone level and emergence of depressive illness in men older than 45 for 2 years. They found that 22% of the hypogonadal men (total testosterone <200 ng/dL) experienced depression, whereas only 7% of the eugonadal men did. Another group looked at the emergence of psychiatric symptoms in men treated for prostate cancer with GnRH

FIGURE 16.13 ● The propeptide POMC is produced in the pituitary gland, where it is cleaved to smaller active peptides such as ACTH, α-MSH, and β-endorphin.

TREATMENT GnRH AGONIST

Clinicians can override the pulsatile nature of a releasing hormone to effectively shut down the production of the sex hormones and treat problems such as endometriosis, prostate cancer, and early-onset puberty.

This treatment has also been used with sex offenders as a form of "chemical castration." In this process, a long-acting GnRH agonist, leuprolide (Lupron Depot), inhibits the release of LH and FSH, although it stimulates the receptor. This effect is achieved because the continuous stimulation—in contrast to the usual intermittent stimulation—causes the desensitization of receptors in the pituitary. As a result, LH and FSH are not produced, which subsequently reduces the production of sex hormones.

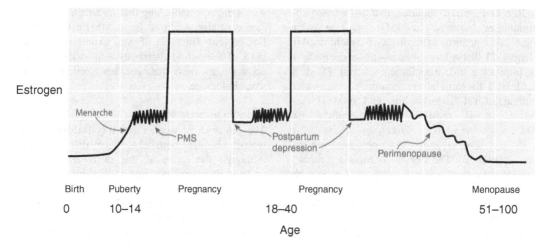

FIGURE 16.14 ● Estrogen levels fluctuate for women from puberty to menopause. The times of greatest vulnerability for depression occur when estrogen levels are changing. (Adapted from Stahl SM. *Essential Psychopharmacology. Neuroscientific Basis of Practical Applications.* 2nd ed. New York, NY: Cambridge University Press; 2000.)

agonists (see sidebar), which causes testosterone to plummet. They reported significant increases in anxiety and depression while the testosterone level was low.

Some of the most convincing data regarding the effects of sex hormones on mood have been treatment studies. With both men and women, positive results have been shown for improving mood when sex hormones were administered. Figure 16.15 shows two representative studies. These studies have many differences, but they both reveal less depression with sex hormones.

The study on the left is with perimenopausal women who have mild or moderate depressive

symptoms. One group was given placebo and the other estradiol. No antidepressants were used. The graph on the right was a study with men. All the men had failed antidepressant therapy and had low or borderline testosterone levels. Everyone remained on his antidepressant while half the group also received supplemental testosterone gel.

These are both small studies and need to be repeated with larger numbers. Likewise, it is important to remember that hormone replacement is not without significant risks. However, the studies demonstrate the powerful effects sex hormones can have on mood.

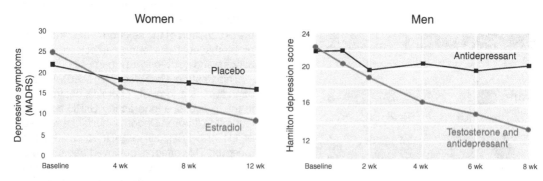

FIGURE 16.15 ● Two studies highlighting the mood-altering effects of sex hormones for women and men with sluggish gonads. (*Left*: Adapted from Soares CN, Almeida OP, Joffe H, et al. Efficacy of estradiol for the treatment of depressive disorders in perimenopausal women: a double-blind, randomized, placebo-controlled trial. *Arch Gen Psychiatry.* 2001;58(6):529-534. *Right*: Adapted from Pope HG Jr, Cohane GH, Kanayama G, et al. Testosterone gel supplementation for men with refractory depression: a randomized, placebo-controlled trial. *Am J Psychiatry.* 2003;160(1):105-111.)

HOT FLASHES AND ANTIDEPRESSANTS

Some women want treatment for the hot flashes associated with menopause, but do not want HRT. The newer antidepressants have been shown to have some benefit. In the best study, the researchers felt that venlafaxine was clearly superior to placebo, but not as effective as estrogen. Their study stands as further evidence that mood and gonadal steroids are linked in ways that we are only beginning to understand.

Traumatic Brain Injury

Traumatic brain injury (TBI) is increasingly recognized as more than just short-term confusion. Soldiers returning from the current wars and football players are reporting enduring problems from the cortical bruising and microscopic tears the brain sustains when it is rattled around inside the hard skull. Memory, cognition, and impulse control in many cases never return to baseline. Although there is currently no medical treatment for TBI, progesterone, often thought of as the "pregnancy hormone," is generating considerable interest. Studies with animals and a few humans suggest that progesterone, administered shortly after the head injury, may have nurturing properties that enable the brain to repair more effectively. A large phase III trial called ProTECT III is underway in the United States with an expected completion date in the middle of 2015.

Pregnancy and Depression

One can get the impression that sex hormones keep people happy. However, it is not that simple. For example, pregnancy, a time of very high estrogen and progesterone levels, has been conceptualized as a period of emotional well-being—even protective against psychiatric disorders. However, a recent study was conducted on women with a history of depression who became pregnant. Some women continued their antidepressants while others stopped them during the pregnancy. The relapse rates for depression during the pregnancy were 26% for those still on their medication and 68% for those who discontinued their antidepressants.

Clearly, pregnancy is not protective against depression for women with a history of depression. Some think the high levels of progesterone during pregnancy may have negative effects on mood. Others speculated about the negative effects of low BDNF during pregnancy. More research is needed to understand this paradoxical finding.

Summary
The sex hormones are not just for fostering the procreation of the species. One focus of this chapter has been on the nourishing capacity the neurosteroids have on the brain cells and subsequently on behavior and emotions. European physicians are more familiar with this body of research and are more comfortable utilizing small doses of hormone replacement to optimize the treatment of mental problems—a perspective we may embrace as the gonads of the baby boomers languish.

QUESTIONS

1. Female gonadal steroids include all of the following, except
   a. Testosterone.
   b. Estradiol.
   c. Progesterone.
   d. GnRH.

2. Many of the androgen effects in the brain are triggered by
   a. 17-β-Estradiol.
   b. 5-α-DHT.
   c. Aromatase.
   d. α-Fetoprotein.

3. Which rat will display lordosis when primed with estrogens and progesterones and paired with a sexually active male?
   a. Males of normal pregnancies.
   b. Males exposed to androgens in utero.
   c. Females of normal pregnancies.
   d. Females exposed to androgens in utero.

4. Known effects of female sex hormones include all of the following, except
   a. Increased spine formation.
   b. Decreased risk of stroke.
   c. Increase γ-aminobutyric acid inhibition.
   d. Gene transcription.

5. Evidence of sexual dimorphism in the vertebrate central nervous system include all of the following, except
   a. SNB.
   b. The robust nucleus.
   c. SDN-POA.
   d. Paraventricular nucleus.

6. As suggested by some research, which area is smaller in homosexual men compared with heterosexual men?
   a. INAH-1.
   b. INAH-2.
   c. INAH-3.
   d. INAH-4.

7. The propeptide POMC is cleaved into all the following active peptides, except
   a. Δ-Fos.
   b. ACTH.
   c. α-MSH.
   d. β-Endorphin.

8. Evidence of the importance of sex hormones and mood includes all of the following except
   a. PMS.
   b. Athletes on anabolic steroids.
   c. Chemical castration for prostate cancer.
   d. Randomized controlled trials.

See Answers section at the end of the book.

CHAPTER 17

Attachment

PARENTAL BEHAVIOR

The goal of reproduction is successful offspring. Parents want offspring who can survive the rigors of the world and produce their own descendents. Many animals produce offspring that require sustained assistance to successfully reach maturity. The particular actions that parents undertake to ensure the growth and survival of their offspring constitute *parental behavior*.

The extent of parental behavior in the animal kingdom occurs along a spectrum ranging from none to helicopter parents. Female salmons lay hundreds of eggs to be fertilized and then swim away. Humans are at the other end of the spectrum—investing many years and enormous resources, and perhaps hoping to be surrounded by their children until the very end.

Females in the animal kingdom do most of the parenting, although there are some exceptions. It is generally believed that males seek to fertilize as many eggs as possible, whereas females seek to successfully raise the few they sire. Parental behavior constitutes any behavior that the parent does for the offspring. For example, a pregnant dog will build a nest a day or two before giving birth. After the delivery, she will lick them clean, eat the placentas, feed them, and keep them warm (and for all this she is called a bitch). Additionally, she will aggressively defend the pups against any suspicious intruders.

The onset of maternal behavior is remarkably precise. An inexperienced mother must immediately perform a full range of new behaviors without much room for error. How does this happen? Terkel and Rosenblatt established that there must be something in the blood that induces maternal behavior. They transfused blood from a female rat that had just delivered to a virgin rat (Figure 17.1). Within 24-hours, the virgin rat was displaying maternal behavior.

Hormones

Biologic endocrinologists have spent considerable time and energy trying to tease out the maternal molecules. Although they have gotten close, there is still no definitive concoction of hormones that will immediately trigger maternal behavior in a nulliparous (virgin) rat. The leading culprits are estrogen, progesterone, and prolactin. An important ingredient appears to be the changing levels of the hormones. In Figure 17.2, note how the progesterone is seen to drop while the estrogen and prolactin rise in a rat just before delivery.

Oxytocin also plays some important role. Traditionally, we conceptualize oxytocin as the neuropeptide released from the posterior pituitary into general circulation, which leads to uterine contractions and milk ejection (see Figure 7.4). Recent research has found receptors for oxytocin within the brain, establishing central actions for this neuropeptide. Indeed, injecting oxytocin directly into the lateral ventricles in a rat will induce maternal behavior in a hormone-primed virgin rat. More recently, it has been shown that oxytocin levels in the paraventricular nucleus (PVN) increase with maternal aggression. Likewise, infusion of synthetic oxytocin into the PVN also increases maternal aggression toward an intruder.

Further complicating this picture is the fact that hormones facilitate maternal behavior but are not required for it. Nulliparous rats will initially avoid new pups placed in their cage. However, if exposed over a series of days (1 hour each day), they will respond maternally to the pups within 5 to 6 days. Pregnant rats will show similar avoidance until after they have delivered. Then they will quickly display maternal behavior to any pup for the rest of their lives, proving that "once a mother, always a mother" (Figure 17.3).

FIGURE 17.1 ● When nulliparous rats are transfused with blood from a new mother, they will display maternal behavior within 24-hours. (Adapted from Nelson RJ. *An Introduction to Behavioral Endocrinology*. 3rd ed. Sunderland, MA: Sinauer; 2005.)

The Brain

Taken together, these studies suggest that the hormonal fluctuations late in pregnancy act on the brain to decrease fear or aversion and increase attraction toward infants. Because maternal behavior persists once it is established, it is likely that the experience permanently changes some regions in the brain. An area that has been intensely studied is the one that we discussed in Chapter 16: the preoptic area (POA) located in the anterior hypothalamus.

The POA is rich in estrogen, progesterone, prolactin, and oxytocin receptors, all of which increase during gestation. Lesions of the POA will disrupt maternal behavior. The POA appears to be a region that receives olfactory and somatosensory input and has projections to midbrain and brain stem nuclei. Numan and Sheehan describe an elegant experiment that demonstrates the central role of the POA with maternal behavior. Postpartum rats were exposed to either pups or candy for 2-hours. Then their brains were analyzed for the presence

FIGURE 17.2 ● Blood levels of progesterone, estradiol, and prolactin in the pregnant rat. The changes that occur prior to delivery may influence maternal behavior. (Adapted from Rosenblatt JS, Siegel HI, Mayer AD. Blood levels of progesterone, estradiol and prolactin in pregnant rats. *Adv Study Behav.* 1979;10:225-311.)

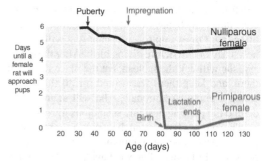

FIGURE 17.3 ● Female rats initially avoid pups. Several days of exposure are required for a nulliparous rat to display maternal behavior. Pregnant rats act similarly until after they deliver. (Adapted from Bridges RS. Endocrine regulation of parental behavior in rodents. In: Krasnegor NA, Bridges RS, eds. *Mammalian Parenting: Biochemical, Neurobiological and Behavioral Determinants*. New York, NY: Oxford University Press; 1990:93-117.)

of the transcription factor Fos. (Fos is used as a general marker of gene expression.)

Figure 17.4 shows the results of the study. This is a slice through the forebrain that includes the anterior hypothalamus on either side of the ventricle. (For a human comparison, see Figure 16.10.) Note the increased activation in the POA as well as other regions of the rat exhibiting maternal behavior.

Dopamine

Up to this point, we have stressed the importance of gonadal steroids and neuropeptides in the development of maternal behavior, but the neurotransmitter dopamine also appears to play an important role. We discussed in Chapter 12 the activation of the orbitofrontal cortex (OFC) and the ventral tegmental/nucleus accumbens area (see Figure 12.3) in the experience of pleasure. As might be expected, these areas are active in mothers.

One study scanned new mothers while they were looking at pictures of their own child and pictures of unfamiliar children. The mothers showed greater activation of the OFC when viewing their own child. With rats, researchers have found that mother rats will press a bar for access to pups the way they will press a bar for amphetamines or electrical stimulation. Additionally, pup exposure increases the release of dopamine at the nucleus accumbens. Alternatively, dopamine blockers will impair maternal behavior (see box). These studies give some neurobiologic explanations for the "joys of motherhood."

Licking and Grooming

This brings us to a series of studies from Michael Meaney's laboratory in McGill University, which may be some of the most important recent neuroscience studies for mental health professionals. These studies tie together maternal behavior with lasting effects on the offspring's behavior, hypothalamic-pituitary-adrenal (HPA) axis, and even their DNA.

The story starts in the 1960s when researchers noted that pups "handled" once a day during the first weeks of life showed a reduced adrenocorticotropic hormone and corticosterone response to stress. Later, it was established that it was not the "handling" per se that produced this effect, but the mother's increased licking of the pups when they

SCHIZOPHRENIA AND DOPAMINE BLOCKERS

Mothers who suffer from schizophrenia are known to be less involved with their children. They are generally more remote and less responsive during mother–infant play. This could be another example of the negative symptoms of the disorder. Worse yet, the problem might be exacerbated by the medications used to treat the patients.

In a recent study, Li et al. looked at the effect of injections of haloperidol, risperidone, and quetiapine on maternal behavior in rats. The antipsychotic medications inhibited maternal behaviors, such as nest building, pup licking, and pup retrieval. The figure shows the results for pup retrieval. Shortly after the injections, mothers failed to retrieve their own pups. Such studies suggest caution when treating human mothers with antipsychotic agents.

Antipsychotic medications disrupt a mother rat's tendency to retrieve her pups. (Adapted from Nelson RJ. *An Introduction to Behavioral Endocrinology*. 3rd ed. Sunderland, MA: Sinauer; 2005; Li M, Davidson P, Budin R, et al. Effects of typical and atypical antipsychotic drugs on maternal behavior in postpartum female rats. *Schizophr Res*. 2004;70(1):69-80.)

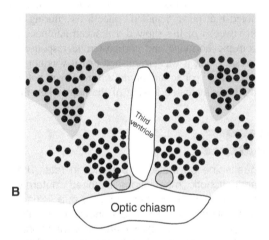

FIGURE 17.4 ● Hypothalamic region of postpartum rats exposed to candy (**A**) or newborn pups (**B**). Each dot represents five cells labeled with Fos activity—a measure of gene expression. VBST, ventral bed nucleus of the terminalis; POA, preoptic area. (Adapted from Numan M, Sheehan TP. Neuroanatomical circuitry for mammalian maternal behavior. *Ann N Y Acad Sci.* 1997;807:101-125.)

were returned to the nest. The mothers were simply trying to get the human odor off their pups and this extra attention to the pups resulted in their improved response to stress when they grew up to be adults.

Meaney discovered naturally occurring strains of rats that licked and groomed their pups at different rates. This particular behavior occurs when the mother rat enters the nest and gathers her pups around her for nursing. She will intermittently lick and groom the pups as they nurse. Meaney named one group the high lick and groom (high L and G) mothers and the other the low lick and groom (low L and G) mothers.

In a flurry of experiments in Meaney's laboratory, it was established that high L and G mothers produced offspring with subtle but significantly different brains. After 20 minutes of restraint (very stressful for a rodent), the rats from high L and G mothers secrete less corticosterone (Figure 17.5A). They also produce less corticotropin-releasing hormone messenger RNA (CRH-mRNA) in the hypothalamus (Figure 17.5B). Additionally, the amount of maternal licking and grooming correlates with the number of glucocorticoid receptors (GRs) in the hippocampus (Figure 17.5C). They literally produce more GRs as a result of enhanced gene expression.

In summary, a mother's increased attention enhances the sensitivity of the HPA axis most likely by turning on the appropriate DNA. Offspring of attentive high-licking mothers demonstrate greater feedback to the hypothalamus by way of the increased GRs, which inhibits CRH production and corticosterone release. Perhaps most significant, the pups from a high L and G mother show a greater willingness to explore novel environments as adults and demonstrate enhanced resilience under duress.

Trading Places
In a follow-up study, Meaney et al. switched some of the mothers and pups. That is, pups from high L and G mothers were raised by low L and G mothers and vice versa. The results were stunning and show how behaviors and patterns emerge from combinations of genetic predisposition and environment. Figure 17.6 shows the behavior of the adopted female rats raised by high L and G mothers once they matured. They were more inclined to explore an open area and provided greater licking and grooming to their own pups. Note how the determining factor is not the genetic makeup, but the nurturing behavior of the mother that raised them. In other words, a low L and G female will become a high L and G mother if she is raised by a high L and G mother. So the behavior can be passed from generation to generation, but it is not genetic—it is epigenetic.

Effect on the DNA
Meaney and his group have taken this line of research to the next level by searching for epigenetic mechanisms that can explain the enduring effects the mother's behavior has on the pups. Briefly, epigenetic molecular attachments on the DNA (see Figures 6.8 and 6.9) affect gene expression, which in turn alters the proteins produced—in this case the GR.

Meaney's group identified a section of the rat DNA that encodes for hippocampal GR. Looking specifically at the promoter region of this DNA—the region where the transcription starts—they analyzed methylation of the cytosine–guanine sites (CG sites).

FIGURE 17.5 ● Rats raised by a mother with a high frequency of licking and grooming behavior show a more modest corticosterone release in response to stress (**A**), less corticotropin-releasing hormone messenger RNA (CRH-mRNA) (**B**), and greater glucocorticoid receptors (GR) in the hippocampus. **C**. The correlation between GRs and licking and grooming by the mother. (Adapted from Liu D, Diorio J, Tannenbaum B, et al. Maternal care, hippocampal glucocorticoid receptors, and hypothalamic-pituitary-adrenal responses to stress. *Science*. 1997;277(5332):1659-1662.)

They found a much greater frequency of methylation for the low L and G group compared with the high L and G group along the GR promoter gene (Figure 17.7). In other words, the mother's attentive behavior reduced the methylation of the gene and allowed for greater production of the GR—which in turn made the rats more resilient. This is an excellent example of the neuroscience model (see Figure 6.13) showing how environment, gene expression, and brain development affect behavior.

The researchers conducted a follow-up study with their rats that is almost unbelievable. They administered directly into the cerebral ventricles an inhibitor (trichostatin A) that results in demethylation of the DNA (Figure 17.8A). These rats displayed less methylation of their DNA and, consequently, greater numbers of GRs. Furthermore, when stressed, these animals showed a modest HPA response (Figure 17.8B); that is, their corticosterone levels became indistinguishable from those of rats raised by a high L and G mother.

The implications from these studies are profound. We can now trace the effects of a mother's behavior down to the offspring's DNA. Furthermore, if we can find ways to cleanse the DNA, we might be able to correct psychiatric problems, not just treat symptoms. However, it is important to note that although demethylation may be the treatment of the future, it is not without risks. Some cancers are believed to result from demethylation of growth promoting genes—genes we do not want to inadvertently turn on.

What about in humans? Meaney and his colleagues recently analyzed the human equivalent of the promoter region of the glucocorticoid gene in cells from the hippocampus in a postmortem study of human brains. They compared suicide victims with a history of childhood abuse to two control groups both without a history of abuse—a control suicide group and a control sudden death, nonsuicide group. The suicide victims with a history of abuse had greater methylation of the glucocorticoid receptor gene compared with the nonabused controls. Additionally, as would be predicted, the mRNA transcribed from the GR gene was reduced in the subjects with a history of abuse. The human findings are consistent with the rat studies.

PAIR BONDING

The attraction between men and women is a special form of social attachment. In the short term, it is required for sexual reproduction; in the long run, bonded parents coordinate the rearing and protection of the offspring. Surprisingly, monogamous pair bonds are rare among mammals: approximately 5%. Monogamy is much more common among birds. The unusual bonding and rebonding that is common with humans might be best described as serial monogamy. The question for us is: what parts of the brain drive the affiliation of men and women?

Romantic Love and Dopamine

Romantic love is a universal human experience. The feeling of attraction that one person may feel for another can be intense, all-consuming, and difficult to control. A person in love feels euphoric. A spurned lover is despondent and even violent. The obsessional thinking and the willingness to "cross

A

Raised by high
L and G mothers

Raised by low
L and G mothers

Born to low
L and G mothers

Born to high
L and G mothers

B

Raised by high
L and G mothers

Raised by low
L and G mothers

FIGURE 17.6 ● Female rats raised by mothers who were high lickers and groomers are less anxious in an open area (**A**) and are more likely to be high lickers and groomers when raising their own pups (**B**)—regardless of their genetic lineage. L and G, lick and groom. (Adapted from Francis D, Diorio J, Liu D, et al. Nongenomic transmission across generations of maternal behavior and stress responses in the rat. *Science.* 1999;286(5442):1155-1158.)

mountains" to be with a lover suggest the activation of the brain's reward system (see Figure 12.6) when one is in love.

Anthropologist Helen Fisher at Rutgers University has spent her career studying the science of love. She and her colleagues scanned the brains of people who were "intensely in love." While undergoing magnetic resonance imaging (MRI), subjects were alternatively shown pictures of their beloved or a neutral individual and the differences were measured. As expected, the images of the beloved lit up the ventral tegmental area (VTA) (Figure 17.9A). The VTA is a dopamine-rich area

with projections to the nucleus accumbens. These are the subcortical regions that mediate motivation and reward.

Another area activated in the study was the caudate nucleus (CN) (Figure 17.9B). This area is also active in obsessive-compulsive disorder (see Figure 22.10). In the Fisher study, activity in the CN correlated with the total score on a test of the subject's feelings: the Passionate Love Scale. Therefore, in simple terms, we can conceptualize love as both an addiction and an obsession.

Growth Factors

A group in Italy—a country that knows a thing or two about romance—studied growth factors in subjects who had recently fallen in love. They speculated that nerve growth factors (NGFs) might be activated when people experience romantic feelings. They drew blood from subjects who recently fell "in love" and couples in long-lasting relationships. They measured the values of four growth factors. Only one—NGF—was significantly higher in the subjects recently in love. Moreover, there was a positive correlation between the level of NGF and the subject's score on the Passionate Love Scale.

Of particular interest, the researchers reexamined the levels of NGF a year or two later in the subjects in love. They found that the levels of NGF had dropped back to the levels seen in the control group (Figure 17.10). This is the neuroendocrine equivalent of what we all know: the honeymoon does not last. It is another example that the brain does not tolerate euphoria for too long. However, if the pleasure wanes, why do we stay in a relationship? In addition to psychological and practical answers, it may be that other neuropeptides kick in. Work with voles may shed some light on this.

Vasopressin

The vole is a rodent that looks like a plump mouse, but is related to the lemming. They are common in the grassy fields of North America. Voles are relevant to our discussion because of their diversity in forming pair bonds. For example, the *prairie vole* will form enduring pair bonds and mutually care for the offspring. In nature, most prairie voles that lose a mate never take on another partner. The closely related *meadow (mountain, montagne) vole*, on the other hand, is socially promiscuous and does not display biparental care.

In the laboratory, researchers have observed that prairie vole males prefer to spend time next to their partners: called *huddling* (see Figure 17.11A). The meadow vole, on the other hand, is more independent. With the proper arrangements, this behavior can be measured and quantitated (Figure 17.11B).

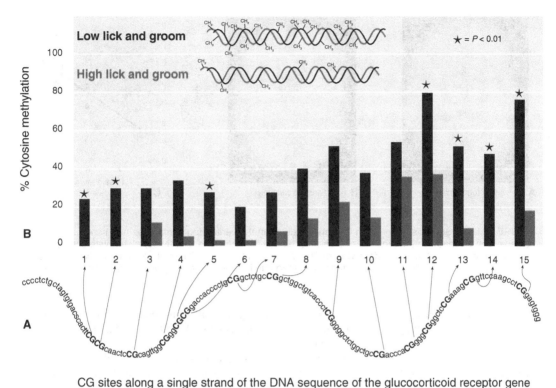

CG sites along a single strand of the DNA sequence of the glucocorticoid receptor gene

FIGURE 17.7 ● The presence of methyl groups attached to cytosine–guanine (CG) sites was assessed along the DNA of the rat glucocorticoid receptor (**A**). Pups from mothers who were high lickers and groomers had significantly less methylation of this section of DNA (**B**). (Adapted from Weaver IC, Cervoni N, Champagne FA, et al. Epigenetic programming by maternal behavior. *Nat Neurosci.* 2004;7(8):847-854.)

Vasopressin has emerged as a critical neuro-peptide mediating the pair bond formation in male voles. Infusion of vasopressin into the male cerebral ventricles accelerated pair bond formation. Likewise, infusion of a vasopressin antagonist prevents pair bond formation. Furthermore, differences in expressions of the vasopressin receptor can be demonstrated in the two species of voles (Figure 17.11C). The prairie vole has significantly more receptors in the ventral pallidum (VP).

FIGURE 17.8 ● Trichostatin A can remove the methyl groups from DNA (**A**). Rats from low L and G mothers who have been treated with trichostatin A display a normal hypothalamic-pituitary-adrenal response to stress (**B**). (**B** Adapted from Weaver IC, Cervoni N, Champagne FA, et al. Epigenetic programming by maternal behavior. *Nat Neurosci.* 2004;7(8):847-854.)

A   Ventral tegmental area   **B**   Caudate nucleus   **C**

FIGURE 17.9 ● Subjects intensely in love show activity in the ventral tegmental area (VTA) and caudate nucleus (CN) when looking at pictures of their lover (**A** and **B**). Activity in the CN correlated with scores on the Passionate Love Scale (**C**). (Adapted from Aron A, Fisher H, Mashek DJ, et al. Reward, motivation, and emotion systems associated with early-stage intense romantic love. *J Neurophysiol.* 2005;94(1):327-337.)

In a study that seems like something out of a science fiction novel, Young et al., through their experiments, have increased partner preference in meadow voles. They used a viral vector to transplant into the VP of meadow voles the segment of DNA that encodes for the vasopressin receptor. This resulted in increased expression of vasopressin receptors. The usually solitary meadow voles now were huddling with their partners. In essence, they

FIGURE 17.10 ● Nerve growth factor in subjects in long-lasting relationships, subjects actively "in love," and these same subjects a year or two later. The hearts on the NGF molecule are the authors' license.

changed a male from being promiscuous into being monogamous. (Won't the social conservatives be thrilled?)

With human men, we know that the endurance of pair bonding runs in families. In some families, the men partner-up for life, while in other families, the men act more like meadow voles. The role of VP in marital commitment is of great interest, but few studies have addressed the issue. One report in 2008 looked at variations of the vasopressin receptor 1a gene in over 500 pairs of Swedish twins, all of whom were married or living with a partner. Everyone answered a questionnaire on the quality of their relationship, which generated a score from 0 to 66 for each person—66 being marital bliss. Men, but not women, with one particular allele (called 334) had lower scores on the Partner Bonding Scale as measured by self-report as well as their wives' score. The results were small but statistically significant and suggest, as with the voles, that the neuropeptide vasopressin influences pair bonding duration in humans.

Oxytocin

Oxytocin and vasopressin are remarkably similar in structure and size (Figure 17.12A). The body and brain, fortunately, recognize the subtle differences and produce distinct responses to these messengers. They are synthesized in the hypothalamus and permeate out into the body and brain by three mechanisms. The best known of these is the release of the molecules into the general circulation from the posterior pituitary (Figure 17.12B). Additionally, the molecules are released from the dendrites of the neurons and diffuse throughout the brain (dashed arrows; Figure 17.12C). Finally, small neurons

Prairie vole

Meadow vole

Time spent huddling (min)

Huddling with partner

Huddling with stranger

VP

FIGURE 17.11 ● The male prairie vole will spend more time huddling with his partner than does the meadow vole (**A** and **B**). The difference in vasopressin receptors (dark areas in (**C**)) in the ventral pallidum (VP) may explain the difference in this behavior. (From Lim MM, Wang Z, Olazabal DE, et al. Enhanced partner preference in a promiscuous species by manipulating the expression of a single gene. *Nature*. 2004;429:754-757.)

project from the hypothalamus to areas such as the anterior cingulate, nucleus accumbens, and amygdala, as well as others. The essential point is that oxytocin and vasopressin are hormones as well as neurotransmitters with diverse methods of transmission and effects on physiology and behavior.

In the lay press, oxytocin is affectionately called the "cuddle hormone" since oxytocin levels are elevated with childbirth, breast-feeding, and an orgasm—all circumstances in which a woman is prone to bond with another human. In one frequently cited study, which may be the source of

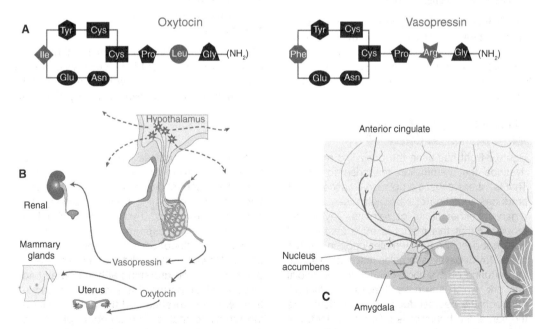

FIGURE 17.12 ● Oxytocin and vasopressin (**A**) are simple proteins consisting of nine amino acids. These neuropeptides are excreted into the pituitary circulation (**B**), diffuse into the brain from the dendrites of the cells (**C**), and are released by small neurons at several locations around the brain.

FIGURE 17.13 ● Oxytocin levels increase in women 7 minutes after cuddling with their partner. (Adapted from Grewen KM, Girdler SS, Amico J, et al. Effects of partner support on resting oxytocin, cortisol, norepinephrine, and blood pressure before and after warm partner contact. *Psychosomatic Med.* 2005;67:531-538.)

the "cuddle hormone" term, oxytocin significantly jumped in women after 10 minutes of "warm contact" with her spouse or partner, but did not change in men (Figure 17.13). Subsequent research using intranasal oxytocin (because it cannot be administered orally) has shown that it:

– improves positive communication between couples,
– increases trusting behavior,
– produces more positive responses of fathers toward toddlers,
– and in general enhances emotional recognition and responsiveness to others.

Brain imaging studies suggest that oxytocin may, in part, improve social interactions by dampening the amygdala/cingulate circuit—a circuit known to be activated in fearful circumstances. It might be that trust and social comfort are increased with less social anxiety.

Enduring Bonds

A simple understanding of human male–female affiliation proposes that it all starts with dopamine and the pleasure centers of the brain. We speculate that other neuroendocrine systems such as oxytocin and vasopressin may then take over to ensure enduring pair bond formation once "the thrill is gone." While there are no data to support this as yet, twin studies suggest monogamy has biological roots. We wonder if those individuals who are prone to stay in one relationship are genetically more endowed with the neuropeptides of attachment.

DISCONNECTED

Affiliation and pair bonding are on one end of the social attachment spectrum. On the other end are those individuals who are isolated and disconnected—individuals who are aloof, distant, and fail to derive pleasure from social interactions. The Unabomber is an extreme example of this sort of person. A graduate of Harvard, with a Ph.D. in mathematics, he lived alone for 16 years in a 10 foot by 12 foot cabin in the woods of Montana without electricity or plumbing. A psychiatrist conducting a court evaluation of the Unabomber gave him a provisional diagnosis of schizophrenia.

The schizophrenic spectrum disorders include the following:

• Schizotypal personality disorder
• Schizoid personality disorder
• Delusional disorder
• Schizoaffective disorder
• Schizophrenia

These comprise a large percentage of the cases of socially disconnected individuals seen in most clinical practices. The impairment in social skills these individuals have, part of the negative signs

TEND-AND-BEFRIEND

Fight-or-flight has been the prevailing model to describe the mammalian response to stress. That is, stress causes a hormonal cascade that produces secretion of catecholamines and the organism either fights or retreats. Taylor has proposed that this model is male centric and does not describe how females cope in difficult times. Taylor believes females respond to stress by nurturing others and enhancing their social network, which she calls "tend-and-befriend." Although the neuroendocrine mechanisms are the same, the behavior is different. In fact, the gender difference in affiliation is one of the most robust findings in human behavioral research.

Engh et al. provide an example from a free-ranging troop of baboons in Africa that they have been following. They have observed and recorded grooming behavior among the females. They found that females who lost a close relative experienced a significant increase in glucocorticoid levels after the death. However, they did not experience a decrease in their grooming although they had lost their close partner. Instead, other associations were established and the rate of grooming remained stable. The authors speculated that this social networking might modulate the stress response.

of schizophrenia, is possibly the most troubling aspect of the illness for unaffected family members—something is missing and no treatment will bring it all back. Very little is known about the neuroanatomic deficits that contribute to the social aspect of the illnesses. However, as we will see in Chapter 23, it has been hard to define any biological deficits that explain the basic condition.

Autism Spectrum

Kanner first described autism in 1943 at Johns Hopkins University. We now envision autism as anchoring the more extreme end of a spectrum of disorders characterized by the following:

• Severe social dysfunctions
• Early communication failure
• Presence of repetitive, rigid, and stereotypic behaviors

Asperger's disorder and childhood disintegrative disorder are other conditions in the autism spectrum, which are believed to share common biologic foundations. These conditions may simply be a less severe form of the underlying disorder.

The social dysfunctions constitute the core deficits of the disorders. The inability to understand other people's feelings and a failure to establish reciprocal relationships emerge early in those with autism.

Robert Schultz et al. at Yale have developed techniques to study this aspect of autism. They used eye tracking technology to study spontaneous viewing patterns while watching video clips of complex social situations. They showed clips from the 1967 movie "Who's Afraid of Virginia Woolf?" to subjects with autism and to age- and IQ-matched normal controls.

Figure 17.14 shows a drawing of one scene from the movie. In the foreground, two adults lean toward each other in a flirtatious interchange. The woman's husband is in the background, silent, but irritated by his wife's behavior. The eye movements from a control (brown) and an autistic subject (black) are collapsed onto this one scene. Note how the healthy control subject focuses on the eyes of the actors. Additionally, the control's focus moves from face to face, literally outlining the charged social triangle.

The autistic subject, on the other hand, attends to less relevant aspects of the scene. This subject displays the following three findings commonly seen in subjects with autism:

• Avoidance of the eyes
• Focus on the mouth
• Preferential attention to objects rather than people

Clearly, this method of observation fails to gather the subtle social cues that are essential to understand

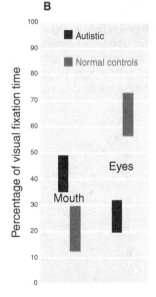

FIGURE 17.14 ● A drawing of a scene from "Who's Afraid of Virginia Woolf" shows the different aspects of the movie that subjects with autism (*black*) and normal controls (*brown*) track with their eyes (**A**). A study comparing 15 patients with autism and 15 controls demonstrated significant differences in time spent observing the eyes and mouths from similar film clips (**B**). (Adapted from Klin A, Jones W, Schultz R, et al. Visual fixation patterns during viewing of naturalistic social situations as predictors of social competence in individuals with autism. *Arch Gen Psychiatry*. 2002;59(9):809-816; Klin A, Jones W, Schultz R, et al. Defining and quantifying the social phenotype in autism. *Am J Psychiatry*. 2002;159(6):895-908.)

the thoughts and feelings of other people. A quantitative assessment of the subject's visual fixation on the eyes and mouths is shown in the graph on the right side of Figure 17.14. Note the dramatic separation between the groups with regard to eye fixation. A finding this large is seldom found in behavioral studies.

Brain Size

The underlying neuroanatomic abnormalities of autism remain unknown. One consistent finding has been enlarged brain volume. In a meta-analysis, Redcay and Courchesne collected studies measuring head circumference and brain size with MRI. They calculated the percent difference from the normal for each study so that the measurements could be compared. The results are plotted by age in Figure 17.15. The authors noted that for autism the brain size is initially reduced, dramatically increases within the first year of life, but then returns to the normal range by adulthood. These findings show a period of pathologic brain growth in autism that is largely restricted to the first 2 years of life.

The phenomenon of abnormal growth in the first years of life mirrors what some parents have reported about their children, namely, that they appeared to be developing normally for the first 15 to 24 months and then showed a regression in social and/or communication skills. In a clever use of technology, Werner and Dawson had blinded observers review home video tapes of autistic children who were reported to have regressed. Indeed, they noted normal social attention and word babble at 12 months of age, but displayed significant impairment by 24 months. This was in contrast to

the group of children with early-onset autism who showed impairment at 12 and 24 months of age.

Medical treatments have failed to provide any consistent benefit for the core features of autism. This is likely true because medical interventions fail to correct the synaptic dysregulation that is believed to be the underlying problem of the disorder. However, intensive behavior modification has been shown to be partially effective. One recent study with children aged 18 to 30 months found that 2 years of 20-hours a week therapist-led treatment (plus homework with the parents on the weekends) resulted in an increase in IQ of almost 18 points compared with 7 for the control group. Additionally, almost 30% in the treatment group were reclassified to a less severe form of autism after 2 years, while only 5% in the control group received a similar upgrade. These results are consistent with a basic tenet of this book—that environmental interactions (in this case B-Mod) can change the brain—possibly "rewire" some of the synaptic errors, especially when the changes are introduced early in life when the brain is more plastic and developing.

Mirror Neurons

Mirror neurons were discovered in one of those beautiful serendipitous scientific moments. Researchers in Italy placed an electrode in a neuron in a monkey's motor cortex and noted that it was active when he grabbed an object. Much to their amazement, it also became active when the monkey watched someone else grabbing the same object. They called these neurons *mirror neurons* and found that they are not uncommon in the brain. Figure 17.16 shows an example of a mirror neuron. Note that the neuron

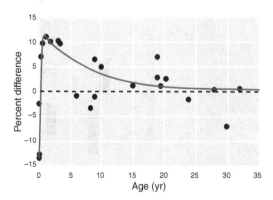

FIGURE 17.15 ● A meta-analysis of brain measurements including head circumference and magnetic resonance imaging scans are plotted by percent difference from norm and age. (Adapted from Redcay E, Courchesne E. When is the brain enlarged in autism? A meta-analysis of all brain size reports. Biol Psychiatry. 2005;58(1):1-9.)

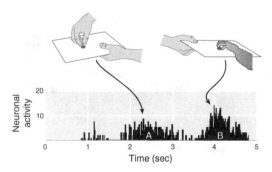

FIGURE 17.16 ● A neuron in the premotor cortex of a monkey is active when it observes a food morsel grasped by a human (**A**). The same neuron is active when the monkey grasps the morsel (**B**). (Adapted from Rizzolatti G, Fogassi L, Gallese V. Neurophysiological mechanisms underlying the understanding and imitation of action. *Nat Rev Neurosci.* 2001;2(9):661-670.)

is active both when a human (A) grasps the object and when the monkey (B) grasps the same object. However, the mirroring does not translate to all actions. If the object is grasped with pliers, the neuron does not become active.

Functional imaging studies on humans have also demonstrated mirroring. For example, a person moving a finger or observing a finger move will show similar activity in the same region of the motor cortex. Another study looked for mirroring with facial expressions. In this study, subjects were shown pictures of people displaying emotional expressions (happy, sad, angry, etc.). The subjects were instructed to either imitate the expression or just observe the picture. Figure 17.17 shows that imitating the expression and just observing it generated similar activity in the premotor region of the cortex, as measured by the functional MRI.

Additional research by this same group has identified a network of neurons connecting the frontal, parietal, and temporal lobes. Furthermore, they found that imitating emotional facial expressions not only activated this network but also activated the emotional centers of the brain, such as the insula and the amygdala. The capacity to reflect another person's emotions may be the neuronal mechanism facilitating empathy. It may be this system that is impaired in disconnected individuals.

Dysfunction of the mirror neuronal network may underlie the lack of empathy in patients with autism. To test this hypothesis, researchers conducted similar facial imitation and observation studies with high functioning autistic children and normally developing children matched for age and IQ. Their results showed a marked decrease in activation of the mirror neuronal network in the children with autism, particularly in the frontal cortex (Figure 17.18A, B). Additional analysis showed that activity in the frontal cortex during the study correlated with the score on the social subscale of the Autistic Diagnostic Interview (Figure 17.18C).

A Normally developing group

B Autistic group

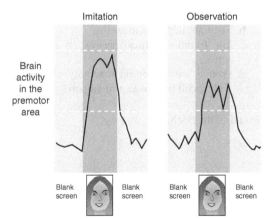

FIGURE 17.17 ● Activity in the facial region of the motor cortex is similar, as measured by functional magnetic resonance imaging, when subjects are imitating a facial expression or just observing it. (Adapted from Carr L, Iacoboni M, Dubeau MC, et al. Neural mechanisms of empathy in humans: a relay from neural systems for imitation to limbic areas. *Proc Natl Acad Sci U S A*. 2003;100(9):5497-5502.)

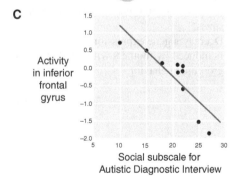

FIGURE 17.18 ● Functional MRI studies for normally developing preteens compared with high functioning age-/IQ-matched subjects with autism while imitating emotional facial expressions. The subjects with autism show less activity of the mirror neuronal network, particularly in the frontal cortex. (Adapted from Dapretto M, Davies MS, Pfeifer JH, et al. Understanding emotions in others: mirror neuron dysfunction in children with autism spectrum disorders. *Nat Neurosci*. 2006;9(1):28-30.)

The propensity to empathize with other's feelings is one of the central features of human social interactions. Individuals with autism are impaired in this ability. Failing to understand the emotions in others may be a result of deficient mirror neurons in patients with autism spectrum disorders. Whether this neuronal failure is the central deficit of the disorder, a downstream effect of some other problem, or just one of a host of deficits remains to be determined.

QUESTIONS

1. Which combination of hormones is believed to trigger maternal behavior in rats just before delivery?
   a. Rising progesterone and rising estradiol.
   b. Rising progesterone and falling estradiol.
   c. Falling progesterone and rising estradiol.
   d. Falling progesterone and falling estradiol.

2. Oxytocin receptors are found in all of the following, except
   a. Uterus.
   b. PVN.
   c. POA.
   d. Optic chiasm.

3. Pups born to mothers who are high lickers and groomers show
   a. Increased reluctance to explore a novel environment.
   b. Increased GRs in the hippocampus.
   c. Increased CRH during stress.
   d. Increased corticosterone when restrained.

4. Lightly methylated DNA
   a. Allows greater access to transcription factors.
   b. Results in greater glucocorticoid response to stress.
   c. Decreases gene expression.
   d. Is induced by mothers with low licking and grooming behavior.

5. Romantic love has a strong correlation with activity in the
   a. VTA.
   b. CN.
   c. Nucleus accumbens.
   d. Amygdala.

6. All of the following are false, except
   a. Vasopressin promotes pair bonding in male voles.
   b. Meadow voles have more vasopressin.
   c. Transplanting oxytocin receptors induces monogamous behavior in male voles.
   d. Tend-and-befriend behavior modulates dips in oxytocin.

7. Eye tracking studies have shown that autistic subjects
   a. Focus on the eyes.
   b. Avoid looking at objects.
   c. Attend to the subtle social cues.
   d. Prefer to look at the lower face.

8. All of the following are true about mirror neurons, except
   a. They play a role in empathy.
   b. They are impaired in autism.
   c. The frontosubcortical network is the most active.
   d. Frontal mirror neuron inactivity correlates with social impairment in autism.

See Answers section at the end of the book.

CHAPTER 18

Memory

The next three chapters review important aspects of cognition. *Cognition* is loosely defined as the ability to do the following:

- Attend to external or internal stimuli
- Identify the significance of the stimuli
- Respond appropriately

This complex processing takes place in the cortices of the brain. It occurs between the arrival of sensory input and the behavioral reaction. In the next two chapters, we discuss intelligence and attention. Here we start with memory.

The ability to store information and access it at some future point is one of the most fascinating aspects of the brain. Indeed, some of the first experiments in psychology were research into learning and memory, which continues to be aggressively studied in modern neuroscience. *Learning* is defined as new information acquired by the nervous system and observed through behavioral changes. *Memory* describes encoding, storage, and retrieval of learned information.

TYPES OF MEMORY

Experts in memory have identified different types and subtypes of memory. Many of these subtle distinctions are not relevant for our purposes. One important distinction is separating memory of details from learning procedures. The facts we learn in school or historic events from our lives are called *declarative memory* (also called *explicit memory*). This is usually what people are referring to when they speak of memory.

Procedural memory is *nondeclarative memory* (also called *implicit memory or somatic memory*). It describes the process of learning a skill or making associations. Examples include learning to ride a bike or playing a musical instrument. This type of memory is outside the conscious thought and

actually can deteriorate if one concentrates too hard. Another example includes the exaggerated startle response seen with post-traumatic stress disorder. This reaction is immediate and takes place before the subject is consciously aware of the stimulus.

The importance of separating declarative from nondeclarative memory is that these two types of memory are encoded through different mechanisms in the brain. Likewise, they are disrupted by different central nervous system lesions or disorders—more on this later.

Immediate, Short, and Long

Memories begin to decay as soon as they are formed. The temporal stages of retention are divided into immediate, short term, and long term (Figure 18.1). These are the stages we test in a comprehensive mental status examination. *Immediate memory* describes the ability to hold a few new facts in mind for a matter of seconds. Looking up a new phone number and successfully dialing the number within seconds is an example of this. We test this function when we ask a person to repeat three objects immediately. Another test of immediate memory is asking a patient to repeat a series of numbers. The average maximum "digit span" is seven numbers plus or minus two.

Short-term memory describes those memories that exist from seconds to minutes. An example of this process is searching the house for a lost item and remembering where you have looked. We test this process when we ask a patient to repeat three objects at 5 minutes. Both immediate and short-term memories are vulnerable to disruption.

Long-term memories are enduring representations that last for days, months, and years: the historic events and facts of our lives. This requires the development of a more permanent form of storage.

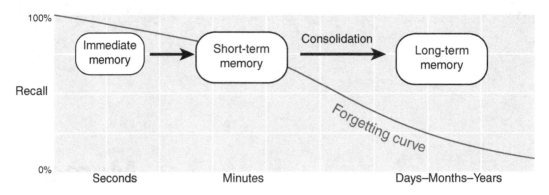

FIGURE 18.1 ● The temporal stages of memory superimposed on a hypothetical curve of memory retention.

The process of moving information from immediate and short-term into long-term memories is called *consolidation*. The physical representation of memories and the areas of the brain dedicated to this function are the focus of this chapter—what do memories look like in the brain, how are they stored, and how do they fade?

CELLULAR MECHANISMS

The Canadian psychologist Donald O. Hebb proposed in 1949 that some changes must take place between two neurons for memories to develop. He wrote as follows:

> When an axon of cell A is near enough to excite a cell B and repeatedly or persistently takes part in firing it, some growth process or metabolic change takes place in one or both cells such that A's efficacy, as one of the cells firing B is increased.

ALCOHOLIC BLACKOUTS

Alcoholic blackouts occur when someone has consumed too much alcohol and awakens without memories of what happened the night before. It is believed that the high blood level of alcohol disrupts the consolidation of short-term memories into long-term memories. The drinker failed to preserve lasting images of the party because long-term memories were never formed. This can happen with short-acting hypnotics and benzodiazepines as well.

Amazingly, memories formed before drinking are actually enhanced by alcohol. That is, drinking after learning improves recall compared with not drinking. It is possible that memories already consolidated remain in a more pristine state, because there is less interference from new memories that are never fully formed during the drinking.

This has come to be called *Hebb's postulate* and can be more easily stated like this: neurons that fire together, wire together. Almost 60 years of research has affirmed that the brain changes with learning and experience.

Long-Term Potentiation

In Chapter 5, we discussed long-term potentiation (LTP), a laboratory procedure with slices of brain tissue that serves as a model for memory formation. In summary:

- A series of rapid signals between two neurons results in a greater stimulus in the postsynaptic neuron when normal activity resumes (see Figure 5.6).
- Increased activity between two glutamate neurons will open the *N*-methyl-D-aspartate (NMDA) receptor, which results in molecular signals to the nucleus that induce gene expression (see Figure 5.7).
- Gene expression results in structural changes on the neuron such as spine formation on the dendrites (see Figure 5.8).

Protein Synthesis

Real memories in mammals, like LTP, require gene expression and protein synthesis for consolidation. For example, a rat can be taught to quickly find a submerged platform in a tub of water—called a *water maze* (see Figure 18.2A, B). However, if one group of rats is given intraventricular injections of the protein synthesis inhibitor *anisomycin* 20 minutes before each test, they cannot remember the location of the submerged platform from one session to the next. These rats spend about the same amount of time each day trying to find the submerged platform (Figure 18.2C). Anisomycin inhibits the production of proteins that are needed to consolidate short-term memories into long-term memories.

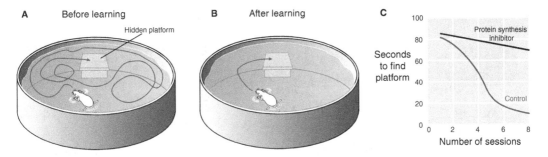

FIGURE 18.2 ● A rat will learn the location of a hidden platform after several sessions in a pool of water. However, rats given a protein synthesis inhibitor fail to learn (**C**). (Adapted from Bear MF, Connors BW, Paradiso MA, eds. *Neuroscience: Exploring the Brain.* 3rd ed. Baltimore, MD: Lippincott Williams & Wilkins; 2007; Meiri N, Rosenblum K. Lateral ventricle injection of the protein synthesis inhibitor anisomycin impairs long-term memory in a spatial memory task. *Brain Res.* 1998;789(1):48-55.)

Epigenetics

A new line of research suggests that epigenetic mechanisms may play a role in memory formation. As discussed in Chapter 6, acetylation of the histones can open up access to the DNA and allow greater gene expression (see Figure 6.9), and we know gene expression is required for protein synthesis. Several laboratories have shown that fear memory, for example, is associated with acetylation of histone H3 in the hippocampus. Likewise, inhibition of the deacetylase enzymes elevated histone acetylation and enhanced long-term memory formation.

In 2009, a group at the Massachusetts Institute of Technology (MIT) established a link among histone acetylase inhibition, memory formation, and synaptic plasticity. They were able to show with mice that overexpression of the inhibitor (so there was less acetylation, more tightly closed DNA, and less gene expression) resulted in decreased dendritic spine density, synapse number, synaptic plasticity, and memory formation. Conversely, deficiencies of the acetylase inhibitor (more acetylation—more gene expression) resulted in increased synapse number and memory facilitation. These studies establish an epigenetic mechanism for the formation of long-term memories and suggest possible future sites for intervention for those with memory impairment.

Extinction

Extinction is the gradual reduction in the response to a feared stimulus when the stimulus is repeatedly encountered without an adverse experience. For example, a person who is afraid of bridges will have a reduction in fear if they repeatedly cross the bridge without falling off or the bridge collapsing. Extinction is the bedrock of behavioral therapy and one of the most effective treatments for anxiety disorders.

Several lines of evidence suggest that extinction is accomplished through the development of new memories rather than erasing the old memories.

Studies have established this by looking at the effect of anisomycin on extinction. Rats given intraventricular injections of anisomycin before repeated exposure to a stimulus (without the negative consequences) fail to show extinction the following day. In other words, the new learning did not erase the old memories.

Faster Extinction?

Would faster learning during extinction therapy improve the effectiveness of exposure and response prevention therapy? A group at Emory University is studying just this possibility. Using the understanding of how memories are formed, they proposed that an NMDA agonist might increase the signal to the nucleus, increase the gene expression, and increase learning. The reader should remember that the glutamate neurons (the most common neurons in the brain) have several different types of receptors. Opening the NMDA receptor as well as the α-amino-3-hydroxy-5-methyl-4-isoxazole propionate receptor increases the excitatory postsynaptic potential and the signal to the nucleus (see Figure 5.2).

Researchers at Emory developed a virtual reality simulator that gives participants the sensation of riding an elevator with a glass floor. Patients with fear of heights can extinguish much of their anxiety with many sessions in this device. D-cycloserine, an antibiotic used to treat tuberculosis, is also a partial agonist at the NMDA receptor. D-cycloserine will open the NMDA receptor and the postsynaptic nucleus will receive a heightened signal (see Figure 18.3). The Emory group gave patients D-cycloserine or placebo before just two sessions in the virtual elevator and found a 50% reduction in fear with those on the active medication (Figure 18.3C).

Further research after this study supports the use of D-cycloserine as a "cognitive enhancer" for psychological treatment of anxiety disorders. Studies with social anxiety disorder and panic disorder have shown that D-cycloserine was superior to

FIGURE 18.3 ● **A.** Activity at the AMPA receptor is insufficient to generate gene expression. **B.** D-cycloserine opens the NMDA receptor and can generate a strong signal to the nucleus. **C.** A study using D-cycloserine and just two sessions of virtual exposure therapy showed a marked reduction in fear of heights. AMPA, α-amino-3-hydroxy-5-methyl-4-isoxazole propionate; NMDA, N-methyl-D-aspartate. (Adapted from Ressler KJ, Rothbaum BO, Tannenbaum L, et al. Cognitive enhancers as adjuncts to psychotherapy: use of D-cycloserine in phobic individuals to facilitate extinction of fear. *Arch Gen Psychiatry*. 2004;61(11):1136-1144.)

placebo when added to cognitive-behavioral therapy. The results for obsessive-compulsive disorder were less impressive. These studies suggest that the right medications administered in conjunction with psychotherapy may improve the learning that seems essential for effective psychological treatment. This may lead to a whole new approach to treating mental illness where exposure, behavior, and cognitive and talking therapies are paired with the appropriate medication or device to produce faster, better, or more durable therapeutic changes.

Structural Plasticity

Some memories last an entire lifetime. These long-term memories persist despite surgical anesthesia, epileptic seizures, and drug abuse. Protein molecules are not stable enough to survive these insults. Therefore, long-term memories must be the result of more stable formations such as structural changes (as seen with LTP) or they might be continuously rebuilt throughout one's life. In Chapter 8, we discussed several examples of cortical strengthening secondary to learning and practicing, for example, monkeys spinning a wheel (see Figure 8.13) and humans playing a

musical instrument (see Figure 8.15). These studies show that the cortex changes with learning.

Synaptogenesis

One mechanism that could explain learning-associated changes in the cortical structure is some type of synaptic growth. Indeed, there is considerable evidence showing that learning increases branching and synapse formation. We have already discussed that rats living in an enriched environment show greater branching and spine formation on their hippocampal neurons (see Point of Interest box page 28).

Spines are the small protrusions on the shaft of the dendrite. They are believed to represent the formation of new synapses, thereby increasing communication between neighboring neurons. It has long been suggested that new spines are involved in memory formation. Leuner et al. tested this theory by teaching rats to blink in anticipation of a puff of air to the eye. Twenty-four hours later, they found that the conditioned rats showed a 27% increase in spine formation on the pyramidal cells from the hippocampus. The reader can perceive the structural difference in the examples in Figure 18.4.

FIGURE 18.4 ● Rats taught to blink when a sound preceded a puff of air to their eyes showed greater spine density 24 hours later. (From Leuner B, Falduto J, Shors TJ. Associative memory formation increases the observation of dendritic spines in the hippocampus. *J Neurosci*. 2003;23(2):659-665.)

Additionally, these changes were blocked with an NMDA antagonist. Therefore, new memories correlate with new spines.

Neurogenesis

Another mechanism that could explain the development of stable memories which can last a human life span is the formation of new neurons. We now know that new neurons are regularly developed throughout adulthood. We have seen that rats exposed to an enriched environment, for example, also showed greater neurogenesis (see Figure 8.5). Are the new neurons produced to hold memories of the enriched environment?

Recently, Leuner et al., again teaching rats to anticipate a puff of air, looked at learning and neurogenesis. They found that those animals that showed a better performance with the task also had more new neurons surviving several days after the instruction. In other words, the greater the mastery of the skill, the greater the number of newly developing neurons that survived.

Perhaps the most compelling data regarding learning and neurogenesis come from Nottemohm and his work with songbirds (see Figure 16.9). We

hope the readers have stored in their long-term memory from Chapter 16 that Nottemohm established that male canaries have a sexually dimorphic brain region called the *high vocal center* (HVC), which is directly involved in song production. Further, the HVC fluctuates in size during the year with seasonal changes in the reproductive hormones.

The relevance of the HVC for this chapter has to do with learning new songs and the changes in the HVC. The male canary changes his song repertoire over the course of 12 months by adding new notes and discarding others. Additionally, the number of new neurons added to the HVC fluctuates throughout the year. Of particular interest, the addition of new song notes and new neurons correlates (Figure 18.5). Although not proven, it appears that the memory of the songs come and go with the development and loss of neurons in the HVC.

Reconsolidation

Until recently, the prevailing belief about memories was that once consolidated they were resistant to change. That is, convulsions, protein synthesis inhibitors, or head trauma cannot erase long-term memories. However, Nader et al. produced a study suggesting that long-term memories can return to a labile state, vulnerable to disruption, before being consolidated again. This phenomenon is called *reconsolidation*. The essential feature of reconsolidation is that the memory must be reactivated for this process to occur.

To understand reconsolidation, it is important to understand the details of the study. First, rats are taught to associate a sound with an adverse stimulation, like a foot shock. When the rats hear the sound again, they "freeze"—a sign of fear in rodents. The researchers can quantify the percent of time the animals spend "frozen." Then the rats are exposed to the sound without the foot shock,

FIGURE 18.5 ● The development of new neurons correlates with the development of new song syllables. (Adapted from Kirn J, O'Loughlin B, Kasparian S, et al. Cell death and neuronal recruitment in the high vocal center of adult male canaries are temporally related to changes in song. *Proc Natl Acad Sci U S A*. 1994;91(17):7844-7848.)

STRESS AND MEMORY

Although not necessarily accurate, singularly traumatic experiences are known to produce long-lasting, intense memories. Chronic stress, on the other hand, corrupts the memory storage process. Humans given stress levels of cortisol demonstrate impaired declarative memory within days. As discussed in Chapter 7, the likely mechanism is excess glucocorticoids causing atrophy of hippocampal dendrites, shrinking the hippocampus, and decreasing hippocampal neurogenesis.

but this time they receive the protein synthesis inhibitor anisomycin injected directly into their amygdala. Amazingly, when tested again, they do not "freeze." In other words, they show no fear. They appear to have forgotten what they learned. By analogy it is as though the long-term memory was ice, which melts to water when reactivated, and then freezes again in the reconsolidation process—but now in a different shape.

While there is still much to be learned about reconsolidation, it provides a possible explanation for some of the healing power of psychotherapy. Do patients reactivate their memories in the course of telling their stories? However, because the patient is now in a safe environment, the memory can be reconsolidated without as much negative effect. Hopefully, this is true and can be further understood in the future as a way to improve the effectiveness of psychotherapy.

ORGANIZATION OF DECLARATIVE MEMORY

One of the great mysteries of neuroscience involves finding the location of long-term declarative memories. Where are they stored in the brain? How are they formed and why do they decay? Unfortunately, there are only basic explanations for these intriguing questions.

Hippocampus

The hippocampus (see Figure 2.6) is crucial for consolidation of long-term memories. The importance of the hippocampus became painfully obvious with the famous case of H.M. H.M. had struggled with minor seizures since the age of 10 and major seizures since the age of 16. Despite aggressive anticonvulsant medications, the seizures increased in frequency and ultimately the patient was unable to work. In 1953, at the age of 27, H.M. underwent a large bilateral resection of the medial temporal lobes

in an effort to remove the nidus of the seizures. Figure 18.6 shows the areas of the brain removed.

The surgery successfully quieted the seizures, but unfortunately left H.M. with profound anterograde amnesia. Although his personality remained the same and his IQ even improved a bit from 104 to 112, he displayed severe and pervasive memory impairments. Specifically, he showed a normal immediate memory, but could not consolidate those memories into enduring traces. For example, when a person exited and reentered his room within a few minutes, H.M. was unaware of that person's earlier visit. However, his remote memories remained intact. In fact, he would frequently speak of events before the surgery, in part because he was not developing new memories. To use a computer metaphor, it is as though H.M. has a "read only" hard drive for memory storage. He can retrieve old memories but cannot write new ones.

This unfortunate outcome for H.M. highlighted the essential role of the medial temporal lobe in forming long-term memories. Subsequent studies with animals and humans have established the hippocampus and the parahippocampal gyrus as crucial for encoding and consolidating memories of events and objects in time and space. For example, numerous studies have shown that lesions of a rat's hippocampus impair its ability to remember the location of the hidden platform in a water maze.

Further studies with H.M. established that the amnesia was not as widespread as initially perceived. For example, H.M. was asked to participate in a mirror tracing task. While viewing his hand in a mirror, H.M. was asked to trace a star while keeping the pencil between the lines. H.M. improved at this task in 10 trials on the first day (Figure 18.7). He did even better on the second and third days. Remarkably, when asked about the task, he stated he had never seen the test before. This highlights what we addressed at the beginning of the chapter:

FAULTY EYEWITNESS IDENTIFICATION AND RECONSOLIDATION

DNA technology has opened a window on some major errors in the criminal justice system. Hundreds of inmates have been released from jails and prisons when the DNA evidence showed that they could not have committed the crime. Eyewitness identification errors account for the largest single cause of wrongful incarcerations. Even more amazing, some eyewitnesses refuse to accept the DNA evidence. They persist in believing their identification.

Although there are many reasons a memory can be wrong, reconsolidation may explain the persistence in maintaining an inaccurate identification. It is possible that the victim, when confronted with the lineup, reactivates the memory of the crime. At that moment the memory returned to a labile state, which was then reconsolidated, but now with the face of the wrong culprit.

FIGURE 18.6 ● Two views of H.M.'s brain identifying the areas that were removed in surgery, which left him with anterograde amnesia. (Adapted from Bear MF, Connors BW, Paradiso MA, eds. *Neuroscience: Exploring the Brain*. 3rd ed. Baltimore, MD: Lippincott Williams & Wilkins; 2007.)

there are different types of memory. H.M.'s explicit memory is disrupted, but his implicit memory remains intact. Consequently, this type of memory must be stored through different mechanisms—ones that are independent of the hippocampus.

H.M. died in December 2008. Studies shortly before his death showed that his declarative memory deficit is not as absolute as previously thought.

For example, he was able to draw a reasonably accurate floor plan of his house, although he had moved there 5 years after his operation. Likewise, when he looked in a mirror he was not startled by his appearance. This suggests that some declarative memories are being stored. Whether this is due to some residual hippocampal tissue or through other mechanisms is not known.

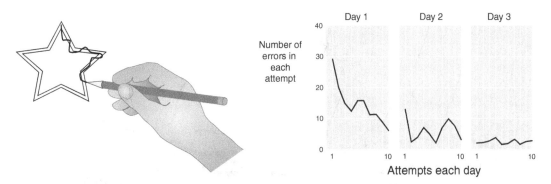

FIGURE 18.7 ● The mirror tracing task asks subjects to trace between two stars while watching their hand in a mirror. The patient H.M. showed improvement at this task although he had no recollection of having taken the test before. (Adapted from Kandel ER, Schwartz JH, Jessell TM, eds. *Principles of Neural Science*. 4th ed. New York, NY: McGraw-Hill; 2000.)

MEMORY AND PLEASURE

We discussed in Chapter 12 that memories associated with getting high could induce cravings in drug addicts. Conversely, it is well documented that pleasure enhances learning. Indeed, dopamine neurons from the ventral tegmental area directly innervate the medial temporal lobe. Recent brain imaging studies have shown simultaneous activation of the ventral tegmental area and medial temporal lobe when subjects are remembering rewarding experiences.

Neocortex

Sensory information comes into the brain and is processed in specific regions of the neocortex. The parahippocampal gyrus receives afferent projections from these cortical areas. The hippocampus has efferent projections back to these cortical regions, which appear to serve as storage sites for long-term memories. Figure 18.8 is a schematic representation of this process.

Damage to the hippocampus impairs the formation of new memories, but what affects remote memories? Bayley et al. examined eight patients with damage to their medial temporal lobes. All patients had problems storing new memories. Then they studied their ability to recall remote autobiographic memories. Only the three patients who also had significant additional damage to the neocortex showed impairment with remote memories.

However, the exact location of long-term memories remains a mystery. It appears that remote memories are stored throughout the cortex rather than in one specific location. Anatomic studies with monkeys have established hippocampal projections to the cortical regions shown in Figure 18.9. These studies suggest that declarative memories are stored in the dorsolateral prefrontal cortex, cingulate gyrus, parietal lobe, and temporal lobe.

System Consolidation

When your computer saves a file to the hard drive, that data are placed in a specific location where it remains unchanged until it is modified. When we put items in our closets, they stay in the same location until we return for them. Storage in the brain, on the other hand, is more dynamic. There is evidence that memories undergo continuing remodeling even weeks and months after they are formed. This process is called *system consolidation*.

Looking at which part of the brain is activated during retrieval of recent and remote memories provides a good understanding of system consolidation. Researchers in France taught mice to navigate a maze. Placing the mice back in the maze at either 5 days or 25 days reactivated those memories. Cerebral metabolic activity was then measured in a functional scanner. At 5 days, the mice had greater activity in their hippocampus. Those tested after 25 days had less activity in the hippocampus and greater activity in the cortical regions such as the cingulate gyrus and frontal cortex. This shows that memories are initially dependent on hippocampus.

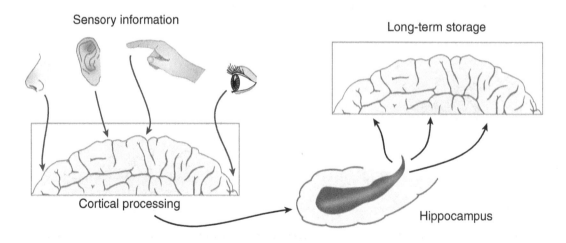

FIGURE 18.8 ● Experiences enter the brain through the senses and are initially processed in the cortex. This information then goes to the hippocampus before being stored in the cortex.

Medial view   Lateral view

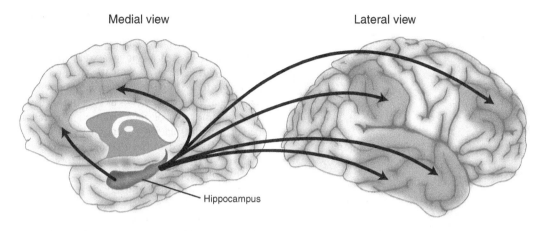

Hippocampus

FIGURE 18.9 ● Efferent projections from the hippocampus go to the cortical areas shaded in gray. It is thought that long-term declarative memories are physically contained within these regions. The exact mechanism remains a mystery. (Adapted from Van Hoesen GW. The parahippocampal gyrus: new observations regarding its cortical connections in the monkey. *Trends Neurosci.* 1982;5:345-350.)

Then, by some process of consolidation that occurs over days, the memories become independent of the hippocampus and reside in a distributed pattern in the cortex.

The same researchers also looked at the remodeling of memories within layers of the cortex. As before, they taught the mice to negotiate a maze and then retested their memory at either 1 day or 30 days. This time they sacrificed the mice and measured Fos (a marker of gene activation) in the parietal cortex. They found that total Fos activity was the same at days 1 and 30. However, the location of activity within the layers of the parietal cortex changed from days 1 to 30. Figure 18.10 shows the change in Fos activity by layer. Note how the

FIGURE 18.10 ● **A.** Micrographs from parietal lobes of mice tested at day 1 (recent) and day 30 (remote). **B.** Percentage of Fos counts per layer. (Micrograph from Maviel T, Durkin TP, Menzaghi F, et al. Sites of neocortical reorganization critical for remote spatial memory. *Science.* 2004;305(5680): 96-99. Reprinted with permission from the AAAS.)

recent memory activates neurons in layers V and VI. Memory after 30 days, in comparison, shows greater activity in layers II and III.

These studies show that memories in the brain are not simply created and stored in a fixed and static receptacle awaiting recall. Memories appear to undergo remodeling as they become independent of the hippocampus and possibly as they are relocated in the layers of the cortex. And all this is done "off-line," without conscious recall of the memory, possibly during sleep.

FORGETTING

From the standpoint of a mental health practitioner, problems with forgetting may be more relevant in day-to-day clinical practice than problems with forming new memories. Sometimes patients forget too much, as with Alzheimer's disease, or, at the other extreme, cannot forget horrific traumatic memories they wish would disappear. While the cellular and molecular mechanisms of learning and memory are becoming clearer, the mechanisms of forgetting remain poorly understood.

The importance of forgetting can be understood from a standpoint of storage. Our brains are simply not large enough to retain all the details of our lives. To further minimize what is retained, it is likely the brain only stores broad outlines of the information. An example of this can be seen in Figure 18.11. Although the reader has seen pennies thousands of times over the past years, it is still hard to correctly identify the accurate drawing of the penny. This example highlights one reason we fail to remember: detailed memories were never stored in the first place. Likewise, any interference at the time of

FIGURE 18.11 ● Because the brain retains so few details about objects, it is hard to identify which penny is an actual representation of the 1-cent coin. Few viewers will recognize that none of the drawings are a good match because Lincoln is facing the wrong direction.

consolidation will impair future recall. However, this is different from forgetting what was once learned.

Numerous experiments have documented a continuous decline for remote memories with the passage of time. The "forgetting curve" in Figure 18.1 shows a hypothetical drop in the ability to recall unrehearsed information with the passage of time. Memories simply grow weaker as we age. How this occurs is poorly understood.

One possible mechanism assumes a passive decay over time. If the connections holding the memory are not used, they become weaker with time. Alternatively, the memory could be overwritten with new information and distorted or lost. Figuratively, it is as though an unused path through the woods is lost as the forest grows over it.

Actively forgetting is another possible mechanism that the brain could use. In this case, it would be more like going through one's closet and throwing away items not worn in the past year or two. Recent research suggests that active forgetting does occur in the brain.

The reader will recall that protein kinases phosphorylate transcription factors such as cAMP response element binding (CREB) to promote gene expression (see Figure 5.5). As is typical in the Yin and Yang mechanisms of the body, different proteins *dephosphorylate* CREB and turn off gene expression. The proteins that dephosphorylate are called *protein phosphatases*, and one of them, called

protein phosphatase 1 (PP1), has been implicated in forgetting. First, the research group established that inhibiting PP1 enhanced learning efficacy.

In a second experiment in a water maze, the researchers tested memory for the location of the hidden platform. Mice with PP1 inhibition remembered equally well at 8 weeks as they did on day 1. However, the control mice showed a decay in memory of the platform location as early as 2 weeks and seemed to have completely forgotten by 8 weeks. These results suggest that forgetting is an active function perpetrated by the brain to clean out memories not being utilized.

Electroconvulsive Therapy

One of the great controversies in psychiatry involves electroconvulsive therapy (ECT) and memory loss. There is no question about loss of memory around the time of the procedure. The electrically induced seizure disrupts formation of new memories so patients never recall details of the treatment or shortly afterward. However, some patient groups have vigorously complained that ECT also erases long-term memories (retrograde amnesia). This was a difficult issue to tease out until the development of autobiographical interviews, which could be individualized to each patient and then administered before and after the ECT.

Harold Sacheim and his group prospectively studied the cognitive effects of ECT on 347 patients at seven hospitals in New York City. At the 6-month follow-up exam, scores on the Mini-Mental Status Exam (as a comparison) had improved from baseline for almost all patients. However, some patients showed persistent deficits for autobiographical memories compared with the pretreatment baseline. Further analysis showed that retrograde amnesia correlated with electrode placement (Figure 18.12). Patients who received bilateral ECT forgot some of their past history, while patients receiving unilateral ECT improved their autobiographical recall.

If long-term memories are a stronger connection between neurons (as we discussed above), then bilateral ECT must in some way disrupt the connections in the cortex. How this happens is a mystery. Some have postulated that the electricity and convulsion induce an outpouring of biochemical molecules such as glutamate and glucocorticoids, which possibly are toxic to the cortical connections. Fortunately, the benefits found with unilateral ECT suggest the problem is not an essential feature of successful treatment. Furthermore, newer developments with shorter pulse widths (ultrabrief right unilateral ECT) have reduced the memory problems even further.

FIGURE 18.12 ● Long-term autobiographical memories deteriorated after electroconvulsive therapy (ECT) for patients who received bilateral ECT, but not for patients receiving unilateral ECT. (Adapted from Sackiem HA, et al. The cognitive effects of electroconvulsive therapy in community settings. *Neuropsychopharmacology*. 2007;32:244-254.)

MIND OF A MNEMONIST

Some people have extraordinary memories. One such person was studied at length in Russia for over 30 years during the time of Stalin. This man, called S. by the psychologist Aleksander Luria, had an unbelievable capacity to accurately recall long lists of words, syllables, or numbers. For example, when shown the nonsense formula in the figure below, S. studied it briefly and then after a few minutes reproduced it without error. Even more remarkable, when spontaneously and without warning asked to recall the formula 15 years later, he did so flawlessly.

$$N \cdot \sqrt{d^2 \times \frac{85}{vx}} \cdot \sqrt[3]{\frac{276^2 \cdot 86x}{n^2v \cdot \pi\,264}}\ n^2b{=}sv\ \frac{1624}{32^2} \cdot r^2s$$

A NONSENSE mathematical formula created to test S.'s memory. (Adapted from Luria AR. *The Mind of a Mnemonist*. New York, NY: Basic Books; 1968.)

S. had an unusual ability to generate vivid enduring images in his mind. When asked to recall the items, he simply recalled the images and read them as one would read symbols on a page. While the stable quality of these images allowed S. to earn a living as a performing mnemonist, it also cluttered his mind. He had trouble forgetting. S. was actually encumbered by past visual images that were activated by similar topics in conversation and reading. The associated images led to mental wanderings taking his mind far from the task in front of him. His gift for details interfered with his grasp of the "big picture."

Was there something different about S.'s brain? Unfortunately, S. lived before the time of brain imaging technology, so any differences in his brain's size or functions that might explain his extraordinary memory remain unknown. He also lived before the revolution in genetics. Might he have had an unusual variant of a protein synthesis gene that allowed for better immediate memory formation?

QUESTIONS

1. Learning to tie shoes is what kind of memory?
   a. Declarative.
   b. Implicit.
   c. Explicit.
   d. Anterograde.

2. Which of the following does not fit with the others?
   a. Short-term memory.
   b. DNA → RNA.
   c. Gene expression.
   d. Protein synthesis.

3. Anisomycin
   a. Enhances extinction.
   b. Accelerates memory formation.
   c. Limits neurogenesis.
   d. Inhibits protein synthesis.

4. All of the following are true about reconsolidation, except
   a. It was an unexpected finding.
   b. It suggests long-term memories are malleable.
   c. Is demonstrated with the use of D-cycloserine.
   d. Helps explain errors in eyewitness identification.

5. The patient H.M. is impaired with which of the following?
   a. Ability to build new long-term memories.
   b. Retrieve long-term memories.
   c. Develop new procedural memories.
   d. Understand explicit instructions.

6. Evidence of system consolidation includes
   a. More mature memories are more dependent on the hippocampus.
   b. Mature memories are more prevalent in the prefrontal cortex.
   c. Cortical layers II and III have less remote memories.
   d. Older memories are more active in the neocortex.

7. All of the following are true about forgetting long-term memories, except
   a. Memories decay with time.
   b. Protein phosphatases have been implicated in forgetting.
   c. Forgetting can be enhanced with anisomycin.
   d. Interference during consolidation increases forgetting.

8. ECT has all of the following effects on memory, except
   a. Inhibits consolidation.
   b. Electrode placement does not affect remote memories.
   c. Erases recent long-term memories.
   d. Some memories are completely lost.

See Answers section at the end of the book.

CHAPTER 19

Intelligence

INTELLIGENCE

The topic of intelligence can generate strong feelings. Specifically, the idea that there is one monolithic kind of intelligence that is reflected by a single number plotted on a bell-shaped curve is hard to accept. Can one number determine a person's life? Other variables such as interpersonal skill, emotional resilience, creativity, and motivation are factors independent of intelligence, which are critical for success in a career or in life. Likewise, a person can show great aptitude in one area, yet struggle in another. Having said that, it is important to acknowledge there is considerable evidence of a general mental ability called *intelligence*, which has a predictive value.

It has been shown that all credible tests of mental ability rank individuals in about the same way; that is, people who do well on one type of test tend to do well on the others and vice versa. Such tests (e.g., the Wechsler Intelligence Scale, which gives an IQ score) are believed to measure some global element of intellectual ability. This global element is called "g" or fluid intelligence; g is conceptualized as reasoning and novel problem-solving ability. Others have described it as the ability to deal with complexity. There is no pure measure of g. An IQ score is an approximation of g.

Some argue that g is only useful to predict academic success or success in situations that resemble school. Arguing against this, others point to data showing the predictive correlates between IQ and employment, marriage, incarceration, and income. From our standpoint, we are interested in the associations between g and the neural substrate of the brain.

Genetics

Before we delve into the neuroscience of intelligence, it is worth discussing some compelling studies on the heritability of cognitive skills. The Colorado Adoption Project that started in 1975 followed up 200 adopted children from childhood through adolescence. They compared the cognitive ability of the children with their adoptive parents and their biologic parents. A control group of children raised by their biologic parents was included for comparison.

Figure 19.1 shows the correlations for verbal and spatial abilities over time between the children and the parents. Note how the adopted children have almost zero correlation between them and their adopted parents. Their cognitive skills more closely match their biologic parents. Another finding of interest is that the correlations improve with age. We become more like our biologic parents as we age—at least with regard to intelligence.

Brain Size

A consistent finding in neuroscience has been the association between brain size and intelligence; that is, all other things being equal, bigger brains really are better. Nottebohm in his work with songbirds found a noteworthy example. The reader will remember that male songbirds have an enlarged high vocal center (HVC), which plays an essential role in his song production. Nottebohm meticulously recorded the diversity of song syllables that each bird produced and then compared this with the size of his HVC. The results are plotted in Figure 19.2 and show a robust correlation.

An extensive song repertoire is not the same as reasoning and problem solving. It is probably closer to having a large fund of knowledge (sometimes called *crystalline intelligence*). However, for our purposes, it shows an association between brain size and a learned task.

With humans, there is a long history of studies comparing brain size and intelligence. In the early

FIGURE 19.1 ● The correlation between children and their biologic parents increases with age for verbal and spatial abilities. The shared environment between adopted children and their parents had little effect on verbal or spatial intelligence scores. (Adapted from Plomin R, DeFries JC. The genetics of cognitive abilities and disabilities. *Sci Am*. 1998;278(5):62-69.)

days, they would simply compare head circumference (hat size) with rough estimates of intelligence. However, there is more to intelligence than just brain size, otherwise whales and elephants would have ruled the world. The important variable is the relative size of the brain to the size of the body.

The Smartest Animal

Why are humans so smart? Or, to put this another way, what features of the human brain distinguish it from the brains of other mammals? If we are so much smarter, one would think it would be easy to spot the differences between our brains and that of our closest animal relatives. Unfortunately, it is hard to find anatomic correlates that explain the significant leap in intelligence we see in humans.

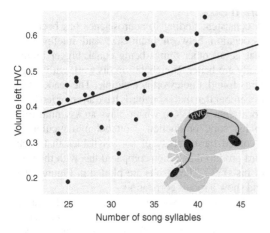

FIGURE 19.2 ● Adult male canaries with a large repertoire of song syllables also tend to have a large high vocal center (HVC), while those with small repertoire have a small HVC. (Adapted from Nottebohm F. The road we travelled: discovery, choreography, and significance of brain replaceable neurons. *Ann N Y Acad Sci*. 2004;1016:628-658.)

There are several variables that have been suggested such as brain size, relative brain weight, or number of cortical neurons, but for almost every variable there is some species that exceeds or is at least equal to humans. A cat has more cortical neurons relative to brain weight than humans and dolphins have almost the same relative brain weight compared with body weight as humans. Cats and dolphins are smart animals, but they cannot design a house, write a play, or solve algebra problems.

There is no single variable that marks the superior human intelligence. The explanation appears to be a combination of relative size and speed of communication:

- Relatively large brain compared with body weight
- Large number of cortical neurons
- Numerous synaptic connections
- Thick, fast axons that transmit signals quickly
- Short distance between neurons

In other words, humans have more cortical neurons with faster conduction velocities that make more connections than elephants, dolphins, or the other great apes.

Our superior intelligence is often attributed to our large prefrontal cortex (PFC)—the locus of executive function. However, comparative studies have found the proportional human PFC to be in line with that of the great apes and maybe smaller than that in elephants and whales. A better explanation may be the proportion of white matter to gray matter in the frontal cortex. Recent magnetic resonance imaging (MRI) studies on humans and other primates compared the relative volumes of white and gray matter in the PFC. The largest difference was found with the PFC white matter (Figure 19.3). The authors suggested that this difference might be a measure of "connectional elaboration." They postulate that

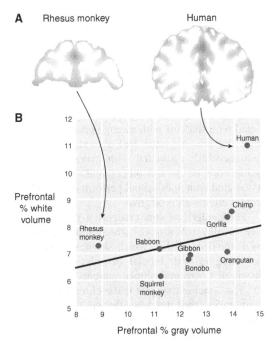

FIGURE 19.3 ● Gray and white matter comparisons in the prefrontal cortex (PFC) for rhesus monkeys and humans (**A**). The proportion of white matter in the PFC (compared with total white matter) is larger for humans than other primates (**B**). (Adapted from Schoenemann PT, Sheehan MJ, Glotzer LD. Prefrontal white matter volume is disproportionately larger in humans than in other primates. *Nat Neurosci.* 2005;8(2):242-252.)

In other words, differences in brain volume may explain some of the differences in IQ, but there is much more that remains unexplained.

Measurements of intelligence remain relatively stable over a person's life span. Yet, we know that the brain is a dynamic organ with more remodeling capability than we could have imagined just a decade ago. Likewise, there is shrinking of the gray matter starting in adolescence. It is unclear how these fluctuations relate to intelligence.

Giedd et al. at the National Institute of Mental Health completed a longitudinal study of cortical thickness and intellectual ability from childhood through adolescence in more than 300 children. The most significant finding was that it was not the absolute thickness of the gray matter that correlated best with intelligence, but rather the rate of change. This was most prominent in the PFC. Figure 19.4 shows the cortical thickness for one location on the right superior frontal gyrus for subjects with superior intelligence and average intelligence. Note how those with superior intelligence have less gray matter when very young, which peaks later, and then shows a more rapid thinning compared with the average children.

These findings are not what were expected. Smart children do not simply have more gray matter. Rather, it is the dynamic properties (perhaps even efficient pruning of unneeded connections) of the cortical maturation that are somehow superior in intelligent children. The significance of this the superior cognitive skills in humans could be a result of more and faster connections, not just more neurons.

The Smartest Humans

Shortly after his death, Einstein's brain was removed by a pathologist at the Princeton Hospital who assumed the world *had* to examine the brain of such a genius. Almost certainly this was not Einstein's last wish. The journey of his brain since 1955 is an entertaining story, but not great science. Most remarkable is the *unremarkable* appearance of the brain of the man who first voiced the theory of relativity. Einstein's brain is just one example of the difficulty of finding neuroanatomical correlates for intelligence.

Modern imaging studies allow the in vivo measurement of brain volume in multiple subjects. McDaniel conducted a meta-analysis of imaging studies comparing brain volume and intelligence. He identified 37 high-quality studies with a total of 1,530 people. The correlation between brain volume and intelligence across the studies was 0.33.

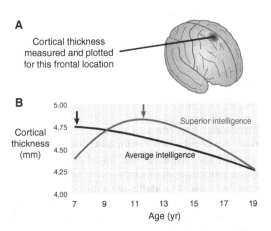

FIGURE 19.4 ● Measurements at the indicated point of the right superior frontal gyrus (**A**). Comparison of the cortical thickness at the point in (**A**) through adolescence for those with superior intelligence compared with those with average intelligence (**B**). (Adapted from Shaw P, Greenstein D, Lerch J, et al. Intellectual ability and cortical development in children and adolescents. *Nature.* 2006;440(7084):676-679.)

finding remains unclear, but suggests that refinement, not size is the hallmark of intelligence.

Parents and their teenage children provide an alternative way to examine the topic of intelligence. We would expect parents and children to have similar intellectual abilities, yet we would seek out the parents if we wanted advice and counsel—not the "know-it-all" teens. However, with almost every anatomical measure of the brain, the teen brain is superior: thickness of gray matter, number of neurons, and number of synaptic connections, for example. It does not make sense—the teens have more brain matter but the adults have more wisdom. The only brain structure that seems to correlate with adult wisdom is frontal lobe white matter, which peaks around 39 years of age (see Figure 8.8). This is further evidence that connectivity may be the secret to intelligence.

The study of patients with brain lesions has been a staple in neuroscience research since the days of Broca. Fortunately, we now have brain imaging capabilities and do not have to wait for patients to die to examine the lesions—which would be particularly problematic for the study of intelligence. A group in California scanned 241 patients with focal brain damage and looked for associations with general intelligence. They discovered a correlation with a "remarkably circumscribed" network in the frontal and parietal cortex including white matter tracts. The authors concluded, "that general intelligence draws on connections between regions that integrate verbal, visuospatial, working memory, and executive processes."

In summary, the essence of intelligence in the brain remains a mystery. The studies mentioned above suggest that numerous neurons, densely packed, with rapid connections between the frontal cortex and other regions of the brain facilitate cognitive performance. More neurons, talking faster to each other, makes for a smarter brain.

Brilliance and Mental Illness

There is a popular belief in the association between "genius" and "madness"—a "fine line" it is often stated. Numerous books have been written on the topic, but these case studies are more anecdote than science. Prospective research is needed. A recent study out of Sweden sheds some much needed light on the issue.

Sweden's social policies and national registries allow for the comparison of academic achievement with later psychiatric hospitalization. All students in Sweden are required to attend school until the summer in which they turn 16. Grades from the final year of compulsory education are normalized based on a national distribution and an average

is calculated for each student. These scores were compared with psychiatric diagnoses for subsequent hospitalization. The results are shown in Figure 19.5.

It appears that exceptional academic achievement is a risk factor for bipolar disorder. For males with excellent grades, there was a fourfold increase in the risk of developing bipolar disorder compared with students with average grades. Students with the lowest grades had a modest (twofold) increased risk compared with average students. Schizophrenia, on the other hand, is uniformly associated with poor school performance and high grades are in fact protective.

The results lend some credence to the book entitled "Brilliant Madness," which was coauthored by Patty Duke and in which she describes about her struggle with bipolar disorder. It certainly seems that activated bipolar patients are thinking too fast—racing thoughts is the clinical term. Are some racing thoughts advantageous? Is a little bit helpful for academic performance, but too much is called mental illness?

Performance Enhancement

There is considerable interest in medications or brain stimulation devices that could enhance cognitive performance. Pharmacologic or device interventions to increase problem-solving skills would be valuable tools in the treatment of such disorders as

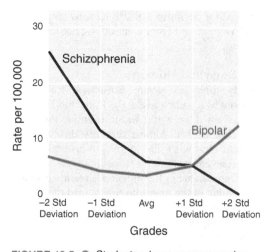

FIGURE 19.5 ● Students whose average grades at 16 were two standard deviations above the norm were more likely to develop bipolar disorder and less likely to develop schizophrenia. (Adapted from MacCabe JH, Lambe MP, Cnattingius S, et al. Excellent school performance at age 16 and risk of adult bipolar disorder: national cohort study. *Br J Psychiatry*. 2010;196:109-115.)

INTELLIGENCE AND ANXIETY

A recent prospective study reported an intriguing association between IQ at the age of 6 and posttraumatic stress disorder (PTSD) symptoms after trauma at the age of 17. Those children with an IQ of 115 or greater were only one-fifth as likely to develop PTSD as similarly traumatized children with an IQ of 100 or less. These results suggest that greater intelligence is in some way protective against the development of secondary anxiety.

DISORDER ADHD

It is not uncommon in clinical practice for a parent to try out their child's stimulant and experience a favorable response. The parent will conclude that they also have attention-deficit/hyperactivity disorder. Often such parents will present with a request for a prescription for themselves. However, improved productivity while taking methylphenidate or amphetamine is a normal response and does not constitute the presence of a disorder.

traumatic brain injury, Alzheimer's disease, and schizophrenia. However, if they worked not only to reverse disease-related deficits but also to enhance healthy brains, there would be a large demand from people without disorders who seek to enhance their cognitive performance. The prospect of "lifestyle" medications for intelligence is worrisome, especially in a meritocracy such as ours where profession and income are largely dependent on school performance and intelligence as measured in school tests.

Although there are no blockbuster treatments in the development pipeline, there are actually several products currently available. The best known agents are the stimulants such as the amphetamines and methylphenidate. Studies have repeatedly shown that these agents will improve cognitive skills in healthy subjects. For example, Figure 19.6 shows how methylphenidate decreased reaction times and errors of omission in healthy subjects in a dose-dependent manner.

Surveys of college students have documented the abuse and misuse of the stimulant medications. Although the estimates vary widely, the practice appears to be common in US colleges. In general, students at more competitive universities, members of fraternities, and those with lower grades are at greater risk for misuse of the stimulants. But misuse is not limited to college students. A recent informal online survey by *Nature* readers found that 20% of the almost 1,500 respondents reported using performance-enhancing medications. The most common was methylphenidate at 62%.

Other pharmacologic agents are also known to enhance cognitive skills. Modafinil marketed for narcolepsy and excessive fatigue has been shown to improve cognitive performance in healthy subjects. Readily available agents such as caffeine and nicotine have also been shown to improve performance. Nature's own performance-enhancing condition (hypomania) is well known to increase productivity (see Figure 19.12). In general, increased energy appears to be the common variable for improved cognitive performance.

DEFICITS

It is beyond the scope of this text to review all known cognitive deficits. However, two topics are worth discussing: mental retardation (MR) and dyslexia. Both have distinct abnormalities that give us greater understanding of the brain.

Mental Retardation
Dendritic Pathology

MR is a nonprogressive developmental disorder affecting global cognitive function. By definition, MR is characterized by an IQ of 70 or below (two standard deviations below the norm of 100). In the United States, this comprises approximately 1% to 2% of the population. There are numerous causes of MR, including genetic aberrations, toxin exposure in utero, and malnutrition.

FIGURE 19.6 ● Healthy men (average age 22) displayed a dose-dependent improvement with methylphenidate, as measured on a continuous performance test. (Adapted from Cooper NJ, Keage H, Hermens D, et al. The dose-dependent effect of methylphenidate on performance, cognition and psychophysiology. *J Integr Neurosci.* 2005;4(1):123-144.)

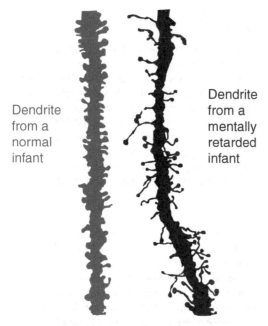

Dendrite from a normal infant

Dendrite from a mentally retarded infant

FIGURE 19.7 ● Dendrites from a healthy child and one with mental retardation (MR), highlighting the abnormal spine morphology in the child with MR. (Adapted from Purpura DP. Dendritic spine "dysgenesis" and mental retardation. *Science*. 1974;186(4169):1126-1128.)

Severe forms of MR often have readily apparent structural abnormalities, for example, microcephaly. However, most subjects with MR show little, if any, obvious changes in brain anatomy. Their brains look roughly normal when examined with MRI. In the 1970s, researchers began postmortem examination of the brains of retarded children and discovered extensive dendritic spine abnormalities (Figure 19.7). Subsequent studies have found aberrant spine morphology and/or reduced dendritic branching as a consistent finding in MR in a variety of syndromes.

The importance of spine architecture for learning and memory has been discussed in several chapters in this book (e.g., see Figures 8.12, 12.13, 16.6, and 18.4). It is reasonable to assert that deficits in spine morphology impair the network connectivity essential for information processing. Likewise, there is only a short step to imagine that problems with information processing play a large role in the cognitive deficits of MR.

Deprivation

Deprivation in early infancy is a well-known cause of cognitive impairment. Studies on animals have established the lasting impact of early environmental

impoverishment. The fall of the totalitarian government ruled by Nicolae Ceaușescu in Romania in 1989 gave the world a group of unfortunate children who could be systematically studied to document the long-term effects of early deprivation.

Under the Ceaușescu regime, orphaned children were raised in institutions under conditions of severe deprivation. When Romania was opened to the world by the new government, the shocking condition of these children was revealed. Most were severely malnourished, with significant developmental delays. European and American families responded by adopting many of these children.

It is assumed that most of these children were put into the institutions as very young babies. Consequently, the age at which they were adopted approximates the length of time they were raised in a deprived environment. Likewise, it is known that these children moved into enriched environments after adoption.

The cognitive skills of 131 of these adoptees have been studied and compared with 50 UK adoptees who were adopted before 6 months of age. IQ tests have been administered to all these children throughout their childhood. Significant improvements were seen during the assessments of 4-year-old and 6-year-old Romanian children. Many children displayed an encouraging "catch up" with the UK adoptees. Recently, the examination results of the 11-year-old Romanian adoptees were reported and are shown in Figure 19.8.

The figure highlights the profound and lasting effects of early institutional deprivation. Of particular interest is the dose–response relationship between IQ and the number of years spent in an

FIGURE 19.8 ● A dose–response effect is shown for different amounts of institutional deprivation on IQ at 11 years of age. WISC, Wechsler Intelligence Scale for Children. (Adapted from Beckett C, Maughan B, Rutter M, et al. Do the effects of early severe deprivation on cognition persist into early adolescence? Findings from the English and Romanian adoptees study. *Child Dev*. 2006;77(3):696-711.)

impoverished environment. Children removed from deprivation before 6 months of age had almost no lasting impairment. However, those children who stayed in the institutions for more than 6 months had 20-point reductions compared with the UK adoptees. These results reiterate the work by Hubel and Wiesel regarding critical periods of development (see Figures 8.10 and 8.12).

Dyslexia

Unlike MR, dyslexia is a localized impairment. Classified as a learning disorder, dyslexia presents as an unexpected difficulty in reading in a person with otherwise normal intelligence and motivation. Dyslexia may be the most common neurobehavioral disorder in children. Estimates of the prevalence range from 5% to 17.5%.

While speech develops naturally, reading is an acquired skill. Children must learn that letters on a page represent the sounds of spoken language. Children with dyslexia have trouble decoding the letters into the sounds of words. Comprehension can be normal once the word is recognized, but sounding out the word is laborious. Reading is effortful and slow for such children. Additionally, the impairment does not spontaneously remit.

The Shaywitzs have been studying dyslexia for almost 20 years at Yale. In a large study, they examined 144 children (70 with dyslexia) using functional MRI (fMRI). The children read real words and pseudowords while being scanned. Figure 19.9 shows the difference in activity in the brains of the normal readers compared with those with dyslexia. Note the increased activity for normal readers at two regions in the left hemisphere: a frontal region and a temporal/occipital region. These regions are thought to be critical for analyzing written words.

In a remarkable application of their findings, Shaywitz et al. conducted a treatment study to see if the dormant regions in the dyslexic children could be awakened. Thirty-seven children, who were second or third graders, with dyslexia received 50 minutes of daily tutoring in their schools for 1 year. They focused on phonics: associating letters and combinations of letters with sounds. Children in the treatment group showed improved reading accuracy, fluency, and comprehension after 1 year.

Of particular interest were the results of the repeated fMRIs 1 year after the study ended (2 years after the start of the study). The baseline scans subtracted from the follow-up scans revealed regions activated in the intervening years. The newly activated regions (Figure 19.10) correspond to the same regions active in fluent readers: frontal and temporal/occipital. This study is further evidence that cognitive exercises can change the brain.

FIGURE 19.9 ● Children with dyslexia and healthy readers were scanned while reading. Normal readers showed greater activation of the frontal region as well as the temporal/occipital region. (Adapted from Shaywitz SE, Shaywitz BA. Dyslexia (specific reading disability). *Biol Psychiatry.* 2005;57(11):1301-1309.)

CREATIVITY

Creativity is conceptualized as the capacity to generate novel approaches to a problem. However, any fool can make a mess and call it art. The talent comes in producing something new that is meaningful and useful. Furthermore, being creative is different from working through a problem and testing all the available solutions. Creative moments seem to come to us in a flash—seemingly out of nowhere—often when the mind appears unfocused, for example, driving in the car or taking a shower. Creative moments feel different, but it has been difficult to identify what happens in the brain when the creative "juices are flowing."

It is a popular belief that creativity is localized to the right brain. Daniel Pink's "A Whole New Mind: Why Right-Brainers Will Rule the Future," a book that was on the New York Times bestseller list for 101 weeks and has been translated into 24 languages, is a good example of this sort of belief.

Dyslexic

A

Frontal

B

Temporal/
occipital

FIGURE 19.10 ● Dyslexic children who received a phonics-based reading intervention over one school year showed increased activation in the regions of the brain associated with fluent reading. (Adapted from Shaywitz SE, Shaywitz BA. Dyslexia (specific reading disability. *Biol Psychiatry.* 2005;57(11):1301-1309.)

Pink argues that the future belongs to people who can utilize their right brain—storytellers, inventors, designers—in general, people who are more creative. Pink and others purport the right brain is the locus for art and creativity, while the left brain is more mathematical and logical. Is this true or just urban legend? What does the science show?

Review of the Literature

Dietrich and Kanso in 2010 reviewed the literature on studies designed to identify the neural underpinnings of creative behavior and found 72 studies reported in 63 articles. They divided the studies into three categories (divergent thinking, artistic creativity, and insight) and looked for patterns in the neuroimaging and neuroelectric findings. Their conclusion is straightforward and robust—it's a mess!

With the possible exception of diffuse prefrontal activation during the creative moment, creativity is not localized to *any* area of the brain. Specifically, they noted that creativity is "not particularly associated with the right brain or any part of the right brain." They concluded that a variety of areas of the brain have been identified in one study or another, but then fail to replicate in numerous other studies. In short, the best we can say at this time is that the creative spirit utilizes the PFC—not a particularly enlightening insight. The problem may be the failure of subdividing creativity into appropriate categories or the limitations of our currently imaging equipment.

Creativity and Mental Illness

Another interesting aspect of creativity is the association with mental illness. Individuals such as artist Vincent Van Gogh, writer Ernest Hemingway, and Nobel laureate John Nash are good case examples of highly imaginative people who also struggled with mental illness. The composer Robert Schumann provides one of the most compelling examples of mental illness and the creation of art (Figure 19.11). Schumann attempted suicide twice and eventually died in an asylum. He had two particularly productive periods of his life during which he also had symptoms of hypomania. Graphing his musical works by the years he created them shows a remarkable fluctuation in productivity with mood.

A larger study supports a correlation between creativity and mental illness. Combing results from two older studies, from a time when people were more likely to have taken the Minnesota Multiphasic Personality Inventory, the authors found that scores for writers and highly creative writers fell between normal controls and patients with psychosis (Figure 19.12). It is important to note that the highly creative writers were not necessarily mentally ill, just sharing some of the traits of the seriously mentally ill.

Recent studies using the current method of systematic structured interviews based on the Diagnostic and Statistical Manual criteria have replicated these findings. That is, successful artists such as writers or visual artists have a high prevalence of mental disorders. The most common disorders are depression and bipolar disorder. It is worth noting that whereas creative artists have a high prevalence of mood disorders, it is likely not the same for creative individuals in other fields

FIGURE 19.11 ● Robert Schumann's works graphed by opus number and year of completion provide a visual display of the creative potential of hypomania and the devastating effects of depression. Robert Schumann, Wien 1839, lithography by Joseph Kriehuber. (Adapted from Jamison KR. Manic-depressive illness and creativity. *Sci Am*. 1995;272(2):627.)

such as science and engineering. It could be that the moody creative individual is not attracted to the hard core sciences.

The similarity between creativity and mental illness may be related to decreased filtering of thoughts and sensations. A good example of unfiltered thoughts occurs when we dream during sleep. In this uninhibited state, we experience a wild variety of thoughts that are—if nothing else—unique and creative. Some think dreaming is similar to psychosis. The important point is that when the inhibitions are off (as with sleep), the mind is open to new associations. Yet, few of the new ideas are useful.

Latent inhibition describes one cognitive mechanism known to filter extraneous sensations during the awake state. *Latent inhibition* is defined as an animal's unconscious capacity to screen out and ignore stimuli that are irrelevant. Specific tests can measure an individual's capacity to ignore irrelevant stimuli. Its significance in our discussions is

that individuals who have reduced latent inhibition have been shown to be more creative. Additionally, this same trait is associated with increased propensity toward psychosis. In other words, a little less inhibition may promote more creative thinking, but too much may be problematic.

A study with Harvard undergraduate students found an intriguing association among latent inhibition, IQ, and creativity. The authors categorized the students by IQ and capacity for latent inhibition. They also determined each student's creative achievement. Students scored high on creative achievement if they had published a book, recorded a musical composition, patented an invention, or won a prize for a scientific discovery. The results of this analysis are shown in Figure 19.13.

The figure reflects that highly creative individuals have a high IQ and are less likely to filter out extraneous stimuli. The authors concluded that such individuals not only have access to

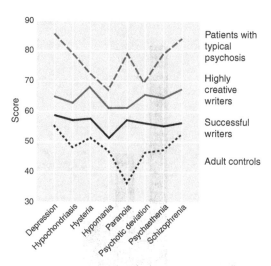

FIGURE 19.12 ● The Minnesota Multiphasic Personality Inventory (MMPI) allows the plotting of symptom severity across a spectrum—the upper graph being more severe symptoms. Highly creative writers and successful writers fall between typical psychotic patients and healthy controls. (Adapted from Simonton DK. Are genius and madness related? Contemporary answers to an ancient question. *Psychiatr Times.* 2005;22(7):23-23.)

more information but also have the brainpower to handle the additional information and are consequently more likely to make original connections. However, the authors agreed with the proposition that too much unfiltered sensory information in lower IQ individuals may be a feature of psychotic thinking.

FIGURE 19.13 ● Undergraduate students with high IQ and low latent inhibition (the ability to filter out irrelevant stimuli) showed greater creative achievement. (Adapted from Carson SH, Peterson JB, Higgins DM. Decreased latent inhibition is associated with increased creative achievement in high-functioning individuals. *J Pers Soc Psychol.* 2003;85(3):499-506.)

Loosening the Frontal Lobes

Artistic expression may be enhanced with loosening of frontal lobe control. Three examples suggest this is true. The first example is of an artist with evolving frontotemporal dementia whose creative expression blossomed as her illness progressed. The patient was a high school art teacher who had been painting since she was a child. In 1986, at the age of 43, she began developing cognitive problems. Grading papers, preparing for class, and remembering students' names became increasingly difficult. In 1995, she took early retirement. By 2000, she required caregiver support for her activities of daily living. An MRI showed moderate bifrontal atrophy along with mild left temporal atrophy.

While she was losing cognitive skills, she was also becoming increasingly uninhibited in her artistic expression. Her paintings, which had been previously more traditional, were now impressionistic, abstract, and emotional. Apparently, the inhibitions within the PFC were removed as the disease progressed and the patient became less constrained in her art. However, when the dementia progressed too far, she was no longer able to paint.

James C. Harris, who writes a commentary each month about the artwork on the cover of *Archives of General Psychiatry* and is also the director of the Johns Hopkins Developmental Neuropsychiatry Clinic, recently wrote about the remarkable drawings discovered in the Chauvet Cave. Dated to approximately 31,000 years ago, the animal drawings have a realistic perspective that seems impossible for Cro-Magnon man (Figure 19.14).

FIGURE 19.14 ● Drawings in the Chauvet Cave made 31,000 years ago. Did the primitive Paleolithic frontal cortex allow for greater artistic expression?

How could these "primitive" people produce such expressive work? Dr. Harris speculates that there is reciprocal relationship between artistic representation and frontal lobe development.

The final example is a longitudinal study of a girl described as an autistic savant whose graphic skills enabled her to draw with amazing perspective as early as 4 years old even though she virtually had no language skills. However, as she matured and her intellectual ability improved, she lost her artistic touch. These three examples, the onset of dementia, the cave paintings, and the autistic savant, highlight a conflicting relationship among the frontal lobes, artistic creativity, and cognitive skills. There is some process or connecting within the frontal lobes in which "more" is better for cognitive skills but "less" is superior for artistic expression.

QUESTIONS

1. All of the following apply to *g*, except
   a. Fund of knowledge.
   b. Novel problem solving.
   c. Fluid intelligence.
   d. Ability to handle complexity.

2. All of the following are true about the male canary's HVC, except
   a. The size is influenced by testosterone.
   b. Greater volume equals greater repertoire of songs.
   c. The size is an indirect measure of *g*.
   d. The size fluctuates with the seasons.

3. Indications that the PFC is a major site of intelligence include all of the following, except
   a. Active during problem solving.
   b. Lesions produce problem-solving deficits.
   c. Larger relative size in more intelligent animals.
   d. Larger proportion of gray matter in humans compared with other primates.

4. Impaired spine formation on dendrites is seen with all of the following, except
   a. Opioid abuse.
   b. Memory formation.
   c. MR.
   d. Impoverished environment.

5. All of the following are true about dyslexia, except
   a. Impaired ability to decode words.
   b. Right hemisphere problem.
   c. Inactive temporal/occipital region during reading.
   d. Increased frontal activity with proper treatment.

6. Most creative individuals in the sciences have the following, except
   a. Active PFC.
   b. Low latent inhibition.
   c. Mental illness.
   d. Above average IQ.

See Answers section at the end of the book.

CHAPTER 20

Attention

INTRODUCTION

The last aspect of cognition that we will review is the ability to attend to external or internal stimuli. Like memory, attention is one of the oldest and most studied areas of cognitive science. One hundred years ago researchers used stopwatches and psychological tests to measure attention. In the latter half of the 20th century, the placement of microelectrodes into the brains of monkeys opened the door to investigating the capacity of individual neurons to attend. Now with brain imaging studies we can observe, in real time, the shifting focus of an awake human solving a puzzle—with or without medication. One hundred years of research has given us a better understanding of the power of the brain to focus on relevant stimuli, although many aspects of the neurobiology of attention remain mysterious.

Attention in a broad sense describes the mechanism that weighs the importance of various stimuli and selects the one that will receive the brain's focus. The brain has limited capacity for attention. Numerous psychological tests have demonstrated the brain's finite capacity to attend as more and more stimuli are added. A relevant example from modern life involves driving while talking on a cell phone. A recent study found that drivers using a cell phone had a fourfold increase in the chance of a serious accident. Handsfree phones were equally problematic. Attending to a conversation detracts the driver from attending to events on the road—contrary to what the driver thinks.

The capacity to concentrate and maintain one's attention is inversely related to the ability to ignore other stimuli. Responding to other stimuli—whether internal or external—changes the brain's focus. The brain cannot attend if it is wandering from one thought to another. The border collie in Figure 20.1 shows an example of highly selective attention. The dog is not only focused on the frisbee but also actively ignoring other objects of potential interest around him. In this state he will ignore female dogs, squirrels, children, and even food. He will not sniff the scent of other dogs or leave his own mark on the shrubbery. He appears to focus solely on the flying sphere.

Athletes provide another example of the intimate relationship between attending and ignoring. The quarterback who has dropped into the pocket and is able to ignore all the noise and violence around him while he searches for an open receiver is an extraordinary example of attending and ignoring.

FIGURE 20.1 ● A border collie ignores everything else around him while focusing on the frisbee.

Likewise, when the artist or the absent-minded professor gets lost in work, they are ignoring most sensory inputs coming into their brain. Treatments that improve attention may be effective because they improve the brain's capacity to screen out the unessential.

Measuring Attention

Continuous performance tasks (CPTs) give an objective estimate of an individual's attention and impulsivity. Subjects watch a computer screen and hit a button or click a mouse whenever a specified sequence of symbols or letters appears (Figure 20.2A). Such tests reflect the subject's capacity to attend as well as the ability to restrain impulsive answers. Results are compared with normative data for individuals in one's age group.

Attention changes across the life span. Figure 20.2B shows the percent errors on one CPT (Test of Variables of Attention) for 1,590 individuals from the ages of 4 to 80+. Note how attention improves with age until the senior years. These findings appear to roughly correlate with the myelination of the white matter in the frontal lobes (see Figure 8.8).

WORKING MEMORY
Prefrontal Cortex

Working memory describes what is actively being considered at any moment. If the conscious brain is actually a tiny person inside a control room orchestrating the body's responses, working memory would be what he sees on the monitors in front of him. It is temporary, limited in capacity, and must be continually refreshed. Traditionally, working memory has been associated with the prefrontal cortex (PFC). It most certainly resides there, but may also include connections with the parietal lobes.

ADHD AND ADULTHOOD

Attention-deficit/hyperactivity disorder (ADHD) was once considered a childhood disorder. More recently, it has become popular for adults to get treatment for this condition. However, a recent meta-analysis of follow-up studies found that most children with ADHD fail to meet the full criteria for the disorder as adults—only 10% to 15%.

Trauma to the PFC impairs working memory. Phineas Gage is the most famous case that shows the effects of frontal brain damage on working memory. He was the young railroad worker who had a tamping iron explode through his frontal cortex (see Figure 14.4). He went from being responsible and organized to impulsive and inattentive. His inability to sustain a thought in his working memory could be considered the root cause of his wandering attention.

Researchers developed a way to test working memory in monkeys, called the *delayed-response task*. In this task, a monkey is shown a piece of fruit being placed in one of two randomly chosen receptacles (Figure 20.3). This is called the *cue*. A screen is then pulled down obscuring the monkey's view and lids are placed over both receptacles. When the screen is lifted, the monkey gets one chance to remove the correct lid and receive his reward. The significance of this test is that the monkey must hold the visual image of the location of the fruit in his working memory during the delay period. Healthy monkeys learn this task quickly. Monkeys with frontal lobe lesions perform poorly.

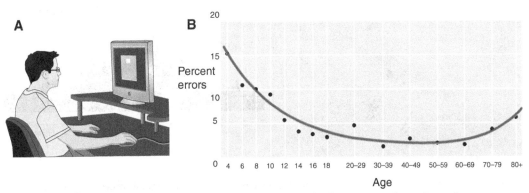

FIGURE 20.2 ● **A.** A continuous performance task provides an objective measure of attention and concentration. **B.** Percent errors as measured by the Test of Variables of Attention are age dependent. (Adapted from Greenberg LM, Crosby RD. *A Summary of Developmental Normative Data on the T.O.V.A. ages 4 to 80+.* Unpublished manuscript available through The TOVA company; 1992.)

FIGURE 20.3 ● The delayed-response task. **A.** The screen is raised and the monkey observes a piece of fruit placed in one of the wells. **B.** The screen is lowered and the wells are covered. **C.** After a specific period of time the screen is raised and the monkey has one chance to remember the correct location of the fruit. (Adapted from Purves D, Augustine GJ, Fitzpatrick D, et al. *Neuroscience.* 5th ed. Sunderland, MA: Sinauer; 2011.)

In the 1970s, researchers began putting microelectrodes into individual neurons in the PFC of monkeys while they participated in the delayed-response task (Figure 20.4A). They found that neurons reacted differently during the task. Some neurons were active only during the cue and response periods, whereas other neurons became active during the delay period (Figure 20.4B).

The delay neurons start firing with the presentation of the cue and stop with the response. These neurons

FIGURE 20.4 ● **A.** Microelectrodes placed into individual neurons in the prefrontal cortex (PFC) and monitored during the delayed-response task. **B.** Neuronal activity in cue neurons (*top*) and delay neurons (*bottom*) during the delayed-response task. **C.** The location of the cue and delay neurons in the right PFC. (Adapted from Fuster JM. Unit activity in prefrontal cortex during delayed-response performance: neuronal correlates of transient memory. *J Neurophysiol.* 1973;36(1):61-78.)

seem to hold the memory of the task—literally the neural equivalent of working memory. When the monkeys incorrectly responded, the delay neurons were usually inactive. If the monkeys were distracted during the delay period, the delay neurons would usually settle down and the monkeys would make incorrect responses or not respond at all.

After the studies, the researchers sacrificed the monkeys and identified the location of the microelectrodes. The results from several of the monkeys from one section of their right PFC are condensed and are shown in Figure 20.4C. The cue neurons and delay neurons are shown in different colors. Note how the delay neurons are more common than the cue neurons and cluster together. It is likely the delay neurons do not work independently but are part of a network that holds the image in working memory.

Catecholamines

Working memory is modulated by the catecholamines: dopamine (DA) and norepinephrine (NE). Pharmacologic interventions that increase DA and NE in the PFC enhance working memory and improve attention. Alternatively, agents that block DA receptors, such as haloperidol, have been shown to degrade performance on delayed-response tasks.

Phillips et al. examined the relationship between accuracy on a delayed-response task and DA release in the PFC. They placed microdialysis probes in the PFC of rats (see Figure 12.4A), which allowed continual analysis of extracellular DA concentrations while the rat performed the task. The rats were tested using an eight-arm radial maze (Figure 20.5A). In the *training* phase, rats were given 5 minutes to explore a radial arm maze that had four randomly chosen arms baited with food. During the *delay*, the rats were confined

at the center of the maze in the dark from 30 minutes to 6-hours. In the *test* phase, food was placed on the opposite arms from the training phase and the rats were given 5 minutes to locate the rewards. Errors were scored as entries into unbaited arms. Extracellular DA was analyzed at baseline and during the testing phase.

The results show an inverse correlation between extracellular DA in the PFC during the testing phase and errors (Figure 20.5B). When the delay was only 30 minutes, the efflux of DA into the PFC increased over the baseline by 75% and the rats made only few error journeys into unbaited arms. However, as the delay was increased, the DA efflux decreased and the errors mounted.

Biofeedback

Neurofeedback (also called *electro encephalogram [EEG] biofeedback*) is a treatment option that

FIGURE 20.5 ● **A.** Radial arm maze with four arms baited. **B.** Percent increase in extracellular dopamine at the testing phase. **C.** Errors at the testing phase. (Adapted from Phillips AG, Ahn S, Floresco SB. Magnitude of dopamine release in medial prefrontal cortex predicts accuracy of memory on a delayed response task. *J Neurosci.* 2004;24(2):547-553.)

allows patients to exercise their brain to improve attention and concentration. The EEG frequencies are divided into four groups (see Figure 15.3). β waves are the frequency pattern produced when a person is alert and concentrating. The goal of neurofeedback is for the patient to generate more β rhythm and less α and θ rhythms.

Neurofeedback utilizes a computer that interprets the EEG frequencies from the user and provides them with feedback through a symbol on the computer screen. For example, the symbol will move up with β rhythm and down with all other EEG frequencies. The user learns to move the image up the screen by producing β rhythms, which in turn strengthens the neurons that focus attention. It is the mental equivalent of lifting weights.

Although there have not been large, randomized controlled trials, results in the literature are about 75% positive. Recently a group in Montreal completed a small controlled trial with functional imaging before and after biofeedback treatment in children with ADHD. Treatment consisted of 40 sessions of neurofeedback, each lasting an hour, over 15 weeks. The neurofeedback group not only improved their scores on measures of attention but also increased the activation of the anterior cingulate cortex (Figure 20.6). Once again, we see that the brain is not a static organ and responds to exercise and training.

The inverse is also true. That is, not exercising the brain—or worse, watching "mindless" television—seems to impair attention. Longitudinal studies have linked childhood television viewing with subsequent attentional problems in adolescence—more TV results in poorer focus. A recent study examined the immediate effects on 4-year-old children of watching a segment of SpongeBob. Children who watched 9 minutes of the cartoon show, as compared with those who spent 9 minutes drawing, showed impairments in executive function (self-regulation, delay of gratification, and working memory) when tested immediately after the intervention. The fast-paced nature of some television fails to train the brain to focus and attend. Is this one reason we are seeing a surge in the diagnosis of attentional disorders?

REWARD AND IMPULSE CONTROL

Sustained attention to a particular task requires an individual to ignore other appealing stimuli. Controlling the impulse to take the immediate, smaller reward and waiting for the larger, delayed reward is essential for completing any project. People who cannot control these impulses are at a disadvantage. In an amazingly simple study, a group at

A Neuropsychological testing

Test	Before	After
Digit span	9.8	11.6*
Continuous performance test	77.5	85**
Conners parent rating scale inattention	71.6	58.9***
Conners parent rating scale hyperactivity	79.4	64.3*

$^*P < 0.05$ $^{**}P < 0.005$ $^{***}P < 0.001$

B Imaging study

FIGURE 20.6 ● **A.** Neuropsychological testing improved after 40 sessions of neurofeedback. **B.** The anterior cingulate cortex showed greater activity after the neurofeedback treatment. (Adapted from Levesque J, Beauregard M, Mensour B. Effect of neurofeedback training on the neural substrates of selective attention in children with attention-deficit/hyperactivity disorder: a functional magnetic resonance imaging study. *Neurosci Lett.* 2006;394(3):216-221.)

Stanford examined the ability of children to wait for the larger reward and then followed up their outcome as adolescents.

In the study, 4-year-old children were sequestered in a room with an assistant who placed a marshmallow on a table. The children were told that the assistant had to run an errand and would be stepping out of the room. They were also told they could eat the one marshmallow, but if they could wait until the assistant returned, they could have two marshmallows. The assistant left the room for approximately 15 minutes and the childrens' response was monitored. Some children ate the marshmallow as soon as the assistant exited the room, whereas the rest showed varying degrees of self-restraint.

The social and academic performance of these children was reassessed in their adolescence. The children who were better at inhibiting the impulse to immediately eat the one marshmallow were more resilient, confident, and dependable as adolescents. Additionally, they were more successful students and even scored higher on the SAT. The SAT scores for the more impulsive children are contrasted with those who showed more self-control. The total scores of the two groups differ by approximately 100 points.

	Impulsive Eaters	Patient Waiters
Verbal	524	610
Math	528	652

Clearly, the ability to suppress the desire to grab the immediate reward was associated with behaviors that have a profound impact on one's life. People who can delay gratification and control their impulses appear to achieve more in the long run.

Nucleus Accumbens and Dopamine

Attention and impulsivity are opposite sides of the same coin. Both are controlled, in part, by DA activity in the nucleus accumbens (NAc). Pleasurable activities increase the release of DA in the NAc (see Figure 12.6). People are less likely to respond to other stimuli if they are engaged in activities they enjoy. Stimulant medications also increase the DA released at the NAc and increase impulse control. People report that stimulants enable them to block out irrelevant stimuli with greater ease.

Clearly, other areas of the brain influence the NAc. For example, the orbitofrontal cortex, the hippocampus, and the amygdala are three regions with important projections to the NAc (see Figure 12.3). However, the NAc is uniquely wired to focus attention on the more favorable rewards.

Other evidence of the role of the NAc in impulsive behavior comes from lesion studies on rats. Rats can learn to choose a larger, delayed reward over a smaller, immediate reward. Lesions of the NAc will reverse this behavior. The rats with damaged NAcs become more impulsive and choose the immediate reward more frequently.

Impulsivity and Youth

Why are adolescents so impulsive and prone to taking risks? One possible explanation is that the frontal cortex has not yet matured—an issue discussed in Chapter 14, in the context of explaining impulsive aggression. Another explanation points to the NAc and dopaminergic tone.

The DA reuptake pump (called the *DA transporter*) has been used as a measure of dopaminergic tone. New technology allows the imaging

BOREDOM

It is no great revelation to say that people have a hard time staying focused on boring tasks. The stimulant medications may improve attention (at least in part) by increasing the level of interest perceived by the brain. Volkow et al. gave methylphenidate or placebo to normal young men and imaged their brains while they solved math problems. When taking methylphenidate, the men found math less boring and more exciting (see figure).

Changes in extracellular dopamine at the striatum correlated with interest in normal adults solving math problems. (Adapted from Volkow ND, Wang GJ, Fowler JS, et al. Evidence that methylphenidate enhances the saliency of a mathematical task by increasing dopamine in the human brain. *Am J Psychiatry*. 2004;161(7): 1173-1180.)

of the DA transporter density. Studies have examined the DA transporter density at the striatum (the region that contains the NAc). Figure 20.7 shows the decline in the DA transporter with age. Note the more precipitous drop in early adulthood.

Other researchers have shown that drug-naïve patients with ADHD have, on average, a slightly higher density in DA transporter at equivalent ages. For example, a 30-year-old patient with ADHD has the DA transporter density of a normal 22-year-old. Therefore, it appears that high DA transporter density (seen with younger individuals and patients with ADHD) correlates with more impulsive behavior, while lower density correlates with better impulse control.

Drug Addiction

The cravings that drug addicts experience at times for their drug of choice might be the most extreme example of seeking immediate gratification. When a drug addict gets this kind of urge, there are few concerns about long-term consequences. Every clinician knows about horror stories of addicts who

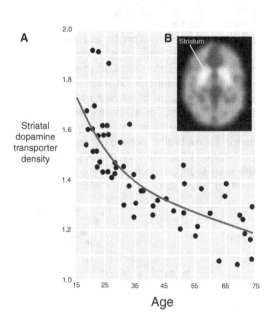

FIGURE 20.7 • **A.** The density of the dopamine transporter at the striatum as a function of age. **B.** Distribution of DA transporter in the human brain. (Adapted from Mozley PD, Acton PD, Barraclough ED, et al. Effects of age on dopamine transporters in healthy humans. *J Nucl Med.* 1999;40(11):1812-1817.)

have squandered the family savings just to get high. What is the role of the NAc in addictive behavior?

We know that chronic cocaine use downregulates the DA receptors at the NAc (see Figure 12.11). Likewise, we have shown that amphetamines and opioids alter the morphology of dendritic spine on neurons in the NAc (see Figure 12.13). These results and the behavior of the addicts suggest that drug abuse damages the NAc. Such an effect might be the pharmacologic equivalent of lesioning the NAc—an effect that enhances impulsive behavior.

ATTENTION-DEFICIT/ HYPERACTIVITY DISORDER
Genetics
ADHD travels in families. It is one of the most heritable psychiatric disorders we know. Pooled analyses of twin studies suggest the heritable rate may be as high as 76%, but the search to identify the specific genes has been disappointing. Pharmacologic and neuroimaging studies suggest a dopaminergic hypothesis for ADHD. Indeed the genes for the DA transporter and the D4 DA receptor have been implicated in numerous studies. However, not all studies are positive and meta-analysis finds only small effects of the individual genes, which explains only a tiny part of the genetic contribution to the disease.

Several genome-wide association studies have been conducted in an unbiased search for candidate genes (five studies as of 2009). Unfortunately, there is little overlap in the findings between the studies, and "classic" transmitters (DA, NE, and serotonin) were not even among the top findings. Other more basic processes such as cell adhesion, neural migration, and neural plasticity have been implicated by the genome-wide studies, but none are statistically significant. Franke concluded, "ADHD is a multifactorial disorder, in which many genes, all with a small effect, are thought to cause the disorder in the presence of unfavorable environmental conditions." Probably not a bad description about the genetics of all psychiatric disorders, as we currently understand them.

Brain Size
As discussed earlier, working memory and impulse control are important features of attention and are usually impaired in patients with ADHD. As would be expected, dysfunction in the PFC and striatum is the most common abnormal brain findings reported for ADHD.

However, the most comprehensive neuroscientific studies on children with ADHD come from Judith Rapoport's laboratory at the National Institute of Mental Health. They have conducted several large prospective case–control magnetic resonance imaging (MRI) studies of the brains of children with ADHD. One study produced multiple MRI scans of 150 children with ADHD and 139 age- and sex-matched controls. Sixty percent of the participants had at least two scans.

The most interesting finding was that children with ADHD had smaller total brain volumes by approximately 5% compared with controls. The difference held true for all four cerebral lobes (including white matter and gray matter), as well as the cerebellum. The trajectory of the total brain volumes did not change as the children aged, nor was it affected by the use of stimulant medication.

Gray Matter Thickness
In a follow-up study, Rapoport's group examined another 300 subjects, half of whom had ADHD.

MINIMAL BRAIN DYSFUNCTION

In the past, ADHD was called *minimal brain dysfunction*, a term now considered derogatory. The findings from Rapoport's laboratory suggest that those older clinicians, without the benefits of modern imaging studies, had a subtle but accurate understanding of the pathophysiology of ADHD.

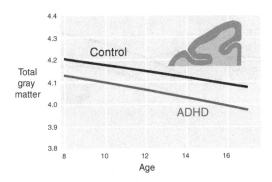

FIGURE 20.8 ● Total gray matter thickness for children with attention-deficit/hyperactivity disorder (ADHD) compared with controls. (Adapted from Shaw P, Lerch J, Greenstein D, et al. Longitudinal mapping of cortical thickness and clinical outcome in children and adolescents with attention-deficit/hyperactivity disorder. *Arch Gen Psychiatry*. 2006;63(5):540-549.)

This time, with better technology, they measured regional gray matter thickness. The most unique feature of this second study was that they followed up the clinical outcome as well as the structural changes in the brain of the children over time. They were able to compare the children who grew out of the disorder with those that did not.

The results showed that children with ADHD had global thinning of all the gray matter compared with the controls, although it was most prominent in the PFC. Additionally, both groups showed the usual pruning of the total gray matter as they grew through adolescence (Figure 20.8). However, two regions were unique when correlated with clinical outcome:

1. Children who remained impaired at follow-up had thinner gray matter in the medial PFC at the beginning of the study.
2. Children who grew out of the disorder showed a normalization of the gray matter thickness in the right parietal cortex.

FIGURE 20.9 ● Regions of significantly greater activation in healthy subjects relative to the attention-deficit/hyperactivity disorder group during a target detection task. (Adapted from Tamm L, Menon V, Reiss AL. Parietal attentional system aberrations during target detection in adolescents with attention-deficit/hyperactivity disorder: event-related fMRI evidence. *Am J Psychiatry*. 2006;163(6):1033-1043.)

These results imply that the normalization of the parietal cortex may be a compensatory activation of the posterior attentional network. Indeed, research suggests that the parietal cortex may play a greater role in attention than previously considered. Imaging studies conducted while the subjects attempted to detect and respond to the presence of an infrequent stimuli (a variation on a CPT) showed greater activation of the bilateral parietal lobes in the controls compared with patients with ADHD (Figure 20.9).

NEGLECT SYNDROME

There is other evidence that the parietal lobes are important for good attention. Parietal lesions can cause a neglect syndrome in which patients ignore objects, people, and even parts of their body that are to one side of the center of gaze. The very existence of parts of the body on the ignored side can be denied. The figure shows an example of a patient after a right parietal stroke attempting to copy some drawings. Note how he fails to copy details from the left side of the drawings. It has been proposed that the parietal cortex is involved in attending to objects at different positions in extracellular space.

A patient after a right parietal stroke attempts to copy the drawings on the left. (From Springer SP, Deutsch G. *Left Brain, Right Brain*. New York, NY: Worth Publishers; 1998.)

Timing and Cerebellum

Some researchers suggest that deficits in time perception are an integral feature of ADHD. Children with ADHD are known to have problems with temporal information processing and the timing of motor tasks. Clinical tests such as estimates of time duration or the reproduction of timed sequences are frequently impaired in children with ADHD. The finger tapping studies by Ben-Pazi provide a specific example of this problem. Children were asked to replicate the same frequency of the presented stimuli by tapping the space bar on a computer. Children with ADHD were less capable of replicating the stimuli and tended to tap faster than the stimulus presentation—getting ahead of themselves.

Figure 20.10A, B shows a comparison between a healthy control and one with ADHD. Note how the healthy control accurately replicates the same frequency of the stimuli, whereas the child with ADHD was responding at a faster frequency. The propensity to hasten the response is greater for children with ADHD (Figure 20.10C). The authors speculate that the rhythmic tapping problems reflect an abnormal oscillatory mechanism for those with ADHD.

These rhythmic motor abnormalities may represent a larger timing problem for patients with ADHD. In other words, the problem is greater than just replicating the tapping of a metronome. The problems with timing may contribute to the impairments seen with higher cognitive skills required to plan and complete a project. Inconsistencies in performance, responding too fast or too slow, and procrastination are behaviors that may be impaired due to temporal processing deficits. For example, patients with ADHD typically overestimate the time left to finish a project. In short, patients with ADHD may have trouble with project planning and completion due to problems getting into a good rhythm and maintaining a consistent pace.

FIGURE 20.11 ● Children with attention-deficit/hyperactivity disorder (ADHD) have smaller total cerebellar volume compared with unaffected controls. (Adapted from Castellanos FX, Tannock R. Neuroscience of attention-deficit/hyperactivity disorder: the search for endophenotypes. *Nat Rev Neurosci.* 2002;3(8):617-628.)

The cerebellum, traditionally conceptualized as controlling motor coordination, has been identified as a possible culprit in the etiology of ADHD. Studies such as those from Rapoport's laboratory have documented smaller cerebellum volumes in patients with ADHD (Figure 20.11). Likewise, stimulant medications are known to activate the cerebellum. Finally, the cerebellum is believed to play an important role in timing responses. Taken together, these findings suggest that patients with ADHD may have impaired timing mechanisms, which may be due to cerebellar dysfunction.

In summary, it is clear that the PFC and striatum play large roles in the pathophysiology of ADHD. More recent studies suggest that the parietal cortex and cerebellum may also contribute to the problems patients experience.

Long-Term Effects of Stimulants

There are two kinds of stimulants widely used in our society. The first, cocaine and methylphenidate, are primarily obtained illegally on the street. The second, methylphenidate and amphetamine, are

FIGURE 20.10 ● The stimulus to replicate is represented by the *black lines* in (**A**) and (**B**). The responses by an unaffected child and one with attention-deficit/hyperactivity disorder (ADHD) are shown with *brown dots*. **C.** The percentage of children who hasten their responses by tapping too quickly. (Adapted from Ben-Pazi H, Shalev RS, Gross-Tsur V, et al. Age and medication effects on rhythmic response in ADHD: possible oscillatory mechanisms? *Neuropsychologia.* 2006;44:412-416.)

FIGURE 20.12 ● Prospective study of cortical thickness at the left middle/inferior frontal gyrus for 43 youths with attention-deficit/hyperactivity disorder. (Adapted from Shaw PS, Sharp WS, Morrison M, et al. Psychostimulant treatment and developing cortex in ADHD. *Am J Psychiatry.* 2009;166(1):58-63.)

available with a prescription. Both classes of medication produce an outpouring of DA. One of the ironies of psychiatry is that the first group is studied by substance abuse clinicians, while the second group of stimulants is studied by clinicians treating ADHD. To a large extent, the two groups are focusing on different aspects of the effects of DA stimulation.

A recent multicriteria decision analysis of drug harm in the United Kingdom compared harm to the user for 20 drugs of abuse. The top three harmful drugs were crack cocaine, heroin, and methamphetamine. The next three were alcohol, cocaine, and amphetamine. Four of the top six harmful drugs are central nervous system stimulants. On the other side of the academic isle is research showing that stimulant medication may actually "normalize" some structural abnormalities in the brain. So on the one hand, stimulants of abuse damage the brain (see Figure 12.11), while on the other hand stimulant medications seem to normalize the brain. How can this be?

The difference appears to be this: when the subjects are analyzed. The substance abusers are evaluated once they are *off* the drugs. The stimulant users—typically patients with ADHD—are usually assessed *on* the medication. Almost no studies in the ADHD literature compare the effects on the brain of subjects who stay on the medication with those who stop it. Figure 20.12 shows the only exception.

Cortical thickness, which we know is thinner for patients with ADHD (see Figure 20.8), is normalized by regular stimulant use as shown in Figure 20.12. However, those patients who stopped the medication between the ages of 12.5 and 16.4 experienced a more rapid thinning of their cortical thickness in the left frontal lobe—an area of importance in ADHD. Clearly the "normalization" is the result of gene expression turned on by the stimulant medication. When the stimulants are stopped, the genes too shut down and the cortex thins. The relevant question is this: what effect have the medications had on the brain in the long term?

This is an important question because more people are taking more stimulant medications for a longer period of time, and what will their brains look like when the medications are discontinued? Will the brain resume the structure it would have had without any exposure to medication—or will it be worse—or will it be better? The importance of this question is highlighted by recent studies finding increased incidence of Parkinson's disease in addicts abusing methamphetamine. And, more troubling is a large, but as yet unpublished analysis looking at the use of diet pills in the sixties and seventies and later problems in the nineties. Patients who had taken benzedrine and/or dexedrine to lose weight were 60% more likely to develop Parkinson's disease as adults. More long-term studies are needed.

QUESTIONS

1. All of the following are true about continuous performance tasks (CPTs), except
   a. They give an estimate of a subject's ability to attend.
   b. Scores change with age.
   c. Treatment will affect the scores.
   d. Elderly subjects perform worst.

2. A delayed-response task measures
   a. The subject's capacity to delay gratification.
   b. Impulsivity.
   c. Working memory.
   d. Relative DA activity at the NAc.

3. The goal of neurofeedback is for the subject to improve their attention by spending more time in which rhythm?
   a. α.
   b. β.
   c. θ.
   d. Δ.

4. Stimulant medications improve attention and concentration through the following mechanisms, except
   a. Increase NE efflux in the striatum.
   b. Increase NE efflux in the PFC.
   c. Increase activity in the cerebellum.
   d. Increase interest in new activities.

5. Activity at the NAc (or striatum) helps explain all of the following, except
   a. Drug addiction.
   b. Impulsivity
   c. Working memory.
   d. Adolescent behavior.

6. Children who fail to grow out of ADHD show all of the following, except
   a. Thinner total gray matter.
   b. Compensatory thickening of the parietal gray matter.
   c. Smaller total cerebellum volume.
   d. Less prefrontal gray matter.

7. Which structure is associated with which finding in ADHD?
   1. PFC   A. Compensatory gray matter thickening
   2. Cerebellum   B. Temporal processing
   3. NAc   C. Working memory
   4. Parietal cortex   D. Delay of gratification

See Answers section at the end of the book.

Disorders

CHAPTER 21

Depression

INTRODUCTION

We wrap up this review of neuroscience by looking closer at the pathophysiology of four common psychiatric disorders. The first will be the depressive disorders. Although we often use the term *depression*, the reader should keep in mind that there are probably a multitude of discrete diseases that all end up with the syndrome we now call depression. For example, psychotic depression, atypical depression, bipolar depression, and pathologic grief may be variants of the same phenomena or they could be different conditions with different mechanisms of action. We have no objective measures to distinguish between the depressive disorders at this time. In the 1920s, we would have talked about pneumonia as one disease, as they all produced coughs and fever, although we now know that there are many different causes of pneumonia (e.g., tuberculosis, pneumococcus, and H. flu).

Depression is a common condition recognized by Hippocrates (melancholia). Yet, in spite of all our technologic advances since the time of the ancient Greeks, we know surprisingly little about the pathophysiology of the disorder. We know even less about bipolar disorder.

Monoamine Hypothesis

The accidental discovery in the 1950s that the tricyclic and monoamine oxidase inhibitor medications could relieve depression symptoms transformed the treatment of the disorder. Numerous spin-off medications have been developed since the 1950s. Most are safer and better tolerated than the earlier medications, but none are more effective. In addition, they all work through the same mechanism: the monoamines. This has driven the common conceptualization of depression as a disorder of serotonin or norepinephrine (NE) or both.

Again, we see that treatment response generates pathophysiology theories. Clinicians call this the *monoamine hypothesis*, and the lay public calls it a *chemical imbalance*. Unfortunately, neither is an accurate description of the biologic mechanisms of depression. At least two factors argue against the monoamine hypothesis as being the only cause of depression:

1. Medications take 6 to 10 weeks to reach full effectiveness, although the neurotransmitter activity at the synapse is altered within a few doses.
2. Studies of neurotransmitter levels in the plasma, cerebrospinal fluid, and brain tissue have failed to find deficiencies in patients who are depressed compared with healthy controls.

Clearly, the depressions are more complex than the simple replacement of an insufficient neurotransmitter.

The Depressed Brain

If you were going to do biopsy on a patient with depression, where would you stick the needle—what would you look for? Structural imaging, functional imaging, and postmortem studies have established five regions that are consistently dysfunctional in most patients with depression. The five regions are shown in Figure 21.1. Note the extensive prefrontal involvement.

It is tempting to match depressive symptoms from the Diagnostic and Statistical Manual of Mental Disorders criteria with specific regions in the brain. For example, anhedonia can be attributed to dysfunction of the nucleus accumbens or cognitive deficits to the anterior cingulate cortex. However, while a few symptoms seem to match up with a brain region, most do not. Most symptoms

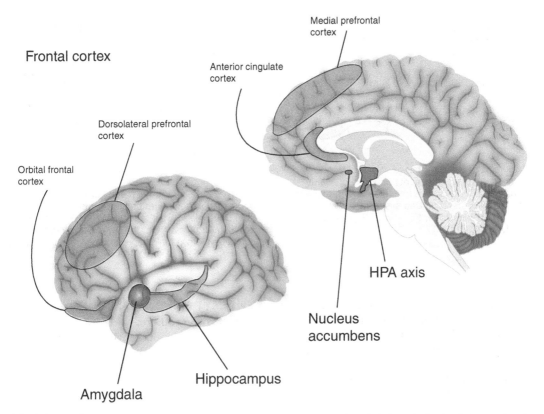

FIGURE 21.1 ● The five major regions of dysfunction in depressed brains. HPA, hypothalamic-pituitary-adrenal.

are likely the product of simultaneous dysfunction in several regions.

Alternatively, it is possible to envision depression as the result of overactivity in some regions and underactivity in others. For example, the hippocampus and nucleus accumbens are considered underactive in depressed patients, whereas the hypothalamic-pituitary-adrenal (HPA) axis and amygdala are overactive. This is appealing because some of the symptoms of depression appear to be caused by loss of function (low motivation, lack of hope, and low appetite), whereas others appear to be caused by hyperactivity (insomnia, anxiety, and suicidal thoughts).

Still, there is no consensus regarding the CNS alterations in the depressed brain. Part of the problem is the manner in which functional imaging studies analyze the brain. Studies that measure regional blood flow such as positron emission tomography (PET) and single photon emission computed tomography (SPECT; see Table 1.2) image the resting or idling brain. Blood oxygen level–dependent functional magnetic resonance imaging (fMRI) compares the brain's activity in response to different stimuli. If the brain is compared with a car, resting PET studies assess the idling car, while fMRI measures the car's performance on the open road—during a task.

A meta-analysis in 2012 of functional neuroimaging studies conducted in patients with major depression may give us the most up-to-date understanding of the dysfunction in the depressed brain. The researchers looked for changes in activity at rest (compared with healthy controls) and the response of the brain to negative stimuli (e.g., viewing pictures of sad faces). They found three differences in the depressed patients relative to the controls:

1. Activation of the pulvinar nucleus of the thalamus.
2. Greater response in the amygdala, insula, and anterior cingulate to negative stimuli.
3. Lower response in the dorsal striatum and dorsal lateral prefrontal cortex (PFC) to negative stimuli.

With these findings, the researchers formulated the following model of depression—heightened activity in the thalamus enhances the response to negative stimuli, which in turn activates the amygdala, insula, and anterior cingulate. Furthermore, there

Decreased metabolism   Increased metabolism

FIGURE 21.2 ● Sagittal views of PET scans on an average group of patients after a successful course of ECT. (Adapted from Nobler MS, Oquendo MA, Kegeles LS, et al. Decreased regional brain metabolism after ECT. *Am J Psychiatry*. 2001;158(2):305-308.)

FIGURE 21.3 ● Diurnal mean plasma cortisol in depressed patients and healthy controls. (Adapted from Deuschle M, Schweiger U, Weber B, et al. Diurnal activity and pulsatility of the hypothalamic-pituitary-adrenal system in male depressed patients and healthy controls. *J Clin Endocrinol Metab*. 1997;82(1):234-238.)

is a failure of the dopamine pathways in the dorsal striatum and dorsal lateral PFC (think pleasure and reason, respectively) to mitigate the impact of the negative stimuli. In essence, patients with depression are excessively responsive to negative information and fail to experience/consider alternative positive explanations.

Frontal Cortex

It all sounds good, but the studies of the prefrontal response to treatment suggest a more confusing model for depression. Looking at just the resting brain—using PET or SPECT scans—we find remarkably differing responses in the PFC to successful treatment. For example, Figure 21.2 shows the effect electroconvulsive therapy (ECT) has on the brain. Note how a successful course of ECT turns *down* the frontal cortex. A study using cognitive-behavioral therapy showed a similar response. However, paradoxically antidepressants, vagus nerve stimulation (VNS), and transcranial magnetic stimulation (TMS) have been shown to *increase* the activity of the PFC.

How can these successful treatments have such disparate effects on the frontal cortex? We think one explanation is that depression results from dysfunction of the frontal cortex and subcortical regions. Successful treatment restores harmony between the regions. A frontal cortex that is organized and more appropriately responsive (whether more active or less active compared with pretreatment) may be less depressed. It may not be the idling rate of activity in the region that is pathological in depression, but rather the relationship between the PFC and the associated other regions in the depression or mood regulating network.

THE HYPOTHALAMIC-PITUITARY-ADRENAL AXIS

Since the 1950s, it has been recognized that depressed patients have excessive activity of the HPA axis. Figure 21.3 shows the increased plasma cortisol levels over 24-hours in patients with depression compared with controls. The hypercortisolemia is stimulated by increased expression of corticotropin-releasing hormone (CRH) and reduced feedback inhibition of the HPA axis (see Figure 7.9). As discussed in Chapter 7, one theory of depression postulates that chronic, unremitting stress leads to the inability of the brain to turn down the HPA axis.

Postmortem studies of depressed patients have shown increased neurons in the paraventricular nucleus of the hypothalamus. The increased neurons are believed to be driving the increased activity in the HPA axis. It is unclear why these patients have more neurons in the hypothalamus. It could be genetic or a reaction to chronic stress.

Some patients with excess cortisol—either taken orally or generated internally—have reduced hippocampal volume. A meta-analysis of MRI studies has confirmed that hippocampal volume is reduced in patients with depression. It is believed that the excess cortisol produced by depressed patients is toxic to the hippocampus and causes the volume loss.

Effective treatments for depression (antidepressants, ECT, and lithium) are known to restore normal HPA function in most patients. It is postulated that this effect is due to increased glucocorticoid receptor production stimulated by the treatments, which has the effect of making the hypothalamus more receptive to negative feedback from cortisol. Finally, effective treatment of depression is believed to preserve and possibly restore hippocampal function (more on this later). A healthy hippocampus provides more inhibitory feedback on the HPA axis, as shown in Figure 7.9.

Consequently, depression appears to result in the breakdown of the normal relationship between the hippocampus and the HPA axis. Increased cortisol from the adrenal gland causes hippocampal damage, which results in decreased inhibitory feedback on the HPA axis—which in turn causes increased cortisol release, and so forth.

Restoring normal functioning of the HPA axis as a treatment focus has generated considerable interest. Several groups have tested CRH receptor blockers as novel treatments for depression. Although the early small studies were favorable, the results were not consistent and were associated with a risk of hepatotoxicity. Research in this area has stalled.

NEUROGENESIS AND BRAIN-DERIVED NEUROTROPHIC FACTOR

As discussed in Chapter 8, the brain is more dynamic than previously thought. The brain contains undeveloped stem cells that can migrate and mature into neurons or glial cells (see Neurogenesis section in Chapter 8). There is compelling evidence that this process is disrupted in depression and corrected with successful treatment.

Volume Loss
Structural imaging studies and postmortem analysis of depressed patients have documented subtle volumetric loss. The findings of a smaller hippocampus (mentioned above) are the best known, but

other findings include smaller PFC, cingulate gyrus, and cerebellum. Additionally, microscopic examinations have shown decreased cortical thickness as well as diminished neural size. One possible explanation is that HPA axis activation is neurotoxic to the brain. Another possibility involves a disruption of normal nerve growth.

The prospect that depression is related to problems with nerve growth factors opens a new way to conceptualize the pathophysiology of the disorder. A failure of neurogenesis and growth factor proteins, such as brain-derived neurotrophic factor (BDNF), may cause subtle shrinkage of the brain in depression.

BDNF is one of a family of neurotrophins that regulate the differentiation and survival of neurons (see Figure 8.9). Most likely, there are a multitude of growth factor proteins maintaining and stimulating nerve growth, but BDNF is the most widely studied at this point. Figure 21.4 shows a dramatic example of the effects of BDNF on serotonergic neurons in the rat cortex. Saline or BDNF was infused directly into the rat frontal cortex for 21 days. Then the animals were sacrificed and the cortex at the site of the infusion was stained for 5-hydroxytryptamine (5-HT) neurons. Note the remarkable arborization of the 5-HT axons in the cortex of the rat exposed to BDNF.

Growth factor proteins such as BDNF provide ongoing maintenance of neurons in the brain. Disruption of these nerve growth factors results in the reduction in the size of neurons, as well as some cell loss. Such reductions and loss may produce psychiatric symptoms.

Saline   BDNF

FIGURE 21.4 ● Brain-derived neurotrophic factor (BDNF) infused directly into the rat frontal cortex results in a supranormal branching of 5-hydroxytryptamine axons. (Adapted from Mamounas LA, Blue ME, Siuciak JA, et al. Brain-derived neurotrophic factor promotes the survival and sprouting of serotonergic axons in rat brain. *J Neurosci*. 1995;15(12):7929-7939.)

It is difficult to assess the quantity and quality of BDNF in living humans, so the evidence connecting BDNF and depression is indirect. A postmortem analysis of suicide subjects found a marked decrease in BDNF in their PFC and hippocampus compared with controls (see Figure 21.5).

FIGURE 21.5 ● **A.** Western blots showing the immunolabeling of brain-derived neurotrophic factor (BDNF) in the prefrontal cortex in three control subjects and three suicide subjects. **B.** Averaged BDNF in the prefrontal cortex and hippocampus for both groups. (Adapted from Dwivedi Y, Rizavi HS, Conley RR, et al. Altered gene expression of brain-derived neurotrophic factor and receptor tyrosine kinase B in postmortem brain of suicide subjects. *Arch Gen Psychiatry*. 2003;60(8):804-815.)

Psychiatric Treatment and Brain-Derived Neurotrophic Factor

Of great interest to psychiatrists are the increases in BDNF and neurogenesis seen with treatments that relieve depression. In rats, the following interventions have been shown to increase BDNF:

1. Antidepressants
2. Lithium
3. Stimulation treatments: ECT, TMS, and VNS
4. Estrogen
5. Exercise

This is a remarkable discovery. It is the first time that one mechanism of action has been found that could explain how all these disparate modes of treatments relieve depression. Presumably, psychotherapy would also increase BDNF, but no one has yet developed a credible animal model that could be tested.

With humans, there are less data on studies following depression treatment and BDNF levels. A recent study from the University of California, San Francisco examined serum BDNF levels in depressed patients before and after the initiation of antidepressant treatment. The results were compared with healthy control subjects. Although serum BDNF levels are not as accurate as direct central measurements, the results are still impressive (see Figure 21.6). The BDNF levels in the depressed patients before treatment were significantly less than the levels in the healthy subjects. After 8 weeks of antidepressant treatment, the serum BDNF levels

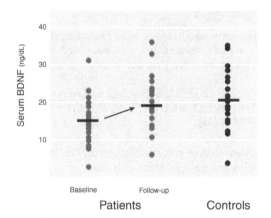

FIGURE 21.6 ● Serum brain-derived neurotrophic factor (BDNF) levels in depressed patients before and 8 weeks after escitalopram or sertraline treatment compared with healthy controls. (Adapted from Wolkowitz OM, Wolf J, Shelly W, et al. Serum BDNF levels before treatment predict SSRI response in depression. *Prog Neuropsychopharmacol Biol Psychiatry*. 2011;35:1623-1630.)

increased significantly and no longer differed from those of the controls.

Neurogenesis

Numerous studies have shown that increased BDNF leads to increased neurogenesis. Therefore, interventions that increase BDNF should also increase the development of new nerve cells. A unique study with rats has demonstrated that fluoxetine stimulates neurogenesis in about the same amount of time it takes humans to respond to the treatment. The rats given fluoxetine did not generate new neurons at a rate any different from placebo after 5 days, but did separate from placebo by 28 days (see Figure 21.7). Of particular interest, it also took 28 days for the rats to change their behavior—demonstrate a greater willingness to move into open, lighted areas to eat.

Scarring the DNA

Nestler et al. at the University of Texas Southwestern Medical Center (he has moved back to New York and is at Mt. Sinai) have taken these ideas one step further. They have looked at the effect of animal models of depression on the DNA that codes for BDNF. First, they stressed mice by placing them in the presence of a different aggressor mouse for 10 consecutive days. The exposed mice—called *defeated mice*—were later socially avoidant with unfamiliar mice. Such a reaction is similar to that of humans with depression and posttraumatic stress disorder. The messenger RNA (mRNA) that encodes for BDNF was analyzed in the defeated mice and comparable controls. As expected, it was greatly reduced in the defeated mice.

The defeated mice were given imipramine, fluoxetine, or placebo for 30 days. The antidepressants not only reversed the avoidant behavior, but also returned the BDNF mRNA to almost normal levels. On the basis of these results, the researchers speculated that depression (or in this case, social defeat) must affect the DNA. What they have found may change the way we view depression.

We discussed in Chapter 6 how DNA must unravel in order for the mRNA to be transcribed (see Figure 6.7). Likewise, we discussed in Chapter 17 the profound effect that a mother rat's behavior has on gene expression (see Figure 17.7). The results from Nestler's laboratory suggest that depression too may be a disorder of gene expression—or what they call *gene silencing*.

The DNA in the region that codes for BDNF was examined in the defeated mice as well as healthy controls. Figure 21.8 shows the results. In the healthy controls, there were a few methyl groups attached to the histones that package the DNA. In the defeated mice, the methyl groups were greatly increased, which had the effect of limiting access to the DNA. The antidepressant-treated group had the addition of many acetyl groups to the histones, although there was no change in the number of methyl groups. The acetyl groups have the effect of opening up the DNA and allowing BDNF mRNA to be transcribed.

Human studies examining methylation of the DNA in depressed patients have not been conducted. Although we would never biopsy the brain of a living depressed person, it would be interesting to compare methylation of the DNA in postmortem studies of depressed patients and nondepressed controls.

In summary, these studies suggest a mechanism for depression. Stress in conjunction with a genetic vulnerability decreases growth factor proteins (such as BDNF) due to "clogging" of the DNA (see Figure 21.9). This leads to thinning of the neuronal structures, which results in depressive symptoms. These structural changes make the prefrontal limbic governing system vulnerable to disruption and dysregulation. Stress, loss, or other processes cause the system to lose self-regulation. Furthermore, it appears that effective treatments such as antidepressants, lithium, ECT, and exercise (and presumably psychotherapy and good social support) will reverse the process. Presumably, the treatment increases the production of growth factor proteins, such as BDNF, that result in renewed neuronal growth, more resilient self-regulating circuits, and a return to healthy mood.

Clearly, this is a simplistic description of what is a very complex and heterogenous process. Much more remains to be discovered.

FIGURE 21.7 ● New neurons (neurogenesis) at 5 days and 28 days on rats given placebo and fluoxetine. (Adapted from Santarelli L, Saxe M, Gross C, et al. Requirement of hippocampal neurogenesis for the behavioral effects of antidepressants. *Science.* 2003;301(5634):805-809.)

A Normal

BDNF mRNA

DNA

Histone

Me

Me

Normal BDNF production

B Chronic defeat

Me Me   Me   Me

Me   Me   Me   Me

Limited BDNF

C Antidepressant treated

BDNF mRNA

Me Me   Me   Me

Acet   Acet   Acet

Acet   Acet

Me   Me   Me   Me

Renewed BDNF production

Me = Methylation of histone   Acet = Acetylation of histone

FIGURE 21.8 ● **A.** DNA must unravel to transcribe messenger RNA (mRNA) needed for protein translation such as brain-derived neurotrophic factor (BDNF). **B.** Chronic defeat (and possibly depression) caused excessive methylation of the histones, which blocks access to the DNA. **C.** Antidepressant treatment renews access to the DNA by adding acetyl groups to the histones. (Adapted from Tsankova NM, Berton O, Renthal W, et al. Sustained hippocampal chromatin regulation in a mouse model of depression and antidepressant action. *Nat Neurosci.* 2006;9(4):519-525.)

GLIAL CELLS

An unexpected finding in postmortem studies of depressed patients has been the reduced number and density of glial cells in the PFC. Subsequent studies have shown that electroconvulsive seizures in rats will increase proliferation of new glial cells but not new neurons in the PFC. Glial cells may play a larger role in depression and its treatment than traditionally believed.

Ketamine

One of the most interesting recent developments in psychiatry has been the use of an old anesthetic drug ketamine—an N-methyl-D-aspartate (NMDA) blocker (see Figure 5.2)—as a rapid treatment for depression. Not only is this a unique approach to the treatment of depression—attacking the glutamate neurons—but also a single IV administration can have a robust response in less than 2-hours in upward of 75% of the subjects—lasting several days to weeks in some patients. There are only a few interventions with such a hearty response—sleep deprivation, intrathecal thyrotropin-releasing hormone, or winning the lottery.

A Normal state **B** Depressed state **C** Treated state

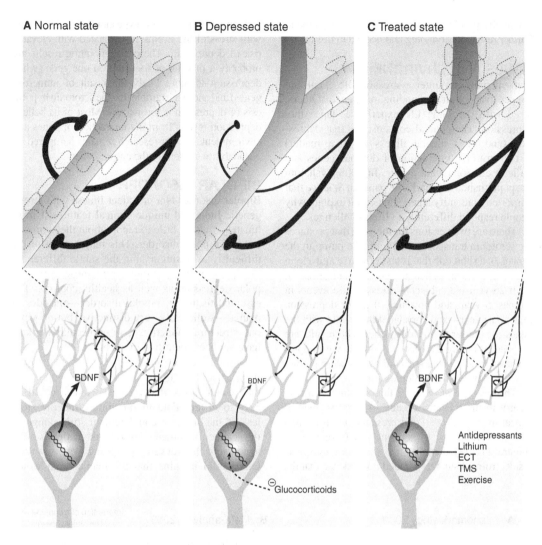

FIGURE 21.9 ● Stress and genetics cause decreased growth factor protein production, which reduces neural substrate. Effective treatment reverses this process. BDNF, brain-derived neurotrophic factor; ECT, electroconvulsive therapy; TMS, transcranial magnetic stimulation. (Adapted from Berton O, Nestler EJ. New approaches to antidepressant drug discovery: beyond monoamines. *Nat Rev Neurosci.* 2006;7(2):137-151.)

Searching for the mechanism of this effect has been a hot topic. Recently, an old friend has emerged: BDNF. Using a mouse model of depression, a group at The University of Texas Southwestern Medical Center found that IV ketamine (as well as another NMDA blocker) induced a behavioral change in the mice within 30 minutes and increased the production of BDNF in their hippocampi. Furthermore, BDNF-knockout mice failed to respond to ketamine. Finally, mice pretreated with protein synthesis inhibitors failed to display antidepressant-like behavioral responses to ketamine—indicating that protein synthesis is required for the antidepressant effect.

The reason this response is so rapid appears to be due to a unique mechanism of action, that is, protein synthesis without gene expression. The ketamine does not turn on the DNA, but rather turns off the suppression of BDNF synthesis from existing mRNA. In other words, ketamine takes the brakes off the mRNA that translates BDNF. All roads lead to Rome—at least for now.

Whether ketamine, or derivatives of it, will turn out to be a treatment for depression is unclear. It is hard to double-blind the studies as the dose needed produces a mild euphoria and dissociated state, and the effects do not appear to last longer than several days. Finally, ketamine can be and is abused (vitamin K), making it potentially problematic for a widespread treatment. Further research is ongoing and needed in this area.

GENES AND ENVIRONMENT

Some people encounter a stressful life event and bounce back with astounding resilience. Others, faced with the same life experience, lapse into depression. The general consensus is that depression (and most mental illness for that matter) results from the interaction of dubious genes and difficult environmental events. In 2003 Avshalom Caspi published a remarkable paper in *Science* that purported to identify a gene that could explain why people respond differently to life's challenges.

There are two versions for the gene that produces the serotonin transporter (the reuptake pump in the synapse): a short one that is less effective and a long one. Caspi and his colleagues collected information from 26-year-old subjects—stressful life events in the past 5 years and presence of major depression in the past year—and correlated these data with the genes for the serotonin transporter. The results are graphed in Figure 21.10A. Individuals with copies of the short allele *and* stressful events were predisposed to develop major depression.

This was one of the most famous studies in psychiatry in the previous decade. A copy seemed to appear in every PowerPoint presentation on depression. Unfortunately, a meta-analysis 6 years later (Figure 21.10B) demonstrated that combining the results from 14 studies "yielded no evidence that the

serotonin transporter genotype alone or in interaction with stressful life events is associated with elevated risk of depression." These disappointing results are probably a product of focusing on one gene (when depression is more likely the result of numerous genes) and another example that the serotonin hypothesis of depression is too narrow. Most of us believe depression results from the interaction of genes and environment, but our research remains hampered by our inability to identify the culprit genes.

BIPOLAR DISORDER

Bipolar disorder is a prevalent illness with strong genetic links and unique clinical features. Unfortunately, there is little to report about the neuroscience of bipolar disorder. This may be due to the difficultly in distinguishing the subtle differences in bipolar patients' brains from those with unipolar depression as well as healthy controls. The essential feature of bipolar disorder—episodes of mania—is clinically very distinctive, but no obvious structural, functional, or molecular markers have yet been identified in the brain.

Global Activation

One would think that manic episodes would be easy to differentiate in functional imaging studies—if the subjects could remain still enough in the scanner. In a manic episode, the patient's brain appears to be revved up—going way too fast. One would imagine that the manic brain would

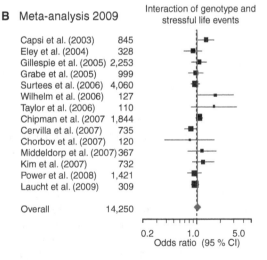

FIGURE 21.10 ● **A.** Individuals with the long allele for the serotonin transporter are less likely to develop depression when dealing with life's stresses. **B.** A meta-analysis (*brown triangle* and *line*) failed to replicate the results. (**A** adapted from Caspi A, Sugden K, Moffitt TE, et al. Influence of life stress on depression: moderation by a polymorphism in the 5-HTT gene. *Science*. 2003;301:386-389. **B** adapted from Risch N, Herrell R, Lehner T, et al. Interaction between the serotonin transporter gene (5-HTTLPR), stressful life events, and risk of depression. *JAMA*. 2009;301(23):2462-2471.)

"light up" in a functional imaging study, but that has not been the case.

The Medical University of South Carolina Functional Neuroimaging Team conducted a prospective fMRI study of six rapid cycling bipolar patients in an effort to identify changes in the brain with different moods. The patients were matched with appropriate controls and asked to call the imaging center whenever in an altered mood. Numerous scans were performed at many unusual hours of the day on each patient and control. The absolute blood flow measures did change over time and were softly, but not significantly, associated with depression and mood. The results from one subject are shown in Figure 21.11. Note how the total brain activity (shown in black) roughly follows the mood changes (shown in brown). Unfortunately, larger studies attempting to show this same phenomenon have been disappointing.

Lithium and Gray Matter

Some imaging studies have found decreased size and activity in the PFC of patients with bipolar disorder—similar to that found in patients with unipolar depression. We mentioned earlier that lithium has been shown to stimulate BDNF synthesis. A group at Wayne State University conducted a clever study matching these two concepts. They examined the gray matter volume changes in bipolar patients after initiating lithium treatment. MRI scans were conducted at baseline and after 4 weeks of lithium. A computer outlined and measured the gray matter

FIGURE 21.11 • Serial functional magnetic resonance imaging of a rapidly cycling bipolar patient. Total brain activity in *black squares*. Mood states in *brown circles*. (Adapted from Kosi S, George MS. Functional magnetic resonance imaging investigations in mood disorders. In: Soares JC, ed. *Brain Imaging in Affective Disorders*. New York, NY: Marcel Dekker; 2003.)

volume in each scan (see Figure 21.12). Eight of the ten patients showed significant increases in total gray matter volume—averaging 3%.

Subsequent studies by other groups have replicated these data. Of interest, valproic acid has not been shown to have the same effect.

Bipolar Summary

Although these studies are interesting, they fail to provide the neuroscientific basis for bipolar

A

Unaltered MRI

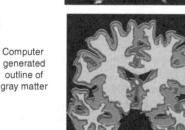

B

Computer generated outline of gray matter

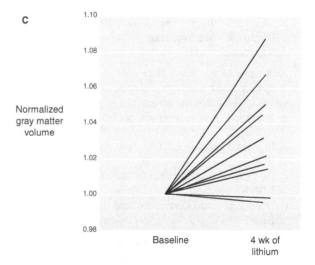

FIGURE 21.12 • Gray matter in magnetic resonance imaging (MRI) (**A**) is outlined and quantified in the computer (**B**). The change in gray matter volume for each subject is shown after 4 weeks of lithium (**C**) (Adapted from Moore GJ, Bebchuk JM, Wilds IB, et al. Lithium-induced increase in human brain grey matter. *Lancet*. 2000;356(9237):1241-1242.)

BDNF UTOPIA?

One can get the impression that nerve growth factors such as BDNF are the solution to all problems. Although future psychiatric treatments may provide better ways to restore nerve growth factor deficiencies in mentally ill patients, it will not be as simple as just finding ways to get more BDNF into the brain. Too much BDNF in some regions of the brain may be detrimental. For example, Nestler et al. using the same "defeated mouse" protocol found that the defeated mice had increased BDNF in the nucleus accumbens. The researchers speculate that the development of the social phobia seen with the defeated mice may be related to too much BDNF in the brain's reward system. Additionally, "too much growth, in an uncontrolled manner" is another way to describe cancer.

disorder that we would like to see. Haldane and Frangou reviewed the literature on imaging studies in patients with bipolar disorder. They suggest that bipolar patients share some features with unipolar depression (reduced activity in the PFC). Yet, other areas such as the amygdala are larger and more active in the bipolar patients. The authors suggest that bipolar disorder may be the result of abnormal interactions between the PFC and subcortical regions such as the amygdala—an abnormality they claim is not seen with unipolar depression. Clearly, more research is needed on this interesting topic.

QUESTIONS

1. All the following are true about the monoamine hypothesis, except
   a. It is often called a *chemical imbalance*.
   b. Explains the delay in response seen with depression treatments.
   c. Proposes deficiencies in 5-HT and NE in depressed patients.
   d. Suffers from a lack of supporting findings.

2. Postmortem studies in depressed patients have found all of the following, except
   a. Reduced neurons in the hypothalamus.
   b. Thinning of the gray matter in certain regions.
   c. Diminished neuronal size.
   d. Reduced glial cells.

3. Antidepressants may decrease depressive symptoms and improve neural survival through which of the following effects?
   a. Increased glucocorticoids and increased BDNF.
   b. Increased glucocorticoids and decreased BDNF.
   c. Decreased glucocorticoids and increased BDNF.
   d. Decreased glucocorticoids and decreased BDNF.

4. Goals for effective treatment of depression include all of the following, except
   a. Decrease HPA activity.
   b. Protect the hippocampus.
   c. Restore normal sleep architecture.
   d. Awaken the PFC.

5. Which intervention has not been shown to increase BDNF in animal models?
   a. Cognitive-behavioral therapy.
   b. Exercise.
   c. TMS.
   d. Estrogen.

6. Possible culprits in the etiology of depression include all of the following, except
   a. Cytotoxic effects of cortisol.
   b. Insufficient limbic activity.
   c. Genetic predisposition for sufficient nerve growth factors.
   d. Disorganized prefrontal activity.

7. One plausible explanation for an antidepressant's effectiveness is
   a. Removing methyl groups from scarred DNA.
   b. Restoring 5-HT and NE to their normal levels.
   c. Restoring access to the DNA.
   d. Neuroprotective effects on mRNA.

8. The pathologic mechanism of bipolar disorder is best described as
   a. Excessive prefrontal activity in manic episodes and decreased activity during depression.
   b. Too much BDNF in subcortical structures.
   c. Cortisol activation of excessive electrical activity.
   d. None of the above.

See Answers section at the end of the book.

CHAPTER 22

Anxiety

INTRODUCTION

Anxiety is part of a mechanism developed in higher animals to handle adverse situations. The anxiety response can be conceptualized as part of the brain's alarm system firing during times of perceived danger. The characteristic responses including avoidance, hypervigilance, and increased arousal are implemented to avoid harm.

The evolutionary drive to survive has invariably enhanced a strong anxiety response. Unfortunately, in many individuals, that mechanism is overactive. The alarm fires too frequently. Such people cannot seem to turn down their internal alarm even when the coast is clear.

Diagnostic and Statistical Manual

The Diagnostic and Statistical Manual (DSM) system categorizes anxiety into a multitude of different disorders (generalized anxiety disorder [GAD], obsessive-compulsive disorder [OCD], post-traumatic stress disorder [PTSD], etc.). Although each disorder has unique clinical features, it is not clear whether they actually describe different pathologic states. The disorders have the following similar characteristics:

1. Most patients with an anxiety disorder will have features of the other disorders.
2. Many of the disorders respond to similar treatment interventions: selective serotonin reuptake inhibitors, benzodiazepines, exposure therapy, and so on.
3. There is little evidence to show that different disorders stem from different regions of the brain.

We believe the reaction to perceived threat is mediated in similar pathways in the brain in patients with various anxiety disorders. The one potential exception is OCD, which has unique mechanisms in the brain and will be reviewed separately.

Acute Stress

The body's reaction to an acutely stressful situation is well known to all of us. The characteristic rapid heart rate, dry mouth, and sweaty palms are the body's response to increased sympathetic activity generated by a stressful situation (see Figure 2.8). Less readily apparent are the endocrine responses to acute stress.

In the late 1970s, Ursin et al. studied the endocrinologic responses of young Norwegian military recruits during parachute training. During the exercise, the recruits repeatedly jumped off a 12 m tower and slid down a long sloping wire to learn the basic skills of parachuting. The training was designed to give the jumper a realistic sensation of the initial free fall. Measures of anxiety and performance skill as well as serum hormone levels were captured at baseline and after each jump.

Initially, anxiety was high and performance was poor. As the days and number of jumps progressed, anxiety subsided and the skills improved. The endocrinologic measures are shown in Figure 22.1. Presumably, the anxiety induces changes in the releasing hormones, which alter the pituitary hormones and ultimately the peripheral hormones (see Figure 7.4). Note how testosterone levels drop with the stress of the jumping, while the other measures increase. Likewise, all return to baseline as the recruits habituate to the task.

While the average individual shows a peak in the endocrine response at the start of a difficult task, which usually subsides as the person gains mastery, this is not true for everyone. Some people have more exaggerated and persistent endocrine reactions. Kirschbaum et al. looked at salivary cortisol levels in 20 men exposed to 5 consecutive days of public speaking. For the total group, the average cortisol levels jumped on the first day and then gradually declined over the following days. However, the men

Cortisol
(µg/100 mL)

Testosterone
(µg/100 mL)

Epinephrine
(µg/100 mL)

Growth hormone
(µg/100 mL)

Jump day

FIGURE 22.1 ● The stress of learning to parachute, on young recruits, results in changes in hormones, which return to baseline as the anxiety decreases. (Adapted from Rosenzweig MR, Breedlove SM, Watson NV. *Biological Psychology.* 4th ed. Sunderland, MA: Sinauer; 2005. Graphs adapted from Ursin H, Baade E, Levine S. *Psychobiology of Stress: A Study of Coping Men.* New York, NY: Academic Press; 1978.)

could be divided into two groups: high responders and low responders. Figure 22.2 shows the cortisol levels for these two groups.

Note how the cortisol in the low responders peaked the first day, but then quickly returned to baseline levels on the following days. These individuals appear to adjust rapidly to the stress of public speaking. The high responders, on the other hand, showed higher, more persistent peaks of cortisol. Such people appear to have a harder time turning off the stress response. Presumably, they have a stronger alarm response originating in the brain, which is driving this endocrine reaction. Alternatively, they have a weak or faulty regulatory system that governs or turns down the response. Or there could be elements of both in some people.

Cortisol has been implicated as a culprit in the development of anxiety after trauma, although not everyone agrees if it is too much or too little. Some researchers believe excess cortisol sensitizes the amygdala and are using mifepristone (RU-486, the "abortion pill") to block the glucocorticoid receptors after a traumatic event. Other researchers believe the traumatic consolidation of memories is enhanced by *insufficient* cortisol and they are giving cortisol to patients acutely after trauma to prevent the development of PTSD. Both groups have produced small pilot studies with positive results. The impending larger trials should clear up this paradox.

NEURONAL CIRCUITRY

Multiple lines of research identify the prefrontal cortex (PFC), amygdala, hippocampus, and hypothalamic-pituitary-adrenal (HPA) axis as the regions involved with anxiety (Figure 22.3). However, if there is one organ that represents an alarm system in the brain, it is the amygdala (see Figure 2.7).

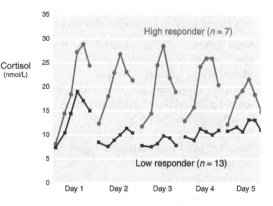

Cortisol
(nmol/L)

High responder (n = 7)

Low responder (n = 13)

Day 1   Day 2   Day 3   Day 4   Day 5

FIGURE 22.2 ● Men stressed by public speaking over 5 consecutive days showed different patterns of adrenocortical response. (Graph adapted from Kirschbaum C, Prussner JC, Stone AA, et al. Persistent high cortisol responses to repeated psychological stress in a subpopulation of healthy men. *Psychosom Med.* 1995;57(5):468-474. Illustration adapted from Images.com.)

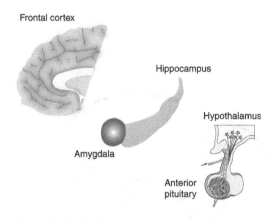

Frontal cortex

Hippocampus

Hypothalamus

Amygdala

Anterior pituitary

FIGURE 22.3 ● The important regions of the brain affecting anxiety.

Amygdala

In their classic studies with rhesus monkeys in the 1930s, Heinrich Klüver and Paul Bucy identified the amygdala as a structure that is essential for the expression of numerous emotions. They removed large segments of the temporal lobes from wild monkeys and transformed the monkey's temperament. Aggressive and easily frightened monkeys were changed into docile, calm creatures.

The monkeys virtually became tame. They did not react fearfully to strange humans or even a snake. Of particular interest, the monkeys failed to learn from negative experience. One monkey, bitten by a snake, later approached a snake again as if nothing had happened—a clear example of the survival value of anxiety. The entire constellation of symptoms is called the *Klüver-Bucy syndrome* and includes a host of other bizarre features, such as hypersexuality and a tendency to transfer objects to the mouth.

In the intervening years, it has been demonstrated that the emotional changes of the Klüver-Bucy syndrome can be elicited with the removal of just the amygdala. Other evidence points to the amygdala as an important region in the recognition and management of fear:

1. Electric stimulation of the amygdala in animals elicits fearful behavior, for example, freezing and tachycardia.
2. Humans with damaged amygdala exhibit impaired fear conditioning.
3. Functional imaging studies of humans show activation of the amygdala during fear learning.

Recognizing Danger

Sensory information enters the brain by way of the thalamus. All neurons carrying auditory and visual information synapse first in the thalamus before being relayed to the appropriate cortical region for analysis. Information about danger is particularly important and needs to be recognized quickly. Work by LeDoux et al. at New York University has shown that the amygdala quickly receives some preliminary information about dangerous events even before it is processed in the cortex.

Figure 22.4 shows an example of a person coming upon a rattlesnake. This life-threatening visual information proceeds from the eyes to the thalamus. However, the thalamus sends fast but rudimentary signals to the amygdala at the same time that the full information is passed back to the visual cortex. The amygdala in turn sends responding signals to the muscles, sympathetic nervous system, and hypothalamus. The person jumps even before being consciously aware of what has been seen. LeDoux has shown with rats that the fear response is preserved even if the neural connections between the thalamus and the cortex are cut. In essence, the animal startles without knowing why.

We all have had the experience of being frightened when seeing something, only to realize that it was just a rope or shadow—not a real threat. It is the fast track from the thalamus directly to the amygdala that causes the false alarm. This is considered to be "unconscious" or preconscious. We jump before we are aware. Patients with anxiety disorders can have exaggerated startle responses. They are burdened with an exaggerated, unconscious reaction to what are actually harmless events.

Anticipatory Anxiety

Some people dread personal interactions in which they will be the focus of attention. Typically, they fear they will embarrass themselves. The anticipatory anxiety can ultimately restrict what they do and limit their social life and career path.

An imaging study looked at the activity in the brain of such patients who were asked to anticipate making a public speech. By subtracting the activity during anticipation from that at rest, they identified the areas of activity. Patients showed greater activity in their amygdala as well as hippocampus and insula. Figure 22.5A shows the functional magnetic resonance imaging (fMRI) slice at the level of the amygdala.

Anticipatory anxiety is not all bad. Figure 22.5B shows the hypothetical upside down U curve that many think represents the benefits and problems with anticipatory anxiety. Some anxiety is beneficial and

FIGURE 22.4 ● Two representations showing the two tracks that emotionally stimulating sensory information takes to the amygdala after entering the brain through the thalamus. HPA, hypothalamic-pituitary-adrenal. (Adapted from LeDoux JE. Emotion, memory and the brain. *Sci Am*. 1994;270(6):50-57.)

actually improves performance; however, too much of it is overwhelming and results in a poorer outcome.

Amygdala Memories

There is evidence that primitive emotionally relevant memories are stored in the amygdala. For example, in rodents:

1. Long-term potentiation (LTP) can be induced in the amygdala;
2. Protein synthesis inhibitors injected directly into the amygdala will prevent the formation of fear conditioning; and
3. Chronic stress will induce increased dendritic branching in the amygdala.

These results suggest that the typical structural changes that are observed with memory formation occur in the amygdala in reaction to fearful circumstances. This may be one reason why traumatic events are so persistent. Fearful experiences form quickly, and enduring memories then reside in both the neocortex and the amygdala.

Prefrontal Cortex

One of the central components of anxiety is the feeling that one is not in control. Patients will complain of increased anxiety when they lose control, for example, when the door closes on an airplane or when their social support drives off—anytime they feel trapped. Feeling in control, on the other hand, calms anxiety. The ability to reappraise a difficult situation into more

TREATMENT   AMYGDALA ACTIVITY

A small study in Sweden looked at the effects of cognitive-behavioral therapy (CBT) and the antidepressant citalopram on brain activity in patients with social phobia. Both treatments were equally effective and both reduced the amygdala activation after 9 weeks of treatment. The degree of amygdala attenuation was associated with clinical improvement 1 year later.

A

B

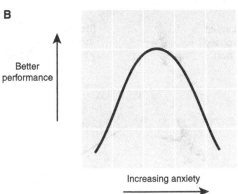

Better performance

Increasing anxiety

FIGURE 22.5 ● **A.** Increased activity at the level of the amygdala when patients with anxiety anticipate making a public speech. **B.** Hypothetical upside down U curve showing benefits and problems of anticipatory anxiety. (Functional magnetic resonance imaging from Lorberbaum JP, Kose S, Johnson MR, et al. Neural correlates of speech anticipatory anxiety in generalized social phobia. *Neuroreport*. 2004;15(18):2701-2705.)

favorable terms is a function of executive control. Rational reappraisal is a central feature of CBT.

The ability to cognitively master difficult circumstances and gain control likely resides in the PFC. Clearly, the PFC plays an important role in managing anxiety. However, the exact prefrontal regions involved (medial, lateral, or orbital) are ill-defined, although the medial PFC gets the most attention. The medial prefrontal cortex (mPFC), which includes the anterior cingulate gyrus, is well connected to the amygdala.

In a simple conceptualization, we can imagine that the mPFC applies the brakes to the amygdala. Several lines of evidence highlight the role of the mPFC in anxiety:

1. Lesions of the mPFC in rats reduce the ability to extinguish fears.
2. Stimulation of the mPFC inhibits a learned fear response; that is, the rat does not show anxiety.

Amygdala activity

Prefrontal cortex activity

FIGURE 22.6 ● In simple terms anxiety disorders may be the result of too much activity in the amygdala and not enough activity in the prefrontal cortex.

3. The mPFC lights up in functional imaging studies when fear is evoked in healthy subjects.
4. Subjects with anxiety disorders have reduced activity in the mPFC.

Taken together, these studies suggest that anxiety in part results from the reciprocal relation between PFC and the amygdala (Figure 22.6). This has been shown clearly in a clever study with traumatized combat veterans and firefighters. The subjects were shown pictures of faces expressing various emotions while in an fMRI (Figure 22.7A). The activity in the brain when the subjects were viewing the happy face was subtracted from the brain activity when viewing the fearful face. The subjects with PTSD were compared with healthy controls.

Figure 22.7B–D shows the results. Note how subjects with PTSD, under the circumstances of the study, show increased activity in their amygdala and decreased activity in their PFC. In essence, their PFC is insufficiently powered and unable to turn down the "alarm" in the amygdala.

Hippocampus

The hippocampus, an area involved with explicit memory acquisition, appears to interact with the amygdala during encoding of emotional memories. Although the exact role of the hippocampus in anxiety disorders remains unclear, it is an area frequently active in imaging studies during fearful situations.

For a number of years, the reduction in volume of the hippocampus in patients with anxiety disorders has been an area of great interest. Several studies have documented smaller hippocampi in anxious patients, presumably due to the toxic effects of an activated HPA axis. However, a unique study with twins provides insight into the cause and effect of hippocampal volume.

Gilbertson et al. recruited 40 pairs of twins, in which one of each pair was exposed to combat in Vietnam and the other had stayed home. (Who knew such a study was possible?) The researchers measured the hippocampal volume of each twin in hippocampal volume of the twin who had *stayed at home* (Figure 22.8B). In other words, the best prediction of a combat veteran's level of PTSD and hippocampal size is not his exposure to trauma, but rather the size of his twin's hippocampus.

This finding brings to light one of the great discoveries in neuroscience. It is the interaction between nature and nurture that results in mental illness (Figure 22.9). In other words, those at increased risk for developing PTSD are those individuals with a small hippocampus and exposure to trauma. Neither alone is sufficient.

FIGURE 22.7 ● **A.** Traumatized subjects and controls are shown pictures of fearful faces and happy faces while in a functional magnetic resonance imaging. The patients show increased activity in the amygdala (**B**) and decreased activity in the prefrontal cortex (PFC) (**C**) compared with controls. Activity in the PFC and amygdala (**D**) has an inverse correlation for the traumatized patients. (**A** Adapted from Calder AJ, Lawrence AD, Young AW. Neuropsychology of fear and loathing. *Nat Rev Neurosci.* 2001;2(5):352-363. **B–D** Adapted from Shin LM, Wright CI, Cannistraro PA, et al. A functional magnetic resonance imaging study of amygdala and medial prefrontal cortex responses to overtly presented fearful faces in posttraumatic stress disorder. *Arch Gen Psychiatry.* 2005;62(3):273-281.)

an MRI. Additionally, the presence and severity of PTSD in the combat-exposed twin was assessed. As with previous reports, the twins who were diagnosed with PTSD had smaller hippocampal volumes (Figure 22.8A). However, the most remarkable finding was that the PTSD score from the combat-exposed twin had a similar correlation with the

FIGURE 22.8 ● **A.** The correlation between hippocampal volume and post-traumatic stress disorder (PTSD) score for the combat-exposed twin. **B.** The correlation between the stay-at-home twin's hippocampal volume and the PTSD score of his combat-exposed twin brother. (Adapted from Gilbertson MW, Shenton ME, Ciszewski A, et al. Smaller hippocampal volume predicts pathologic vulnerability to psychological trauma. *Nat Neurosci.* 2002;5(11):1242-1247.)

Hippocampus size   Combat   Risk of PTSD
                    exposure

Twin A

Normal

Twin B   None →   Low

Twin A   ——   High risk
                      for PTSD
Small

Twin B   None →   Low

FIGURE 22.9 ● The risk of developing post-traumatic stress disorder (PTSD) is highest among individuals with a small hippocampus and exposure to trauma.

Taken together, these findings suggest an important role for the hippocampus in the development of anxiety. These early preliminary data suggest that there is something neuroprotective about a large hippocampus that mitigates the development of PTSD, even when someone is exposed to unimaginable trauma. Possibly, a large hippocampus is better able to limit the acquisition of haunting memories or more efficient at extinguishing them once they develop.

Two recent twin studies published in 2012 corroborated the Gilbertson findings. In one study with women, a smaller hippocampus correlated with a diagnosis of GAD. In a large study with male twins, hippocampal volume correlated with self-esteem.

NEUROTRANSMITTERS AND CELL BIOLOGY

γ-Aminobutyric Acid

GABA is the major inhibitory neurotransmitter in the brain. Activating GABA neurons calm down the brain. Too much GABA activation causes sluggishness and even coma. The GABA receptor has several sites that bind with other substances, which has the effect of enhancing the inhibitory activity of the GABA neurons. Figure 5.3 shows that ethanol, barbiturates, and benzodiazepines are known to bind with the GABA receptor. It is no wonder that people use and abuse these substances to calm down and reduce anxiety.

ALCOHOLISM AND ANXIETY

There is controversy about the relation between alcoholism and anxiety. Acute alcohol intoxication reduces anxiety. Many clinicians believe that substance abusers are self-medicating their anxiety with alcohol and other calming agents. Longitudinal and genetic studies support this perception for some patients.

However, there is compelling evidence that chronic alcohol exposure induces long-term central nervous system adaptations that cause anxiety. For example, the following have been observed:

1. Withdrawal from alcohol increases anxiety.
2. The anxiety of withdrawal decreases as abstinence persists.
3. Studies on twins have shown that anxiety disorders are common in the alcoholic twin but not the sober twin.
4. Rats exposed to chronic alcohol show alterations in γ-aminobutyric acid (GABA) receptors.

5. Abstaining alcoholics showed a decreased benzodiazepine receptor distribution (see figure).

Abstaining alcoholics show decreased benzodiazepine receptor distribution in frontal cortex and cerebellum compared with controls.

Frontal cortex

Cerebellum

Adapted from Abi-Dargham A, Krystal JH, Anjilvel S, et al. Alterations of benzodiazepine receptors in type II alcoholic subjects measured with SPECT and [123I]iomazenil. *Am J Psychiatry.* 1998;155(11):1550-1555.

Abnormalities in the benzodiazepine GABA receptor have been implicated as a possible cause of anxiety disorders. Results of the original imaging studies and more recent genetic studies suggest that alterations in the structure or concentration of the benzodiazepine GABA receptor may predispose individuals to anxiety. However, the hypotheses have not been consistently or conclusively established.

Norepinephrine

The norepinephrine (NE) neurons with cell bodies in the locus coeruleus (shown in Figure 4.5) are believed to be part of the stress response system and play an important role in anxiety. The following evidence supports this belief:

1. NE neurons project to the amygdala.
2. Stressed rats show increases in NE release.
3. NE stimulates the release of corticotropin-releasing hormone, which in turn activates the HPA axis.
4. Peripheral NE (the sympathetic branch of the autonomic nervous system) produces somatic symptoms of anxiety: racing heart, sweating, dry mouth, and so on.

With this in mind, blocking NE with the beta-blocker propranolol has been proposed as a treatment to prevent the development of PTSD. That is, giving a beta-blocker in the acute aftermath of trauma (in the ER, on the battle field, etc.) to inhibit the NE stimulation and limit the development of haunting memories. Early small studies reported mild to moderate effects. Subsequent larger, controlled trials have been disappointing.

Brain-Derived Neurotrophic Factor

This brings us back to a topic we first addressed in Chapter 5—LTP. Figures 5.5 to 5.8 show how excessive stimulation alters the signals to the nucleus, which affects gene expression and ultimately changes the structure of the neurons. LTP is an analogy for trauma-induced anxiety (PTSD). With anxiety, we see heightened activity in the amygdala and reduced activity in the PFC and hippocampus. Clearly, something changes in the traumatized anxious brain. The missing ingredient may be growth factor proteins (such as brain-derived neurotrophic factor [BDNF]) that can alter the structure and function of the neural networks.

Animal studies have shown that BDNF is essential for the acquisition and extinction of anxiety:

1. BDNF transcription is increased in the amygdala after fear conditioning.
2. When BDNF is selectively deleted from the hippocampus in mice, they show impaired ability to extinguish conditioned fear.
3. BDNF in the lateral part of the dorsolateral prefrontal cortex (DLPFC) appears to control fear memory formation, while BDNF in the medical DLPFC is necessary for fear extinction.

In summary, this research implies that the development of anxiety and the failure to extinguish it likely occur through the production of growth factor proteins in specific regions of the brain. These conflicting roles for BDNF show how difficult it would be to develop an effective antianxiety treatment, which manipulates the expression of BDNF.

OBSESSIVE-COMPULSIVE DISORDER

OCD is classified as an anxiety disorder in the DSM nomenclature. However, some clinicians conceptualize OCD as a different kind of disorder. They see OCD as one extreme of a spectrum of repetitive behavioral problems: body dysmorphic disorder, certain eating disorders, gambling, and even autism. These conditions are frequently called *OC spectrum disorders*.

Regardless of the nomenclature controversy, OCD is unique among the anxiety disorders because it is driven by a different neural activity. This was first noticed in the 1930s by the behavioral sequela after von Economo's encephalitis pandemic from 1917 to 1926. Patients who had

THE PARADOX OF ANTIDEPRESSANTS AND ANXIETY

If the NE system is part of the anxiety response, why does blocking NE reuptake, and consequently increasing NE at the synapse, relieve anxiety? How can more be less? For example, antidepressants such as the highly noradrenergic imipramine and the NE reuptake inhibitor reboxetine are known to reduce panic attacks. This does not make sense.

This paradox highlights that our understanding of anxiety and how the antidepressants calm the nervous system are in need of further study. Most likely, the antidepressants reduce anxiety by growth or increased strengthening of inhibitory networks.

EARLY ADVERSITY

Early adverse experiences have a significant impact on the later development of anxiety. Harry Harlow established with monkeys the profound negative impact of being raised without a mother or peer relationship. He replaced the mother of infant rhesus monkeys with an inanimate surrogate object during the first months of life. The infant monkeys displayed long-term deficits in social adaptation as well as increased anxiety-related behaviors.

We have discussed examples in which early experience changes neural structures. For example, the following have been observed:

1. Rats raised in standard wire cages have less dendritic branching than those raised in an enriched environment (see Point of Interest, page 90).
2. Licking and grooming by the rat mother effects the pup's response to stress (see Figure 17.5).
3. Children raised in Romanian orphanages have lower IQs (see Figure 19.8).

A recent study looked at the effect of breast-feeding on anxiety in humans. Children whose parents separated or divorced when the children were between the ages of 5 and 10 years were assessed for anxiety when they turned 10. The children who were breast-fed had less anxiety and more resilience in response to the difficult circumstances. Although there are no details about the effects of breast-feeding on the brain, the results of this study seem strikingly similar to what Michael Meaney found with his high lick and groom mother rats (see Figure 17.8). Extra attention at an early stage of life may be neuroprotective.

recovered from the original infection were often inflicted with OCD or parkinsonism. The basal ganglia were implicated. Symptoms of OCD are also seen with other disorders that affect the basal ganglia: Tourette's syndrome, Parkinson's disease, Sydenham's chorea, and so on.

Basal Ganglia

The basal ganglia are subcortical structures that are usually associated with movement and motor control. Disruption of the basal ganglia leads to such disorders as Huntington's disease, Parkinson's disease, and hemiballismus. However, the exact function of the basal ganglia in OCD remains unclear.

The basal ganglia are made up of interconnected nuclei—the caudate, putamen, and globus pallidus (Figure 22.10). The caudate and putamen together are called the *striatum* and contains the nucleus accumbens (NAc). Many areas of the cerebral cortex send signals to the basal ganglia, which are relayed to the thalamus, which in turn sends an impulse back to the cortex. This loop is called the cortico-striatal-thalamic-cortical circuit.

Functional imaging studies of obsessing OCD patients have repeatedly shown increased activity in the orbitofrontal cortex, anterior cingulate gyrus, and basal ganglia. It is presumed that these areas light up due to looping signals within the cortico-striatal-thalamic-cortical circuit. However, the particular circuit may depend on the particular

ritual: washing, checking, or hoarding seem to activate slightly different regions. Likewise, treatment interventions, whether with psychotherapy or medications, show decreased activity in the basal ganglia for those who respond.

Psychosurgery

There is a long and troubling history of attempts to treat mental illness with neurosurgical interventions (see page 166). Understandably, many are reluctant to even consider neurosurgery as a treatment option for psychiatric diseases. However, there is good evidence that some limited procedures with treatment-resistant patients can diminish OCD symptoms.

Different techniques are preferred in various regions of the world. In the United States, the popular technique is anterior cingulotomy, which is based on the concept of interrupting the circuit between the anterior cingulate gyrus and basal ganglia. Figure 22.11 shows the location of the lesions in postsurgical MRI scans.

Follow-up studies have found that approximately 30% of the anterior cingulotomy patients have a 35% or greater reduction on the Yale-Brown Obsessive Compulsive Scale. Complications include urinary incontinence and seizures, but appear to be infrequent. A different technique used more regularly in Europe is anterior capsulotomy. Although this procedure appears to be more effective, it is also associated with more complications, for example, cognitive and

FIGURE 22.10 ● The structures of the basal ganglia and how they reside within the brain.

affective dysfunction. More recently, deep brain stimulation has been studied as a way to treat severe and intractable OCD in a manner that is reversible and more flexible. The Food and Drug Administration (FDA) has issued a humanitarian device exemption to allow psychiatrists to treat treatment-resistant OCD patients with deep brain stimulation. The bilateral leads are implanted in a manner to interrupt this pathological cortico-subcortical circuit.

FIGURE 22.11 ● Three views of anterior cingulotomy for treatment-resistant obsessive-compulsive disorder (OCD). The white *arrows* show the location of the lesions. The white rings around the lesions are secondary edema from the procedure. (Redrawn from Richter EO, Davis KD, Hamani C, et al. Cingulotomy for psychiatric disease: microelectrode guidance, a callosal reference system for documenting lesion location, and clinical results. *Neurosurgery.* 2004;54(3):622-628.)

DOES MEDICATING ANXIETY PREVENT LEARNING?

Medication and psychotherapy alleviate anxiety through different mechanisms but with equal effectiveness. Combining the two treatment modalities is generally believed to be more efficacious than either of them alone, although this has not been conclusively established. However, some clinicians wonder whether medications limit the learning that is essential for effective psychotherapy.

There are only three large, combined psychotherapy/medication studies for the treatment of anxiety disorders that have long-term follow-up after stopping the medications:

1. Alprazolam and exposure therapy, alone and in combination, for panic disorder
2. CBT, imipramine, or their combination for panic disorder
3. Exposure therapy and sertraline in social phobia

In all three trials, one outcome was the same. When the medication was stopped, the group that received a combination of medication and psychotherapy deteriorated relative to the group that received psychotherapy alone. The figure shows the result for the CBT/imipramine study for panic.

Studies have shown that extinction results from the development of new memories rather

than the erasure of the old fearful memories. Does medication limit the development of new memories that are required for effective, enduring psychotherapy? These studies suggest that some therapeutic changes that usually occur in the brain with psychotherapy are impeded by the presence of the psychoactive medication.

When treatment was stopped after the 6-month maintenance period, the group receiving imipramine (Imp) and cognitive-behavioral therapy (CBT) failed to sustain the benefits of psychotherapy.

1. Marks IM, et al. *Brit J Psych*. 1993;162:776-787.
2. Barlow DH, et al. *JAMA*. 2000;283:2529-2536.
3. Haug TT, et al. *Brit J Psych*. 2003;182:312-318.

QUESTIONS

1. Which hormone initially drops owing to the stress of parachute jumping?
   a. Glucocorticoids.
   b. Gonadotropins.
   c. Growth hormone.
   d. Mineralocorticoids.

2. All of the following are true about Klüver-Bucy syndrome, except
   a. Made aggressive monkeys tame.
   b. Induced hypersexuality.
   c. Identified the hippocampus as important for anxiety.
   d. Was elicited through removal of most of the temporal lobe.

3. Evidence that the amygdala is important for experiencing fear
   a. Ischemic damage increases fear response.

   b. Electric stimulation reduces freezing and heart rate.
   c. Emotional trauma has no effect on the amygdala.
   d. Treatment reduces activity in the amygdala.

4. The recognition of a threatening object includes all of the following, except
   a. The brain reacts once all the signals are analyzed.
   b. Signals from the amygdala stimulate heart rate.
   c. Auditory and visual information proceed to the thalamus.
   d. Memories modulate the amygdaloid response.

5. Stimulation of the medial PFC has what effect on a rat's fear response?
   a. Inhibits the expression of anxiety.

b. Impairs extinction.

c. Increases the activity in the amygdala.

d. Decreases activity in the anterior cingulate gyrus.

6. The best estimate of the volume of a combat veteran's hippocampus is

a. The total duration of trauma he experienced.

b. The intensity of combat trauma he experienced.

c. The level of glucocorticoids in the morning at rest.

d. The size of his twin's hippocampus.

7. Medications decrease anxiety in all the following ways, except

a. Increase the GABA inhibitory signal.

b. Increase BDNF production at the NAc.

c. Modulation of the NE neurons.

d. Quieting the amygdala.

8. Imaging studies show increased activity in all the following regions in OCD patients, except

a. Orbitofrontal cortex.

b. Anterior cingulate gyrus.

c. Amygdala.

d. Basal ganglia.

See Answers section at the end of the book.

CHAPTER 23

Schizophrenia

HISTORIC PERSPECTIVE

Over 100 years ago, Emil Kraepelin, a German psychiatrist, described the syndrome now called *schizophrenia*. Bleuler actually coined the term *schizophrenia*. Kraepelin called it *dementia praecox*. Kraepelin's major contribution to psychiatry was recognizing that schizophrenia and manic depression are different disorders. The patient with schizophrenia has a persistent deteriorating course in mental functioning, whereas the patient with manic depression will experience periods of remission. Figure 23.1 shows a modern interpretation of the clinical course of schizophrenia.

Kraepelin was convinced that schizophrenia was an organic disease of the brain and spent considerable time and energy conducting postmortem studies on the brains of patients with schizophrenia. They had a good track record of identifying pathology, as one of his colleagues was the neuropathologist Alois Alzheimer. Unfortunately, Kraepelin

was never able to discover a specific abnormality in the brains of schizophrenic patients. This pattern was to continue for a long time.

Numerous postmortem studies were conducted over the next 70 years comparing the brains of schizophrenic patients with healthy controls. Still no distinguishing pathology was isolated. The absence of gliosis in the tissue was of particular interest. Gliosis, sometimes called the *glial scar*, is considered the hallmark of neurodegenerative disorders and is found with such conditions as Huntington's or Alzheimer's diseases as well as with trauma and ischemia.

The absence of any significant neuropathology along with the burgeoning interest in psychoanalytic theory led to psychosocial explanations for schizophrenia. Terms such as the *refrigerator mother* and the *double-bind* were developed to explain the psychological turmoil that caused schizophrenia. Some clinicians even speculated

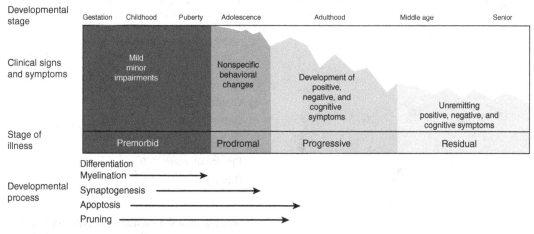

FIGURE 23.1 ● The typical clinical course of schizophrenia includes a relatively normal childhood interrupted in late adolescence or early adulthood by a dramatic deterioration from which few remit. (Adapted from Lewis DA, Lieberman JA. Catching up on schizophrenia: natural history and neurobiology. *Neuron*. 2000;28(2):325-334.)

that patients voluntarily chose to be psychotic to avoid conflict in their lives.

Although the development of chlorpromazine (Thorazine) in the early 1950s dramatically changed the treatment of schizophrenia, the identification of biologic abnormalities remained elusive. In 1972, Plum summarized the frustration when he called schizophrenia the *graveyard of neuropathologists*. Schizophrenia was actually dropped from the preeminent neuropathology textbook (Greenfield's Neuropathology) for the next two editions and only added back in 1997. It was the emergence of significant findings on brain imaging studies that finally ended the debate about whether there are quantifiable (measurable) changes in the brain (more on this in the next section).

Although we follow convention and use the term "schizophrenia," many researchers are struck by the variations between patients. For example, some patients have no hallucinations and mostly struggle with negative symptoms, while other patients have chronic hallucinations and few negative symptoms. To remind readers of this heterogeneity, some use the term "the schizophrenias." In this book we will use the standard term schizophrenia.

MODERN EPIDEMIC?

E. Fuller Torrey calls schizophrenia an invisible plague. He believes that schizophrenia is a modern illness that has increased so gradually that the change is not perceptible during any single person's lifetime. Additionally, the changes in diagnostic criteria that occur over the decades make comparisons between generations difficult. In spite

of these difficulties, there is evidence to support Dr. Torrey's belief.

The ancient Greeks and Romans were astute observers of human behavior. Reviews of the writings from ancient times provide the following descriptions of conditions that we easily recognize:

1. Epilepsy
2. Migraine headache
3. Melancholia
4. Anxiety
5. Chronic alcoholism
6. Delirium

The ancient writers did describe psychotic symptoms including hallucinations and delusions. However, in almost every case the psychosis cleared. There are no reports that describe an initial psychotic break in late adolescence or early adulthood with a chronic unremitting course. The absence of a condition that looks like schizophrenia stands in contrast to the good clinical descriptions of other neuropsychiatric syndromes. This softly suggests that the illness was not present in ancient Greece or Rome.

The 19th and 20th centuries saw an explosion in the institutionalization of patients with chronic mental illness. Many of these patients had schizophrenia. Figure 23.2 shows the growth in institutionalized patients as a percentage of the total population in four countries. There are many reasons for confining the seriously mentally ill: industrial revolution, changes in social norms, lack of effective treatments, and so on. An additional explanation is the emergence of a psychiatric epidemic.

POINT OF INTEREST

There is considerable evidence that people born and/or raised in urban settings are at greater risk for developing schizophrenia. For example, a Danish study compared the diagnosis of schizophrenia with where the patient resided on his/her 15th birthday.

Denmark

■ Copenhagen	6.5	
■ Copenhagen suburb	4.1	The incidence of schizophrenia per 1,000
■ Provincial city	3.5	
■ Provincial town	3.0	
■ Rural area	2.6	

What is it about urban life that increases the risk of developing schizophrenia?

Denmark segregated by population density.

Adapted from Pedersen CB, Mortensen PB. Urbanization and traffic related exposures as risk factors for schizophrenia. *BMC Psychiatry.* 2006;6:2.

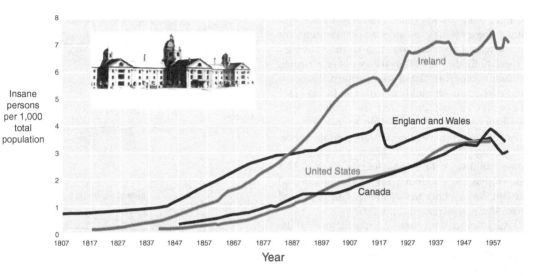

FIGURE 23.2 ● The epidemic of mental illness in the last two centuries. (Adapted from Liberman RP, Musgrave JG, Langlois J. Taunton State Hospital, Massachusetts. *Am J Psychiatry*. 2003;160(12):2098; Torrey EF, Miller J. *The Invisible Plague: The Rise of Mental Illness from 1750 to the Present*. New Brunswick, NJ: Rutgers University Press; 2001.)

Although we may never know for sure whether schizophrenia is a modern epidemic or has been around for ages, the topic raises the issue of etiology. What causes schizophrenia? We will start with what is known about the brain of patients with schizophrenia.

GRAY MATTER

The development of brain imaging techniques provided a way to examine schizophrenic brains in live people. The first computed tomography scans in schizophrenia were published in 1976 and showed enlarged lateral ventricles in a group of patients with chronic schizophrenia. Others quickly replicated this study. However, it was magnetic resonance imaging (MRI), with its ability to differentiate gray and white matter, that finally provided irrefutable evidence of the biologic nature of schizophrenia.

The most famous MRI studies were the original studies on twins. E. Fuller Torrey and Daniel Weinberger et al. at the National Institute of Mental Health recruited monozygotic twins from the United States and Canada. They originally studied 15 sets of twins who were discordant for schizophrenia: one had the illness, whereas the other was unaffected. MRI was done in all 30 participants. The most remarkable finding was that in 12 of the 15 sets of twins the affected individual was easily identified by visual inspection of corresponding coronal scans (Figure 23.3).

The results of the twin study have been replicated and extended. The most common finding remains enlarged ventricles, but better technology

has allowed more detailed analysis. Patients with schizophrenia show consistent but subtle decreases

35-year-old female identical twins

28-year-old male identical twins

FIGURE 23.3 ● Coronal magnetic resonance imaging of two sets of twins discordant for schizophrenia. The enlarged lateral ventricles are readily apparent in the subjects on the right. (Courtesy of Drs. E. Fuller Torrey and Daniel Weinberger.)

in total brain volume and total gray matter volume. These results provide an explanation for the increased ventricle size; that is, the ventricles expand to fill the void left by the loss of gray matter.

Judith Rapoport's laboratory performed sequential MRI scans on children with childhood-onset schizophrenia and compared the findings with age-matched controls in an effort to follow up the changes in the brain that occur during adolescence. They found that the rate of change was greater for those children with schizophrenia. Figure 23.4 shows that the children with schizophrenia had striking loss of gray matter along with decreased brain size and increased ventricles.

Adolescence is a time of remodeling of the connections in the brain to create a more efficient organ. Processes such as pruning, apoptosis, and synaptogenesis are accepted features of the maturing brain (see Figures 8.8, 19.4, and 20.8). Studies such as the one described here suggest that schizophrenia may be the result of overly exuberant remodeling of the gray matter.

Certainly, the process of gray matter reduction occurs in the same time frame as the usual onset of schizophrenic symptoms. Although no definitive evidence exists to prove this theory, some genetic studies suggest that altered expression of genes that control synaptic plasticity contributes to the development of schizophrenia.

Reduced Neuropil Hypothesis

As stated before, traditional microscopic examination of the gray matter of schizophrenics will not identify anything unusual. So it has been difficult to explain the gray matter loss. Investigators at Yale utilized labor-intensive three-dimensional analytic tools to estimate cellular densities. They compared neuronal density in three regions of the

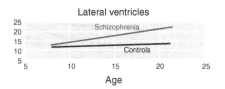

FIGURE 23.4 ● Children with schizophrenia have loss of brain volume and gray matter as well as enlargement of lateral ventricles through adolescence. (Adapted from Gogtay N, Sporn A, Rapoport J. Structural brain MRI studies in childhood-onset schizophrenia and childhood atypical psychosis. In: Lawrie S, Johnstone E, Weinberger D, eds. *Schizophrenia: from Neuroimaging to Neuroscience.* New York, NY: Oxford University Press; 2004.)

brain from patients with schizophrenia and from healthy controls. The regions were Brodmann's areas 9 and 46 in the prefrontal cortex (PFC) and area 17 in the visual cortex. They found increased density of neurons but not glial cells in the gray matter of schizophrenic patients (Figure 23.5).

It appears that schizophrenic patients have the same number of neurons as healthy controls, but they are packed together in less space—called the *reduced neuropil hypothesis.* The tighter packaging of the schizophrenic neurons results from reduced cell

FIGURE 23.5 ● Patients with schizophrenia have increased neuronal density in all three areas of the brain tested. Glial density was no different. (Adapted from Selemon LD, Goldman-Rakic PS. The reduced neuropil hypothesis: a circuit based model of schizophrenia. *Biol Psychiatry.* 1999;45(1):17-25.)

size, less branching, and decreased spine formation. Figure 23.6 shows a drawing of this process. Figure 23.7 shows examples of actual spine formation from schizophrenic patients and controls. The key point is that it is not neuronal loss, but rather the loss of the richness of the dendritic connections that causes the reduced gray matter in schizophrenia. Presumably, this also results in deficient information processing.

Although the underlying cause of neuronal atrophy remains unknown, recent evidence suggests a role for altered neuronal apoptosis. Apoptosis is usually associated with programmed cell death (see Figure 8.9). However, sublethal apoptotic activity may result in synaptic elimination without frank cell death. Apoptosis is controlled by pro- and antiapoptotic proteins, which may be disturbed in schizophrenia.

One further point worth mentioning is that these studies highlight the extensive whole brain involvement of schizophrenia. That is, it is not a disorder of just one region of the brain. Rather, schizophrenia seems to affect almost the entire cortex.

A

Healthy control gray matter

Schizophrenic gray matter

B

Healthy neuron

Schizophrenic neuron

Reduced:
Soma size
Spine formation
Dendritic branching

FIGURE 23.6 ● **A.** Schematic representation of the increased density but decreased size of schizophrenic gray matter. **B.** Suspected neuronal atrophy of schizophrenic pyramidal neurons, which results in defective connectivity. (**A** adapted from Selemon LD. Increased cortical neuronal density in schizophrenia. *Am J Psychiatry*. 2004;161(9):1564.)

Functional Brain Imaging

Traditionally, the hallmark of schizophrenia has been hallucinations and delusions. In actuality, the symptoms of schizophrenia are made up of the following three categories of impairment.

1. Positive symptoms: hallucinations and delusions
2. Negative symptoms: lack of motivation, apathy, and so on
3. Cognitive impairment

The cognitive dysfunction, which includes problems with attention, memory, and executive function, may be the most detrimental aspect of the illness. They have a greater negative impact on the individual than the positive symptoms. Likewise, cognitive functioning is the best predictor of long-term outcome from the disorder.

The pattern of cognitive impairment in schizophrenia implicates the frontal cortex. *Hypofrontality* is a term sometimes used to describe this problem. However, functional imaging studies have given inconsistent results. Weinberger et al. recognized that the function of the frontal lobe must be measured when it is engaged in a cognitive challenge.

To test this theory, patients and healthy controls underwent xenon XE 133 inhalation procedure for regional cerebral blood flow measurements while they were performing the Wisconsin Card Sorting test (Figure 23.8). The control subjects showed increased activation of their frontal lobes while performing the test, but the schizophrenic patients did not. Furthermore, there was a good correlation between the change in blood flow in the frontal cortex and percent errors on the test.

Control   Schizophrenic

Mean spine density

Area 46   Area 17

FIGURE 23.7 ● **A.** Drawings of actual dendrites and spines from pyramidal neurons in the dorsolateral prefrontal cortex of controls and schizophrenic patients. **B.** Mean spine density in frontal cortex and visual cortex from controls and schizophrenic patients. (Adapted from Glantz LA, Lewis DA. Decreased dendritic spine density on prefrontal cortical pyramidal neurons in schizophrenia. *Arch Gen Psychiatry*. 2000;57(1):65-73.)

FIGURE 23.8 • **A.** Subjects were scanned while performing the Wisconsin Card Sorting task. **B.** Healthy subjects displayed increased blood flow to the prefrontal cortex (PFC), whereas those with schizophrenia did not (*arrow*). **C.** Percent errors on the task correlated with change in PFC blood flow. (Adapted from Weinberger DR, Berman KF, Zec RF. Physiologic dysfunction of dorsolateral prefrontal cortex in schizophrenia. I. Regional cerebral blood flow evidence. *Arch Gen Psychiatry*. 1986;43(2): 114-124.)

In summary, these results suggest that the cognitive impairment in patients with schizophrenia comes from impaired frontal lobes. Atrophic, disconnected neuronal cells presumably cause the PFC dysfunction.

Inhibitory Neurons

The activity of the large pyramidal neurons in the gray matter is modulated by smaller local interneurons (see Figure 2.3). Most of the interneurons are γ-aminobutyric acid (GABA) neurons and hence are inhibitory. There are several types of GABA neurons. Figure 23.9A shows two of them: parvalbumin and calretinin. The location of their inhibitory input seems to have different effects on the pyramidal neuron.

The GABA interneurons are important in the discussion of schizophrenia because there is evidence that the parvalbumin neurons are impaired in patients with the disorder. GABA is synthesized from a number of enzymes, one of which is called *glutamic acid decarboxylase* (GAD). One form of messenger RNA (mRNA) that encodes for GAD (GAD67) has been shown repeatedly to be decreased in patients with schizophrenia. It is one of the most consistent findings in postmortem studies. Figure 23.9B, C shows the results of a study comparing the expression of GAD67 in patients and controls.

Of particular interest, the deficiency in GAD67 expressing interneurons seems to be limited only to the parvalbumin neurons and is not found in other GABA neurons. Furthermore, the number of parvalbumin neurons is not reduced in patients with schizophrenia. So the GABA neurons that are implicated in schizophrenia are not limited in number, but have decreased expression of important genes that might impair the function of the cortex.

Working memory depends on the coordinated firing of pyramidal neurons in the PFC. The inhibitory interneurons are essential for the synchronization of the output from the pyramidal neurons. Tasks such as the delayed response task (see Figure 20.3) require inhibitory control to bridge the time between stimulus presentation and behavioral response. The cognitive impairment in patients with schizophrenia may be due to a failure to properly coordinate the pyramidal neurons.

WHITE MATTER

Schizophrenia also appears to be a disorder of disrupted connectivity. The white matter tracks that connect different regions of the cortex, as well as the cortex with the deeper brain structures, may also play an important role in the disruption of good connections. White matter is composed of the myelinated axons that transport the signals generated by the neurons. Figure 23.10 shows a drawing of some of the long and short white matter tracks. Disruption of the integrity of the white matter tracks leads to degradation of the neuronal signal.

Imaging

MRI studies on patients and controls have found a small but nonsignificant trend toward reduced white matter in schizophrenia. Other studies using the more recently developed diffusion tensor imaging (DTI) technology (see Figure 3.13) have found abnormalities in patients with schizophrenia compared with healthy controls. Some insight into the significance of these findings can be gleaned from comparing the result of DTI studies in other

FIGURE 23.9 ● **A.** γ-Aminobutyric acid (GABA) interneurons have inhibitory input on the pyramidal neurons in the prefrontal cortex. **B.** Glutamic acid decarboxylase (GAD)67 expression cells from the prefrontal cortex of a control and a patient with schizophrenia. **C.** Mean number of GAD67 messenger RNA (mRNA) expression neurons by gray matter layer. PFC, prefrontal cortex. (**A** Adapted from Tamminga C, Hashimoto T, Volk DW, et al. GABA neurons in the human prefrontal cortex. *Am J Psychiatry*. 2004;161(10):1764. **B, C** Adapted from Akbarian S, Kim JJ, Potkin SG, et al. Gene expression for glutamic acid decarboxylase is reduced without loss of neurons in prefrontal cortex of schizophrenics. *Arch Gen Psychiatry*. 1995;52(4):258-266.)

demyelinating diseases. For example, multiple sclerosis and human immunodeficiency virus (both known to induce cognitive impairment and hallucinations with some patients) also produce changes in the DTI analysis. These results suggest that all three diseases may share some similar white matter degradation.

Myelin
Oligodendrocytes
Oligodendrocytes are one of the glial cells that support the neurons. Specifically, the oligodendrocytes provide layers of myelin that insulate the axons and enhance the speed of transmission of neural impulses (see Figure 3.10). Diseases that affect the integrity of the myelin sheath impair the function of the brain and can cause psychotic symptoms in some cases. One particular disease—metachromatic leukodystrophy—usually begins with demyelination of the frontal lobes.

The rare late-onset form of metachromatic leukodystrophy occurs in about the same time frame as schizophrenia—from adolescence to young adulthood. Reviews of such cases have noted that over half the individuals had psychotic symptoms including auditory hallucinations and bizarre delusions.

Others have looked at the oligodendrocyte population in patients with schizophrenia. Hof et al. counted the number of oligodendrocytes in the white matter of Brodmann's area 9. They found that there was a 27% decrease in the number of oligodendrocytes in patients with schizophrenia compared with the controls (see Figure 23.11).

The application of microarray analysis (see Figure 1.11) has further implicated the involvement of myelin in schizophrenia. Hakak et al. applied postmortem tissue from patients with schizophrenia and controls to microarray chips to identify gene expression. In other words, they wanted to see which genes were active in which subjects.

More than 6,000 genes were compared between the schizophrenic and control subjects. Only 17 genes were significantly downregulated in the schizophrenic patients. Of these, six were myelin related. The other 11 showed no particular pattern. The authors concluded that the results gave a clear indication that deficient oligodendrocytes and myelination are involved in schizophrenia.

FIGURE 23.10 ● A drawing of the white matter tracks connecting various regions in the brain. (Adapted from Gray's Anatomy of the Human Body as displayed at Bartleby.com.)

FIGURE 23.11 ● **A.** One oligodendrocyte can provide the myelin covering over many axons. **B.** Patients with schizophrenia have less oligodendrocytes in their white matter. (Graph adapted from Hof PR, Haroutunian V, Friedrich VL Jr, et al. Loss and altered spatial distribution of oligodendrocytes in the superior frontal gyrus in schizophrenia. *Biol Psychiatry.* 2003;53(12):1075-1085.)

AUDITORY HALLUCINATIONS

In 1863, Broca described lesions of the left frontal cortex in patients with language expression deficits (see Figure 1.3). Roughly 10 years later, Wernicke described a different language deficit associated with lesions of the superior temporal lobe. The region Wernicke described was a part of what is now called the *auditory cortex*. The perception of sound starts in the ear, then proceeds through the brain stem and thalamus before reaching the auditory cortex on the superior aspect of the temporal lobe (see Figure 23.12). White matter tracts called the *arcuate fasciculus* connect the auditory cortex with the frontal cortex.

Wernicke and later Kraepelin both postulated that auditory hallucinations were due to temporal lobe abnormalities since neurologic causes of auditory hallucinations pointed in that direction. Indeed, an auditory aura preceding a seizure suggests the temporal lobe as the nidus of the electric activity. Likewise, hallucinations can result from strokes that involve the temporal lobes. However, until recently the neuronal correlates of auditory hallucinations for schizophrenia were unknown.

A group in Switzerland has done extensive imaging studies of schizophrenic patients when they were hallucinating. In the past, the time it took to scan a person was so long it obscured the difference between the hallucinating state and the nonhallucinating state. Now with rapid functional MRI scans, the differences can be detected. Patients were asked to press a button with the onset of hallucinations and keep it pressed for as long as they lasted. Images during hallucinations were compared with images when the voices were silent. Figure 23.13A shows the activity in the gray matter of the auditory cortex during hallucinations for one patient.

POINT OF INTEREST

Numerous researchers have documented a correlation between auditory hallucinations and the size of the temporal lobe; that is, a smaller temporal lobe predicts more hallucinations. This seems counterintuitive. Why does less brain tissue produce positive symptoms?

FIGURE 23.12 ● **A.** Pathways from the ear to the cortex. **B.** Auditory signals synapse in the thalamus before reaching the auditory cortex. **C.** The Arcuate fasciculus is composed of white matter tracts that connect the auditory cortex with the frontal cortex.

A   **B**

FIGURE 23.13 ● **A.** Functional magnetic resonance imaging (fMRI) showing the gray matter regions activated when schizophrenic patients are experiencing auditory hallucinations (*arrows*). **B.** Diffusion tensor imaging showing the areas of altered white matter tracts for patients who hear auditory hallucinations compared to healthy controls. (**A** from Dierks T, Linden DE, Jandl M, et al. Activation of Heschls gyrus during auditory hallucinations. *Neuron.* 1999;22(3):615-621. **B** from Hubl D, Koenig T, Strik W, et al. Pathways that make voices: white matter changes in auditory hallucinations. *Arch Gen Psychiatry.* 2004;61(7):658-668.)

Recently, this same research group used DTI to look at white matter tracts in schizophrenic patients with hallucinations compared with patients without hallucinations and healthy controls. Remarkably, they found that patients with hallucinations have significantly more alterations of the white matter tracts of the arcuate fasciculus (Figure 23.13B).

Taken together, these studies suggest that auditory hallucinations are derived from abnormalities in the regions that register external sounds. The patient with auditory hallucinations may misidentify inner speech as coming from an external source due to lack of integrity of the system. It is reminiscent of a phone or television picking up other signals and playing more than one sound track at a time.

These studies highlight the complexity of schizophrenia (or the schizophrenias). For just one symptom, abnormalities have been identified in both the gray matter and white matter for patients with schizophrenia. Clearly, schizophrenia is a confusing disorder with diverse and numerous effects on multiple areas of the brain.

ETIOLOGY

We have tried to establish that schizophrenia appears to be a disorder of disconnectedness. There is no specific brain region affected, but rather a dysfunction of circuits within and between regions. Additionally, the onset of the full disorder suggests a neurodevelopmental disruption. It is plausible to envision that schizophrenia results from the abnormal expression of genes that govern maturational processes. However, what goes wrong and how does all this occur?

Genetics

One of the most consistent findings in schizophrenia research is the heritable nature of the illness and related illnesses. Figure 1.1 shows the striking power of the genes with this disorder. The closer one is related to someone with schizophrenia, the more likely that person is to get the illness. However, even the monozygotic twin of a person with schizophrenia only has approximately a 50% chance of getting the illness. Furthermore, patients with schizophrenia are less likely to procreate. If this is a genetic disorder with Mendelian properties, we would expect it to decline in frequency over many generations. Clearly, there is more involved than just genes in the traditional sense.

Environment

Prenatal Complications

Adverse environmental events are known to be potential triggers for developing schizophrenia. Maternal infection is one well-known risk factor for schizophrenia. Obstetric complications are also associated with schizophrenia. A large prospective study that followed up children from birth through adulthood found that the odds of schizophrenia increased linearly with increasing number of hypoxia-associated obstetric complications.

Famine

Two large epidemiologic studies of in utero exposure to maternal starvation have shown an increased risk of schizophrenia among the off-spring. In October 1944, a Nazi blockade of the western Netherlands precipitated a famine that did not remit until liberation in May 1945. During the blockade, daily food rations fell to <500 calories per person per day. In follow-up studies, the risk of developing schizophrenia in exposed children had doubled. Additionally, there was also a significant increase in births with neural tube defects.

The second study looked at the effects of famine caused by the Great Leap Forward in China during 1960 to 1961. Similar results were found (Figure 23.14). In both situations, the birth rate dropped during the famine. Some speculate that the lack of folate in the diet had a detrimental effect on the developing fetal brain. Folate is needed for DNA synthesis and repair. Its absence can lead to chromosomal instability. (Is this why the Irish, with their interminable famines, experienced a greater epidemic of mental illness? See Figure 23.2.)

Finnish Adoption Study

Many people conceptualize schizophrenia as resulting from some interaction between genes and the environment, but it has been hard to tease out the relation between these factors. The Finnish Adoption Study provides some interesting data to help understand this interaction. Researchers collected the names of all women who were hospitalized in Finland from 1960 to 1979 and diagnosed with schizophrenia. Then they identified the children from these women who were adopted away. They collected a similar number of adopted children as matched controls.

Detailed and blinded assessments were made of the adoptive families by experienced psychiatrists. Using specific scales, they divided families into those that were more healthy and those that

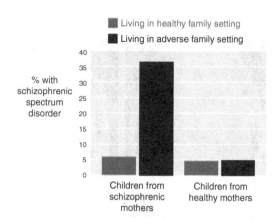

FIGURE 23.15 • Children born to schizophrenic mothers and raised in more dysfunctional family environments were at increased risk for developing schizophrenic spectrum disorders.

were more dysfunctional. Additionally, each child was assessed for a schizophrenia spectrum disorder based on the *Diagnostic and Statistical Manual of Mental Disorders-Third Edition-Revised* (DSM-III-R) criteria, for example, schizophrenia, delusional disorder, depressive disorder with psychotic features, and schizotypal personality disorder.

The remarkable results of this study are shown in Figure 23.15. Only the children born to mothers with schizophrenia and raised in an adverse family household showed an increased risk of developing schizophrenic spectrum disorders. This is an example of a genetic–environment interaction. Children at genetic risk for schizophrenia appear to be more sensitive to problems in the environment.

Gene Expression

In several chapters of this book, we have discussed the enduring effects that life events can have on the DNA. Environmental events change the genes—a cardinal feature of the neuroscience model (see Figure 6.13). Enhancing or silencing specific genes changes behavior. This enables animals to adapt their behavior to their particular environment. However, some events seem to silence important genes and have devastating effects on behavior. Schizophrenia may be such a condition.

Researchers are starting to look at changes in gene expression in patients with schizophrenia as a way to better understand the disorder. To proceed with such an examination, an important protein must first be identified and then the DNA that encodes for that protein must be analyzed.

FIGURE 23.14 • The relative rate of developing schizophrenia doubled for those born during the famine during 1960 to 1961 in one region of China.

Although we imagine there are numerous such proteins, one that has been identified is reelin, a protein expressed by GABA interneurons. Reelin is recognized as crucial for neuronal migration, axonal branching, and synaptogenesis throughout brain development. Additionally, reelin and its mRNA have been found to be reduced in postmortem brains of schizophrenic patients.

We have previously discussed that the addition of methyl groups to the DNA limits gene expression—the methyl groups prevent the transcription factors from "zipping" off some mRNA. Tsuang et al. at the University of California in San Diego recently looked at the methylation of the reelin DNA from gray matter from postmortem brains of patients with schizophrenia. Not surprisingly, they found a distinct methylated signal in 73% of the schizophrenic samples but only in 24% of the control samples. To put it another way, the reelin DNA of the schizophrenic patients was three times more likely to be methylated.

Not only does this give a possible mechanism to explain the failure of gene expression in patients with schizophrenia but also fits with known environmental events that increase the risk of developing the disorder. For example, transient ischemia is known to increase DNA methylation. Likewise, folate is necessary for normal DNA methylation. This may explain why fetal hypoxia and maternal famine predispose some individuals to develop schizophrenia.

This is not to say that DNA methylation is the only mechanism to explain schizophrenia. Spontaneous mutation during spermatogenesis is another possible cause. It is known that schizophrenia is associated with increased paternal age, and older fathers are more likely to have increased de novo germline mutations. A recent analysis of genome-wide sequencing of DNA from 78 Icelandic families (219 individuals) found that it is the age of the father that determines the number of de novo mutations in the child (Figure 23.16). The important point is that changes to DNA—particularly vulnerable DNA—can be a way for us to understand the genetic/environmental etiology of schizophrenia.

The take-home message is this: There are likely to be multiple genetic vulnerabilities to schizophrenia, which are rarely expressed but not uncommon. Insults from the environment, such as diet, infection, and ischemia, have detrimental and lasting effects on the DNA. Those individuals having

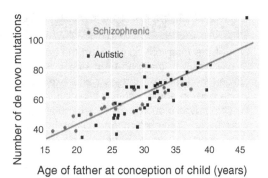

FIGURE 23.16 ● As the father's age at conception of the child increases, the number of single nucleotide polymorphisms (SNPs) increases. A father at 20 years passes along on average 25 mutations, while a 40-year-old father passes on about 65. (Adapted from Kong A, Frigge ML, Masson G, et al. Rate of *de novo* mutations and the importance of father's age to disease risk. *Nature*. 2012;488:471-475.)

both genetic vulnerability and environmental insult are the ones who develop schizophrenia.

Dopamine Hypothesis

It does not seem proper to write an entire chapter on schizophrenia without mentioning dopamine. The dopamine hypothesis is an old and enduring theory purporting that overactivity of the dopamine system is part of the pathogenesis of schizophrenia. It was first proposed in 1966 on the basis of pharmacologic studies. Dopamine blocking agents provided the first effective treatment for the positive symptoms of schizophrenia. Furthermore, amphetamines, which increase dopamine at the synaptic cleft, can induce psychosis.

Although the popularity of the dopamine blocking agents is at an all-time high, the belief that dopamine overactivity causes schizophrenia has dwindled. Modulation of dopamine activity may be effective in diminishing psychotic symptoms, but there is minimal evidence to implicate the dopamine neurons in the pathogenesis of the disorder. Howes and Kapur put it nicely in their review of the dopamine hypothesis when they proposed that dopamine dysregulation is the final common pathway of psychosis that is manipulated by "upstream factors." Most likely it is the disconnections among the glutamate and GABA neurons that are the etiopathogenesis of schizophrenia.

ANTIPSYCHOTICS AND THE SHRINKING BRAIN

One of the foremost concerns in the treatment of psychosis is the long-term effect of medication. Medication changes gene expression, which can, in some instances, propagate irreversible adverse outcomes, for example, tardive dyskinesia. While medications can be beneficial in the short run, we do not know the effects on the brain in the long run. A recent decadelong study out of Nancy Andreasen's lab in Iowa produced unsettling results on this issue.

MRI scans were performed every three years on 211 first-episode patients treated with antipsychotic medication. On average, patients had three scans over 7.2 years. The investigators found that gray matter volumes decreased over time in all brain regions except the cerebellum. Patients who received the higher lifetime doses of medication had less gray matter. These results are consistent with controlled antipsychotic treatment studies in animals.

The potential neurotoxicity of antipsychotic medications reminds us to avoid unnecessary treatment and use the lowest dose possible, until more information is available.

QUESTIONS

1. Neurodevelopmental causes that could explain schizophrenia include excessive amounts of all of the following, except
   a. Pruning.
   b. Synaptogenesis.
   c. Apoptosis.
   d. Myelination.

2. Evidence that schizophrenia is a biologic disorder includes all of the following, except
   a. The difference in lateral ventricles in the twin study.
   b. Gliosis in the PFC.
   c. Gray matter reduction in childhood-onset schizophrenia.
   d. Hypofrontality.

3. All of the following support the reduced neuropil hypothesis, except
   a. Oligodendrocyte dysfunction.
   b. Reduced neural cell size.
   c. Limited spine formation on the dendrites.
   d. Increased density of gray matter.

4. Evidence that GABA interneurons are impaired in schizophrenia
   a. Increased methylation of calretinin DNA.
   b. Reduced parvalbumin neurons.
   c. Reduced GAD67.
   d. Increased reelin.

5. All of the following suggest white matter impairment in schizophrenia, except
   a. Microarray analysis.
   b. DTI.

   c. Oligodendrocyte cell counts.
   d. Significantly reduced white matter volume.

6. Auditory hallucinations have been shown to activate which region on fMRI?
   a. Superior temporal lobe.
   b. Broca's area.
   c. Wernicke's area.
   d. Arcuate fasciculus.

7. All are plausible theories on the etiology of schizophrenia, except
   a. Methylation of DNA.
   b. Spontaneous mutations.
   c. Dopamine hypothesis.
   d. Genetic/environmental interactions.

8. Match the following:
   1. Bleuler
   2. E. Fuller Torrey
   3. Kraepelin
   4. Plum
   5. Refrigerator mother
   6. Wisconsin Card Sorting

   A. Psychoanalytic theory
   B. Distinguished schizophrenia from bipolar disorder
   C. Hypofrontality
   D. Invisible epidemic
   E. Coined the term schizophrenia
   F. Graveyard of neuropathologists

See Answers section at the end of the book.

CHAPTER 24

Alzheimer's Disease

HISTORIC PERSPECTIVE
Human Longevity

Although historic records indicate that older people have always existed, old age was once rare. Before the 20th century, few people lived beyond 50 years. Now, 95% of the children born in developed countries live past that age (Figure 24.1). Changes in health care, sanitation, and nutrition (to name a few) have had a profound impact on life expectancy. The ultimate result is that more and more people are living to ripe old ages. With more people living into their geriatric years, the aging-related central nervous system (CNS) disorders are becoming common.

All nerve cells are affected by aging. Sensory and motor skills decline with age. Neurodegenerative disorders such as Parkinson's disease, amyotrophic lateral sclerosis, and Huntington's disease become more prevalent as people get older. Cellular and molecular changes that accumulate over time

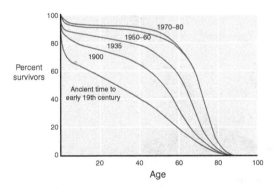

FIGURE 24.1 ● The percentage of people living beyond the age of 60 years has increased dramatically in the last two centuries. (Adapted from Kandel ER, Schwartz JH, Jessell TM, eds. *Principles of Neural Science*. 4th ed. New York, NY: McGraw-Hill; 2000.)

The maximum human life span is approximately 125 years and has not changed in over 100,000 years. Cell culture studies suggest that each species has a biologic clock that influences its life span. For example, fibroblasts will only divide a limited number of times before dying. The number of divisions is related to life span (see table).

Lifespan and Cell Division of Different Species

Species	Maximum Life Span (y)	Maximum Fibroblast Doubling
Galapagos tortoise	175	125
Man	125	60
Mouse	4	28

The important point is that life span and age-related illnesses such as dementia are likely to be controlled by different mechanisms.

render neurons vulnerable to damage. Most likely, the damage results from a combination of genetic vulnerability and environmental hits.

Dementia, the progressive deterioration of cognitive skills, is perhaps the most worrisome development for all of us. There are numerous causes of dementia, including cerebral vascular accidents, alcoholism, and infections. Alzheimer's disease (AD) is the most common cause of dementia. The surge in dementia cases as the baby boomers age is expected to overwhelm the health care system unless some intervention is discovered.

Alois Alzheimer

The disease we now call Alzheimer's was first discussed when Alois Alzheimer presented a case in 1906 of a woman with the early onset of dementia. Her symptoms started in middle age with a change in personality and mild memory impairment. She was institutionalized when she became paranoid and unmanageable. Alzheimer repeatedly examined the woman as he followed up her deteriorating clinical course. Four and a half years after her initial symptoms, she was bedridden in a fetal position until she died.

The autopsy revealed gross atrophy of the cortex without localized foci. With the application of the new staining methods (see Figure 1.4), Alzheimer found sclerotic plaques scattered throughout the cortex, especially in the upper layers. Additionally, he noted that many of the cortical neurons were reduced to dense bundles of neurofibrils. Alzheimer thought that his description of plaques and neurofibrillary tangles in a patient with "presenile dementia" was a new and unique condition.

In fact, Alzheimer's finding was cognitive loss associated with the following:

1. Cortical atrophy
2. Plaques outside the neurons
3. Tangles inside the neurons

These findings have become the description of the dementia that bears his name. Figure 24.2 shows a schematic representation of what Alzheimer might have seen when he looked through his microscope.

ALZHEIMER'S DISEASE

Surprisingly, what Alzheimer saw roughly a 100 years ago remains the focus of current research. However, the application of modern technology has greatly advanced the understanding of the pathophysiology of atrophy, plaques, and tangles.

Cortical Atrophy

The most striking feature of the Alzheimer's brain is the dramatic shrinkage of the cortical tissue secondary to neuronal cell death. AD is a bit like losing hair. It starts years before it is actually noticed and progresses slowly. In some people, it starts sooner and proceeds faster. Furthermore, almost everyone experiences some hair loss with aging.

Brain volume loss is also a "normal" feature of aging. Brain volume peaks in adolescence and then declines as much as 0.2% to 0.5% per year. Patients with AD experience accelerated neural loss. Likewise, some people are genetically predisposed to early-onset AD.

Examination of the AD brain at autopsy shows extensive atrophy. Figure 24.3 compares two views of normal brains with AD brains. The enlargement of the ventricles and sulci in combination with the decreased tissue is easily recognized—and a bit unsettling for those of us in middle age.

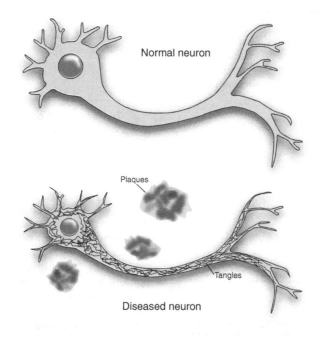

FIGURE 24.2 ● Alzheimer's disease includes the constellation of neuronal shrinkage, plaques, and neurofibrillary tangles.

Normal brains   Alzheimer's brains

FIGURE 24.3 ● Gross examination (A) and coronal slices (B) show the extensive shrinkage of the brain from Alzheimer's disease. (A courtesy of George Grossberg and the St. Louis University Alzheimer's Brain Bank.)

FIGURE 24.5 ● Positron emission tomography (PET) images showing glucose metabolism in a normal brain compared with an Alzheimer's disease brain. Note the reduced activity in the frontal and temporal regions of the AD brain. (Adapted from Mattson MP, Magnus T. Ageing and neuronal vulnerability. *Nat Rev Neurosci.* 2006;7[4]:278–294.)

Brain imaging, although not yet diagnostic for early AD, can document the volume loss and contrast the changes for those with and without AD. Figure 24.4 shows the results of sequential magnetic resonance imaging on one patient destined to develop familial AD. Note how his brain atrophy proceeds faster than in a healthy elderly control. It is also of interest that the symptoms of AD did not appear until significant brain tissue was lost.

The decrease in energy metabolism secondary to the extensive neuronal damage can be seen in functional imaging studies such as positron emission tomography (PET). Figure 24.5 shows the marked reduction in glucose metabolism in a patient with AD compared with a healthy control. The difference is so prominent that some have suggested that

PET could be used to differentiate patients with AD from those normally aging. A large European study including more than 500 subjects found a 93% sensitivity and specificity for separating mild to moderate AD from normal controls. Unfortunately, they were not as effective at separating AD from other forms of dementia, and PET is even less helpful in diagnosing patients with mild cognitive impairment and determining whether they will go on to develop AD.

Amyloid Plaques

The extracellular deposits that Alzheimer saw are called *amyloid plaques*, which is a bit of a misnomer. They are actually aggregates of fibrous protein and not amyloid at all. It was not until 1984 that the primary component of the plaques was found to be a small protein called *amyloid-β or A-β*. (To add to the confusion, the most common term used in the literature is beta-amyloid or β-amyloid.) Specifically, it is a long 42-amino-acid chain called A-β-42 that seems to be the real culprit, although there may be others that are more noxious.

FIGURE 24.4 ● A. Sequential magnetic resonance imaging (MRI) scans show the aggressive brain atrophy in a patient with Alzheimer's disease (AD) compared with healthy geriatric controls. B. MRI in a patient with AD at baseline and 4 years later (C). Brown overlay represents tissue loss compared with baseline. (Adapted from Fox NC, Schott JM. Imaging cerebral atrophy: normal ageing to Alzheimer's disease. *Lancet.* 2004;363(9406):392-394.)

FIGURE 24.6 ● Amyloid plaques are formed from the cleavage of amyloid-β precursor protein into smaller proteins that clump together. (Adapted from Wolfe MS. Shutting down Alzheimer's. *Sci Am*. 2006;294(5):72-79.)

A-β is cleaved from a larger molecule called *amyloid-β precursor protein* (APP). APP is a large protein protruding through the cell wall (Figure 24.6). It is found in cells throughout the body, but is prominent in neurons. The functions of APP are not fully understood, but may include regulating neuronal survival, neural neurite outgrowth, and synaptic plasticity.

APP is cleaved into smaller portions by at least two enzymes called *β- and γ-secretase*. The final cleavage results in the generation of A-β-42 (and others) that coalesces into long filaments. It is the clumping of the filaments that forms the "amyloid" plaques. Pharmacologic inhibition of the activity of the secretase enzymes has been of interest to those seeking ways to slow down the development of plaques.

Amyloid Hypothesis

Many believe that amyloid plaques are the source of the problem with AD. Two lines of reasoning suggest this is true. First, some people carry a genetic predisposition for early-onset AD usually developed before the age of 65 years. In all cases where they have identified the gene, the genetic abnormality causes an increased production of A-β. The toxicity of A-β is the other evidence that supports the amyloid hypothesis. A-β is toxic to neurons grown in Petri dishes. Furthermore, A-β can impair the development of long-term potentiation as well as the memory for a maze in rodents.

Recently, researchers from England have reported the results of a long-term study with marmoset monkeys. The monkeys received cerebral injections of A-β or other brain tissue that did not contain β-amyloid. Because the monkeys died, their brains were analyzed for amyloid plaques (Figure 24.7). Monkeys that were injected with A-β were much more likely to have cerebral amyloidosis at autopsy. These results not only show the toxic effects of A-β but also imply that the presence of A-β seeds the progression.

The exact mechanisms of the toxicity of A-β remain murky. Some research suggests that it is the soluble form of the protein that causes the damage. Other research suggests that it is not the A-β-42

GENE EXPRESSION

In previous chapters we have discussed how the addition of methyl groups to the DNA structure can silence gene expression, which, in turn, can produce psychiatric symptoms. The opposite may be happening with AD; that is, the awakening of improper gene expression through demethylation. There is some indirect evidence that demethylation of the DNA sequence coding for β-secretase results in increased production of that enzyme. This could result in greater production of A-β and a faster progression of the disease.

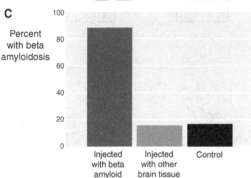

FIGURE 24.7 ● Marmoset monkeys (A) can develop cerebral amyloid plaques (B). Monkeys injected with A- were much more likely to develop amyloidosis in the next 3 to 4 years (C). (Adapted from Ridley RM, Baker HF, Windle CP, et al. Very long-term studies of the seeding of beta-amyloidosis in primates. *J Neural Transm*. 2006;113:1243–1251.)

protein, but different A-β proteins as yet unidentified. Furthermore, it is not clear why the plaques coalesce in the first place. Some evidence hints that the genetic forms of AD result from an overproduction of APP, whereas the more common sporadic cases result from the failure to clear the excess A-β. Clearly, efforts to treat the disorder would benefit from better understanding of these issues.

Imaging Amyloid

The first step in any treatment approach is an accurate diagnosis of the condition. Historically, the gold standard for the diagnosis of AD has been at autopsy—a bit late to start treatment. As noted earlier, imaging studies are poor at differentiating AD from other forms of dementia. More recently, researchers have been looking at ways to detect the presence of amyloid deposits in subjects even before symptoms appear. In 2012, the FDA approved florbetapir F18 (Amyvid) for PET imaging of the brain in cognitively impaired adults. Florbetapir binds to amyloid in the brain and gives an estimate of the density of the plaques. Figure 24.8 shows the results of a scan comparing a healthy control with a patient with AD. With this scan, unlike the PET scan in Figure 24.5, the subject with the disease lights up when the florbetapir attaches to the amyloid deposits.

The usefullness of a florbetapir PET scan is to identify reversible causes of cognitive decline, other than AD, such as depression. The ultimate utility of such a scan—identifying early stages of the disease so that treatment can be started prior to substantial neural cell loss—awaits the development of effective treatments.

Neurofibrillary Tangles

The final major pathology of AD is the intracellular neurofibrillary tangles. The neurofibrillary

FIGURE 24.8 ● A positive scan (left) shows high uptake of florbetapir F18 in the cortical gray matter, indicating the presence of amyloid plaques. A negative scan (right) is paradoxically a healthier brain. (Images courtesy of Avid Radiopharmaceuticals, a wholly owned subsidiary of Eli Lilly and Company. © Eli Lilly and Company.)

tangles come from the proteins on the microtubules of the neuron. The microtubules are the internal cytoskeleton that provides structure for the cell and, more importantly, transports essential molecules and organelles from the cell body to the synapses. Damage to the microtubules causes the peripheral aspects of the neuron to effectively starve.

The tau proteins bind to the microtubules and provide stability. The problem seems to start with the hyperphosphorylation of the tau proteins (Figure 24.9). Too many phosphates attached to the tau proteins cause them to detach from the microtubules. It is these detached proteins that clump together and form the neurofibrillary tangles, which in turn clog the neuron's axons and dendrites and cause the cell to die. What causes the hyperphosphorylation remains unclear but seems to be initiated by β-amyloid—possibly soluble A-β that diffuses across the cell wall.

Alzheimer's Disease Progression
AD is a relentlessly progressive disorder. There are no remissions. The first signs are marked by subtle decline in memory. As the disease advances, changes in personality and language skills develop. Eventually even motor functions are impaired. Understanding the spread of the pathology of AD gives a greater appreciation of the changing clinical picture.

The progression of the disease can be staged by the development and progression of neurofibrillary tangles. In a landmark analysis of more than 2,500 brains in Germany over 10 years, Braak documented the insidious evolution of AD shown in Figure 24.10. The initial stages start in the entorhinal cortex of the hippocampus. From there the disease spreads into the temporal and frontal cortex. The final stages involve the entire brain, with the greatest deposits remaining in the regions where it all started.

PREVENTION AND TREATMENT
The number of cases of AD is expected to quadruple in the next 40 years if nothing is done to prevent or treat the disease. Current treatments can temporarily improve cognition in those affected,

CEREBRAL SPINAL FLUID

Tau protein is increased in the cerebral spinal fluid (CSF) of patients with AD. The diagnostic accuracy of the disease may be enhanced from measurements of specific proteins in the CSF, as well as better imaging studies—in patients with signs of cognitive decline.

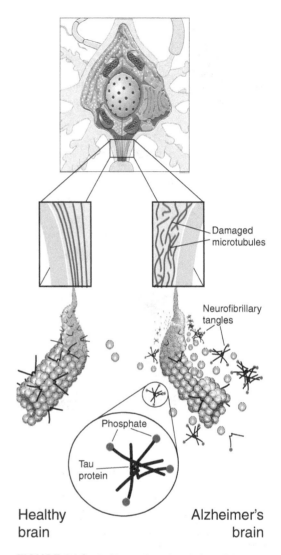

FIGURE 24.9 ● Hyperphosphorylation of the tau proteins produces neurofibrillary tangles that damage the microtubules. The result is impaired axonal transport and ultimately cell death.

but do nothing to alter the underlying pathophysiology of the condition. Recent studies have been disappointing. Encouraging preliminary studies have failed in larger trials. The optimistic predictions of just a few years ago have not borne fruit.

Perhaps even more discouraging is that we do not even know which pathology of AD is most detrimental: amyloid plaques, neurofibrillary tangles, or some upstream event that precedes the development of plaques and tangles. Those of us on the other side of our life curve hope that the scientific community will develop effective interventions in the near future. We will review several of the favorable prospects.

A Preclinical   **B** Initial clinical symptoms   **C** Fully developed AD

Stages I and II   Stages III and IV   Stages V and VI

FIGURE 24.10 ● The spread of neurofibrillary tangles in Alzheimer's disease (AD). (Adapted from Braak H, Braak E. Frequency of stages of Alzheimer-related lesions in different age categories. *Neurobiol Aging*. 1997;18(4):351-357.)

Vaccine

Immunizations against childhood diseases have transformed the risks of growing up. The possibility of using vaccines to treat and/or prevent AD is an exciting application of this old intervention, which could likewise revolutionize growing old. The trick is to get the immune system to attack the amyloid plaques without irritating other parts of the brain or inciting an inflammatory response in the CNS.

The basic plan is laid out in Figure 24.11. Peripheral injections of A-β-42 are ingested by antigen-presenting cells. A-β antigens are presented to T cells, which in turn activate B cells. Anti-Aβ antibodies produced by the B cells attack the amyloid plaques as well as soluble Aβ. Microglial cells then clean the plaques through phagocytosis.

The vaccine was initially tested in mice genetically engineered to overexpress APP (APP mice). Such mice will develop amyloid plaques and memory loss by the age of 12 months. They have become the accepted animal model of AD. Immunotherapy with APP mice has produced extraordinary results (Figure 24.12). Clearing of amyloid plaques and

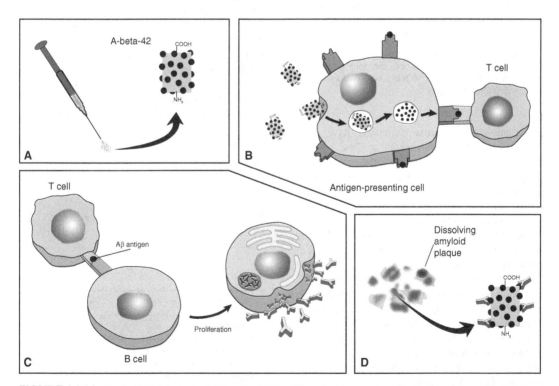

FIGURE 24.11 ● **A.** Aβ is injected peripherally. **B.** The Aβ molecules are ingested and presented to T cells by the antigen-presenting cells. **C.** T cells activate B cells, which produce anti-Aβ antibodies. **D.** The anti-Aβ antibodies attack Aβ in the amyloid plaques and are cleared by microglia. (Adapted from Schenk D, Hagen M, Seubert P. Current progress in beta-amyloid immunotherapy. *Curr Opin Immunol*. 2004;16(5):599-606.)

FIGURE 24.12 ● A. Slices of amyloid-β precursor protein (APP) mice hippocampi show the accumulation of amyloid plaques without and with the Aβ vaccination. **B.** Vaccinated mice display memory similar to control mice and superior to the APP mice. (A from Lemere CA, Maier M, Jiang L, et al. Amyloid-beta immunotherapy for the prevention and treatment of Alzheimer disease: lessons from mice, monkeys, and humans. *Rejuvenation Res.* 2006;9(1):77-84, courtesy of Cynthia A. Lemere. B adapted from Morgan D, Diamond DM, Gottschall PE, et al. A beta peptide vaccination prevents memory loss in an animal model of Alzheimer's disease. *Nature.* 2000;408(6815):982-985.)

preservation of cognitive functions have been repeatedly documented in animal studies.

In 2001, clinical trials of a synthetic version of the β-amyloid protein for use as a vaccine were started in humans. Preliminary safety studies were completed without a hitch. Unfortunately, the larger phase II study had to be stopped after several months when 6% of the participants developed an excessive inflammatory response (meningoencephalitis). Further analysis has suggested that T-cell activation may have been the problem.

Follow-up studies on the 372 subjects who were immunized have found some encouraging results. Those individuals who did mount an antibody response to A-β showed subtle signs of improved memory and cognitive skills. Furthermore, postmortem studies of a few patients have documented clearing of the amyloid plaques in some regions of their brains.

In 2012, a group in Sweden published what appears to be the next step in the vaccine story.

The vaccine, called CAD106, is designed to mount an antibody response against a small portion of the Aβ molecule without activating the T cells (humeral response but not cellular). A small double-blind phase 1 study of 58 patients with mild to moderate AD was conducted to establish safety and tolerability. While almost every patient developed minor side effects (sore throat, headache, fatigue, etc.), none developed meningoencephalitis. (Whew!) The ultimate effects on cognition or amyloid deposits will need to be measured in larger studies. Furthermore, there are other vaccines also in development, so this exciting treatment option continues to move forward.

The neuronal loss from AD might be prevented or at least limited with appropriate stimulation from growth factor proteins. Animal studies suggest that growth factor proteins may be useful for treating neurodegenerative diseases such as AD. Specifically, nerve growth factor (NGF, see

ANTIPSYCHOTICS

Alzheimer's original patient was ultimately admitted to his ward because of her uncontrollable psychotic symptoms. Currently, most clinicians would quickly place such a patient on a new-generation antipsychotic medication. Yet, the use of antipsychotic medications for AD is not without problems. A meta-analysis looked at the effect of second-generation antipsychotic medications on cognitive decline in patients with AD. They found that the medications actually worsened the cognitive decline when compared with placebo (see table).

Meta-Analysis of Cognitive Decline in Patients Treated with Second-Generation Antipsychotic Medications

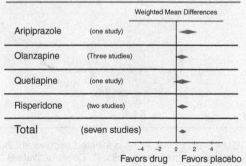

Adapted from Schneider LS, et al. *Am J Ger Psych.* 2006:14:19–210.

Figure 1.9) has been shown to prevent cholinergic degeneration and improve memory in animals. The problem arises in choosing a method to deliver the NGF to the brain. The molecule is too large to cross the blood–brain barrier. Likewise, direct infusion into the ventricles results in excessive stimulation and intolerable side effects, for example, pain and glial cell infiltration.

An alternative method of delivery entails hijacking the DNA in autologous fibroblasts using retroviral vectors. Such fibroblasts can be induced to express NGF. In turn, they can be placed directly into the brain of the subject and deliver NGF within a few millimeters of the nucleus basalis of Meynert, where cholinergic neuronal degeneration occurs. Because the fibroblasts are autologous, they do not activate an immune response.

Researchers at the University of California in San Diego completed a phase I trial with eight patients with probable AD. Fibroblasts producing NGF were injected into the subjects' cholinergic basal forebrain. Two patients had significant complications from the surgery, but with five of the remaining six, cognition stabilized or improved during the 6 to 18 months after injection. PET scans showed increased activity.

Although this treatment will not halt the development of amyloid plaques or neurofibrillary tangles, it does show that NGFs may play a role in reducing the symptoms of AD. Additionally, the study highlights that unique mechanisms can be utilized to deliver NGFs to specific regions of the brain.

A larger randomized, double-blind, placebo-controlled phase 2 trial commenced in 2009 seeking to recruit 50 patients. Patients in the placebo arm of this ambitious study are required to undergo sham neurosurgery. As much as we would not wish to inflict sham neurosurgery on anyone, this is no other way to accurately assess the efficacy of the treatment. The study should be completed in 2014.

Brain Reserve

Postmortem studies have found that a substantial proportion of people have the histopathology of AD, but not the cognitive failings of dementia. Prospective studies suggest the number may be as high as 40%. Some believe that this is due to *brain reserve*; that is, greater neural substrate buffers against the clinical expression of the disease (similar to starting with more adipose tissue during times of famine). Indeed, prospective studies have found that individuals who have the plaques and tangles at death, but were not demented, had greater number of neurons in the frontal, parietal, and temporal cortices.

One of the most remarkable studies on this topic was the Nun Study, in which the correlation between early verbal skills and later cognitive impairment was determined. The researchers completed extensive cognitive assessments of the nuns older than 75 years in their retirement. In their early 20s, the nuns had completed an autobiographic essay when they entered the order. These essays were blindly graded for linguistic ability. The nuns with low idea density and low grammatical complexity in their autobiographies written 50 years earlier were 15 times more likely to have low cognitive scores in late life. In other words, cognitive skills in early life prevent cognitive impairment later on.

A follow-up study has taken this analysis one step further by including postmortem brain examination. This study included 156 individuals in whom the researchers could correlate educational background, level of cognition before death, and amyloid load in the brain at autopsy. The results are shown in Figure 24.13. The individuals with greater years of education had less cognitive impairment even with increasing amyloidosis. The authors concluded that education is associated with factors that somehow reduce the effect of amyloid on cognition. They estimated that the difference between 15 and 22 years of education is equivalent to approximately 2.6 years of amyloid progression. We hope this information provides some relief for the sort of person reading this book.

"Use it or lose it" is one of the mantras resulting from this line of research, the implication being that exercising the brain is neuroprotective against the pathology of AD. Clearly, the research

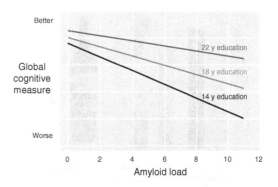

FIGURE 24.13 ● The cognitive impairment associated with amyloidosis is reduced in people with more education. (Adapted from Bennett DA, Schneider JA, Wilson RS, et al. Education modifies the association of amyloid but not tangles with cognitive function. *Neurology.* 2005;65[6]:953–955.)

described here shows that smarter, more educated people have greater brain resilience. What we do not know is whether these people were born with a larger reserve of neural substrate or whether a lifetime of cognitive enrichment–stimulated neuronal growth protected their brains from the effects of AD.

Caloric Restriction

Caloric restriction is known to enhance longevity (see LONGEVITY, page 158). Dietary restriction may also retard the effects of AD. Studies with animals suggest that low-calorie diets may protect the brain in the following ways:

1. Limiting oxidative stress
2. Reducing DNA damage
3. Increasing brain-derived neurotrophic factor production

A recent study shows the profound effects that calorie restriction can have on amyloid deposits in nonhuman primates. A colony of squirrel monkeys was raised on a diet reduced by 30% and compared with a freely eating control group. As the monkeys died of natural causes, their temporal cortical tissues were measured for β-amyloid, APP, and the secretase enzymes.

The monkeys on dietary restriction showed no change in the amount of APP molecule, but a remarkable reduction in A-β. The activity of β- and γ-secretase enzymes (Figure 21.6) was no different between the two groups. However, α-secretase was almost 100% more active in the diet-restricted group. α-Secretase is an enzyme that cuts the APP molecule in a manner that limits the production of β-amyloid. In other words, caloric restriction enhances the activity of an enzyme that prevents the buildup of amyloid plaques.

Although caloric restriction may be effective in altering the buildup of β-amyloid, it seems unlikely to be utilized by the large number of people at risk for AD. Indeed, the industrial societies that are at most risk for AD are also the ones struggling with the obesity epidemic. However, if treatments that reduce hunger or enhance satiety can be developed, these could be reasonable pharmacologic approaches to forestalling AD.

Exercise

Four clinical trials presented at the Alzheimer's Association International Conference in 2012 suggest that regular exercise can improve memory and preserve brain functions in the elderly. One such study from the University of Pittsburgh randomized 120 sedentary elderly adults to aerobic exercise or a stretching control group. Both groups demonstrated improvements in spatial memory at 6 months and 1 year. However, the exercise group had a 2% increase in their hippocampal volume at 1 year while the stretching group showed a slight decline.

Exercise is a low-cost, easily accessible treatment intervention that may preserve brain structures and maintain memory. Apparently, what is good for the heart is also good for the brain.

CABERNET SAUVIGNON

Alzheimer's modeled mice showed significant reductions in cortical β-amyloid with daily Cabernet Sauvignon. (Adapted from Wang J, Ho L, Zhao Z, et al. Moderate consumption of Carernet Sauvignon attenuates AB neuropathology in a mouse model of Alzheimer's disease. *FASEB J.* 2006;20:2313-2320.)

It is with great pleasure that we report the results of a study showing the cerebral benefits of moderate doses of red wine. Mice altered to overexpress APP were given daily supplements of California Cabernet Sauvignon, ethanol, or water. The wine group had not only superior memory function but also less β-amyloid in their cortex (figure).

We think that anyone who has finished reading every word of this book should celebrate with a little California Cabernet Sauvignon. Heck, it will give a little tweak to the nucleus accumbens, as well as promote β-amyloid clearance—all in moderation of course.

QUESTIONS

1. One hundred and twenty-five years
   a. Life expectancy.
   b. Fibroblast duration.
   c. Maximum cell divisions.
   d. Life span.

2. Alzheimer's identified all of the following, except
   a. Cortical atrophy.
   b. Amyloid plaques.
   c. β-Amyloid.
   d. Neurofibrillary tangles.

3. All of the following are increased in AD, except
   a. Amyloid-β precursor protein (APP).
   b. A-β-42.
   c. Ventricular size.
   d. CSF tau protein.

4. Neurofibrillary tangles are composed of
   a. Damaged microtubules.
   b. Extracellular protein tangles.
   c. Excessively phosphorylated tau.
   d. Untransportable cellular products.

5. The goal of Alzheimer's vaccine is to increase which of the following?
   a. A-β-42.
   b. T-cell activation.
   c. Memory performance.
   d. Anti-Aβ antibodies.

6. Increases with calorie restriction
   a. Amyloid-β precursor protein (APP).
   b. α-Secretase.
   c. β-Secretase.
   d. γ-Secretase.

See Answers section at the end of the book.

Bibliography

CHAPTER 1

1. Bailey CH, Chen M. Morphological basis of long-term habituation and sensitization in Aplysia. *Science.* 1983;220:91-93.
2. Bear MF, Connors BW, Paradiso MA, eds. *Neuroscience: Exploring the Brain.* 3rd ed. Baltimore, MD: Lippincott Williams & Wilkins; 2007.
3. Bouchard TJ. Twin studies of behavior: new and old findings. In: Schmitt A, Atzwanger K, Grammer K, et al. eds. *New Aspects of Human Ethology.* New York, NY: Plenum Publishing; 1997:121-140.
4. Finger S. *Minds Behind the Brain: A History of the Pioneers and Their Discoveries.* New York, NY: Oxford University Press; 2000.
5. Friend SH, Stoughton RB. The magic of microarrays. *Sci Am.* 2002;286:44-53.
6. Gottesman II. *Schizophrenia Genesis.* New York, NY: WH Freeman; 1991.
7. Hodgkin AL, Huxley AF. Action potentials recorded from inside a nerve fibre. *Nature.* 1939;144:710-711.
8. Illing R-B. Humbled by history. *Sci Am Mind.* 2004;14:86-93.
9. Ioannidis JPA. Excess significance bias in literature on brain volume abnormalities. *Arch Gen Psychiatry.* 2011;68:773-780.
10. Kandel ER. *In Search of Memory: The Emergence of a New Science of Mind.* New York, NY: WW Norton & Co.; 2006.
11. Levi-Montalcini R. The nerve growth factor. *Ann N Y Acad Sci.* 1964;118:149-170.
12. Ramón y Cajal S. *Recollections on My Life. Transactions of the American Philosophical Society.* Vol 8, Part 2. Philadelphia, PA: The American Philosophical Society; 1937.
13. Rorden C, Karnath HO. Using human brain lesions to infer function: a relic from a past era in the fMRI age? *Nat Rev Neurosci.* 2004;5:813-819.
14. Zimmer C. *Soul Made Flesh: The Discovery of the Brain—And How It Changed the World.* New York, NY: Free Press; 2004.

CHAPTER 2

1. Abbott NJ, Ronnback L, Hansson E. Astrocyte-endothelial interactions at the blood-brain barrier. *Nat Rev Neurosci.* 2006;7(1):41-53.
2. Bear MF, Connors BW, Paradiso MA, eds. *Neuroscience: Exploring the Brain.* 3rd ed. Baltimore, MD: Lippincott Williams & Wilkins; 2007.
3. Behrstock S, Ebert A, McHugh J, et al. Human neural progenitors deliver glial cell line-derived neurotrophic factor to parkinsonian rodents and aged primates. *Gene Ther.* 2005;13(5):379-388.
4. Bower JM, Parsons LM. Rethinking the "lesser brain". *Sci Am.* 2003;289(2):50-57.
5. Cowan WM. The development of the brain. *Sci Am.* 1979;241(3):113-133.
6. Fuster JM. *The Prefrontal Cortex: Anatomy, Physiology, and Neuropsychology of the Frontal Lobe.* 3rd ed. Philadelphia, PA: Lippincott-Raven Publishers; 1997.
7. Gabathuler R. Blood-brain barrier transport of drugs for the treatment of brain diseases. *CNS Neurol Disord Drug Targets.* 2009;8(3):195-204.
8. Kandel ER, Schwartz JH, Jessell TM, eds. *Principles of Neural Science.* 4th ed. New York, NY: McGraw-Hill; 2000.
9. Lewis DA. Structure of the human prefrontal cortex. *Am J Psychiatry.* 2004;161(8):1366.
10. Mashour GA, Walker EE, Martuza RL. Psychosurgery: past, present, and future. *Brain Res Brain Res Rev.* 2005;48(3):409-419.
11. Nestler EJ, Hyman SE, Malenka RC. *Molecular Neuropharmacology. A Foundation for Clinical Neuroscience.* 2nd ed. New York, NY: McGraw-Hill; 2009.
12. Salloway SP, Malloy PF, Duffy JD, eds. *The Frontal Lobes and Neuropsychiatric Illness.* Washington, DC: American Psychiatric Publishing, Inc; 2001.
13. Snell RS. *Clinical Neuroanatomy: A Illustrated Review with Questions and Explanations.* 3rd ed. Philadelphia, PA: Lippincott Williams & Wilkins; 2001.
14. Welch MJ, Meltzer EO, Simons FE. H1-antihistamines and the central nervous system. *Clin Allergy Immunol.* 2002;17:337-388.

CHAPTER 3

1. Bear MF, Connors BW, Paradiso MA, eds. *Neuroscience: Exploring the Brain.* 3rd ed. Baltimore, MD: Lippincott Williams & Wilkins; 2007.
2. Breedlove SM, Watson NV, Rosenzweig MR. *Biological Psychology.* 6th ed. Sunderland, MA: Sinauer; 2010.
3. Fields RD. The other half of the brain. *Sci Am.* 2004;290(4):54-61.
4. Haydon PG. GLIA: listening and talking to the synapse. *Nat Rev Neurosci.* 2001;2(3):185-193.
5. Insel TR. Faulty circuits. *Sci Am.* 2010;302(4):44-51.

6. Kaufmann WE, Moser HW. Dendritic anomalies in disorders associated with mental retardation. *Cereb Cortex.* 2000;10(10):981-991.
7. Kolb B, Forgie M, Gibb R, et al. Age, experience and the changing brain. *Neurosci Biobehav Rev.* 1998;22(2):143-159.
8. Tian GF, Azmi H, Takano T, et al. An astrocytic basis of epilepsy. *Nat Med.* 2005;11(9):973-981.

CHAPTER 4

1. Bear MF, Connors BW, Paradiso MA, eds. *Neuroscience: Exploring the Brain.* 3rd ed. Baltimore, MD: Lippincott Williams & Wilkins; 2007.
2. Breedlove SM, Watson NV, Rosenzweig MR. *Biological Psychology.* 6th ed. Sunderland, MA: Sinauer; 2010.
3. Cooper JR, Bloom FE, Roth RH. *The Biochemical Basis of Neuropharmacology.* 8th ed. New York, NY: Oxford University Press; 2003.
4. Goff DC, Coyle JT. The emerging role of glutamate in the pathophysiology and treatment of schizophrenia. *Am J Psychiatry.* 2001;158(9):1367-1377.
5. Holmes A, Heilig M, Rupniak NM, et al. Neuropeptide systems as novel therapeutic targets for depression and anxiety disorders. *Trends Pharmacol Sci.* 2003;24(11):580-588.
6. Iversen L. Cannabis and the brain. *Brain.* 2003;126 (pt 6):1252-1270.
7. Nestler EJ, Hyman SE, Malenka RC. *Molecular Neuropharmacology. A Foundation for Clinical Neuroscience.* 2nd ed. New York, NY: McGraw-Hill; 2009.
8. Purves D, Augustine GJ, Fitzpatrick D, et al. *Neuroscience.* 5th ed. Sunderland, MA: Sinauer; 2011.
9. Snyder SH, Ferris CD. Novel neurotransmitters and their neuropsychiatric relevance. *Am J Psychiatry.* 2000;157(11):1738-1751.
10. Stahl SM. *Stahl's Essential Psychopharmacology. Neuroscientific Basis of Practical Applications.* 3rd ed. New York, NY: Cambridge University Press; 2008.
11. Strand FL. *Neuropeptides: Regulators of Physiological Processes.* London: MIT Press; 1999.
12. Tsen G, Williams B, Allaire P, et al. Receptors with opposing functions are in postsynaptic microdomains under one presynaptic terminal. *Nat Neurosci.* 2000;3(2):126-132.

CHAPTER 5

1. Bear MF, Connors BW, Paradiso MA, eds. *Neuroscience: Exploring the Brain.* 3rd ed. Baltimore, MD: Lippincott Williams & Wilkins; 2007.
2. Breedlove SM, Watson NV, Rosenzweig MR. *Biological Psychology.* 6th ed. Sunderland, MA: Sinauer; 2010.
3. Engert F, Bonhoeffer T. Dendritic spine changes associated with hippocampal long-term synaptic plasticity. *Nature.* 1999;399(6731):66-70.
4. Huang YZ, Edwards MJ, Rounis E, et al. Theta burst stimulation of the human motor cortex. *Neuron.* 2005;45: 201-206.
5. Kroeze WK, Hufeisen SJ, Popadak BA, et al. H1-histamine receptor affinity predicts short-term weight gain for typical and atypical antipsychotic drugs. *Neuropsychopharmacology.* 2003;28(3):519-526.
6. LeDoux J. *The Synaptic Self. How Our Brains Become Who We Are.* New York, NY: Viking; 2002.
7. Nestler EJ, Hyman SE, Malenka RC. *Molecular Neuropharmacology. A Foundation for Clinical*

Neuroscience. 2nd ed. New York, NY: McGraw-Hill; 2009.
8. Purves D, Augustine GJ, Fitzpatrick D, et al. *Neuroscience.* 5th ed. Sunderland, MA: Sinauer; 2011.
9. Ressler KJ, Rothbaum BO, Tannenbaum L, et al. Cognitive enhancers as adjuncts to psychotherapy: use of D-cycloserine in phobic individuals to facilitate extinction of fear. *Arch Gen Psychiatry.* 2004;61(11):1136-1144.
10. Rogawski MA, Loscher W. The neurobiology of antiepileptic drugs. *Nat Rev Neurosci.* 2004;5(7):553-564.
11. Strohle A, Romeo E, di Michele F, et al. Induced panic attacks shift gamma-aminobutyric acid type A receptor modulatory neuroactive steroid composition in patients with panic disorder: preliminary results. *Arch Gen Psychiatry.* 2003;60(2):161-168.
12. Tecott LH, Smart SL. Monoamine neurotransmitters. In: Sadock BJ, Sadock VA, eds. *Kaplan and Sadock's Comprehensive Textbook of Psychiatry.* 8th ed. Philadelphia, PA: Lippincott Williams & Wilkins; 2005:49-60.
13. Victor M, Ropper AH. *Adams and Victor's Principles of Neurology.* 7th ed. New York, NY: McGraw-Hill; 2001.

CHAPTER 6

1. Cook EH, Scherer SW. Copy-number variations associated with neuropsychiatric conditions. *Nature.* 2008;455:919-923.
2. Dick DM, Riley B, Kendler KS. Nature and nurture in neuropsychiatric genetics: where do we stand? *Dialogues Clin Neurosci.* 2010;12:7-23.
3. Higgins ES. The new genetics of mental illness. *Sci Am Mind.* 2008;19:40-47.
4. Jirtle RL, Skinner MK. Environmental epigenomics and disease susceptibility. *Nat Rev Genet.* 2007;8:253-262.
5. Lincoln T, Joyce GF. Self-sustained replication of an RNA enzyme. *Science.* 2009;323:1229-1232.
6. Kananen L, Surakka I, Pirkola S, et al. Childhood adversities are associated with shorter telomere length at adult age both in individuals with anxiety disorder and controls. *PLoS One.* 2010;5:e10826.
7. Kendler KS, Prescott CA. *Genes, Environment and Psychopathology: Understanding the Causes of Psychiatric and Substance Use Disorders.* New York, NY: Guilford Press; 2006.
8. Maher B. The case of the missing heritability. *Nature.* 2008;456:18-21.
9. Mattick J. Deconstructing the dogma: a new view of evolution and genetic programming of complex organisms. *Ann N Y Acad Sci.* 2009;1178:29-46.
10. Miller BH, Wahlestedt C. MicroRNA dysregulation in psychiatric disease. *Brain Res.* 2010;1338:89-99.
11. Pennisi E. Shining a light on the genome's "dark matter". *Science.* 2010;330:1614.
12. Psychiatric GWAS Consortium Coordinating Committee. Genome wide association studies: history, rationale and prospects for psychiatric disorders. *Am J Psychiatry.* 2009;166:540-556.
13. Strachan T, Read A. *Human Molecular Genetics.* 4th ed. New York, NY: Garland Science; 2011.
14. Waterland RA, Jirtle RL. Transposable elements: targets for early nutritional effects on epigenetic gene regulation. *Mol Cell Biol.* 2003;23:5293-5300.
15. Williams NM, Zaharieva I, Martin A, et al. Rare chromosomal deletions and duplications in attention-deficit hyperactivity disorder: a genome-wide analysis. *Lancet.* 2010;376:1401-1408.

CHAPTER 7

1. Azukizawa M, Pekary AE, Hershman JM, et al. Plasma thyrotropin, thyroxine, and triiodothyronine relationships in man. *J Clin Endocrinol Metab.* 1976;43(3): 533-542.
2. Bauer M, Heinz A, Whybrow PC. Thyroid hormones, serotonin and mood: of synergy and significance in the adult brain. *Mol Psychiatry.* 2002;7(2):140-156.
3. Bauer M, London ED, Silverman DH, et al. Thyroid, brain and mood modulation in affective disorder: insights from molecular research and functional brain imaging. *Pharmacopsychiatry.* 2003;36(suppl 3): S215-S221.
4. Bauer M, Whybrow PC. Thyroid hormone, neural tissue and mood modulation. *World J Biol Psychiatry.* 2001;2(2):59-69.
5. Bear MF, Connors BW, Paradiso MA, eds. *Neuroscience: Exploring the Brain.* 3rd ed. Baltimore, MD: Lippincott Williams & Wilkins; 2007.
6. Bradley RG, Binder EB, Epstein MP, et al. Influence of child abuse on adult depression. *Arch Gen Psychiatry.* 2008:65:190-200.
7. Breedlove SM, Watson NV, Rosenzweig MR. *Biological Psychology.* 6th ed. Sunderland, MA: Sinauer; 2010.
8. Constant EL, de Volder AG, Ivanoiu A, et al. Cerebral blood flow and glucose metabolism in hypothyroidism: a positron emission tomography study. *J Clin Endocrinol Metab.* 2001;86(8):3864-3870.
9. Fava M, Labbate LA, Abraham ME, et al. Hypothyroidism and hyperthyroidism in major depression revisited. *J Clin Psychiatry.* 1995;56(5):186-192.
10. Forrest D, Reh TA, Rusch A. Neurodevelopmental control by thyroid hormone receptors. *Curr Opin Neurobiol.* 2002;12(1):49-56.
11. Gordon JT, Kaminski DM, Rozanov CB, et al. Evidence that 3,3′,5-triiodothyronine is concentrated in and delivered from the locus coeruleus to its noradrenergic targets via anterograde axonal transport. *Neuroscience.* 1999;93(3):943-954.
12. Kim JJ, Diamond DM. The stressed hippocampus, synaptic plasticity and lost memories. *Nat Rev Neurosci.* 2002;3(6):453-462.
13. Lupien SJ, de Leon M, de Santi S, et al. Cortisol levels during human aging predict hippocampal atrophy and memory deficits. *Nat Neurosci.* 1998;1(1): 69-73.
14. Marangell LB, Ketter TA, George MS, et al. Inverse relationship of peripheral thyrotropin-stimulating hormone levels to brain activity in mood disorders. *Am J Psychiatry.* 1997;154(2):224-230.
15. McEwen BS. Protective and damaging effects of stress mediators. *N Engl J Med.* 1998;338(3):171-179.
16. Nestler EJ, Hyman SE, Malenka RC. *Molecular Neuropharmacology. A Foundation for Clinical Neuroscience.* 2nd ed. New York, NY: McGraw-Hill; 2009.
17. Raison CL, Miller AH. When not enough is too much: the role of insufficient glucocorticoid signaling in the pathophysiology of stress-related disorders. *Am J Psychiatry.* 2003;160(9):1554-1565.
18. Rupprecht R, Holsboer F. Neuroactive steroids: mechanisms of action and neuropsychopharmacological perspectives. *Trends Neurosci.* 1999;22(9):410-460.
19. Sapolsky RM. *Why Zebras Don't Get Ulcers: An Updated Guide to Stress, Stress-Related Diseases, and Coping.* New York, NY: Barns & Noble Books; 1998.
20. Sapolsky RM. Stress and plasticity in the limbic system. *Neurochem Res.* 2003;28(11):1735-1742.
21. Shelton R, Osuntokun O, Heinloth AN, Corya SA. Therapeutic options for treatment-resistant depression. *CNS Drugs.* 2010;24:131-161.
22. Snell RS. *Clinical Neuroanatomy: A Illustrated Review with Questions and Explanations.* Philadelphia, PA: Lippincott Williams & Wilkins; 2001.
23. Starkman MN, Giordani B, Gebarski SS, et al. Decrease in cortisol reverses human hippocampal atrophy following treatment of Cushing's disease. *Biol Psychiatry.* 1999;46(12):1595-1602.
24. Starkman MN, Giordani B, Gebarski SS, et al. Improvement in learning associated with increase in hippocampal formation volume. *Biol Psychiatry.* 2003;53(3):233-238.
25. Vaidya VA, Castro ME, Pei Q, et al. Influence of thyroid hormone on 5-HT(1A) and 5-HT(2A) receptor-mediated regulation of hippocampal BDNF mRNA expression. *Neuropharmacology.* 2001;40(1):48-56.
26. Wolkowitz OM, Rothschild AJ. *Psychoneuroendocrinology: The Scientific Basis of Clinical Practice.* Washington, DC: American Psychiatric Publishing, Inc; 2003.
27. van Zuiden M, Geuze E, Willemen HL, et al. Pre-existing high glucocorticoid receptor number predicting development of posttraumatic stress symptoms after military deployment. *Am J Psychiatry.* 2011;168: 89-96.

CHAPTER 8

1. Antonini A, Stryker MP. Rapid remodeling of axonal arbors in the visual cortex. *Science.* 1993;260(5115): 1819-1821.
2. Bartzokis G, Lu P, Tinqus K, et al. Lifespan trajectory of myelin integrity and maximum motor speed. *Neurobiol Aging.* 2010;31:1554-1562.
3. Bear MF, Connors BW, Paradiso MA, eds. *Neuroscience: Exploring the Brain.* 3rd ed. Baltimore, MD: Lippincott Williams & Wilkins; 2007.
4. Bhardway RD, Curtis MA, Spalding KL, et al. Neocortical neurogenesis in humans is restricted to development. *Proc Natl Acad Sci U S A.* 2006;103(33): 12564-12568.
5. Breedlove SM, Watson NV, Rosenzweig MR. *Biological Psychology.* 6th ed. Sunderland, MA: Sinauer; 2010.
6. Brown J, Cooper-Kuhn CM, Kempermann G, et al. Enriched environment and physical activity stimulate hippocampal but not olfactory bulb neurogenesis. *Eur J Neurosci.* 2003;17(10):2042-2046.
7. Elbert T, Candia V, Altenmuller E, et al. Alteration of digital representations in somatosensory cortex in focal hand dystonia. *Neuroreport.* 1998;9(16):3571-3575.
8. Gage FH. Mammalian neural stem cells. *Science.* 2000;287(5457):1433-1438.
9. Gage FH. Brain, repair yourself. *Sci Am.* 2003;289(3): 46-53.
10. Gogtay N, Thompson PM. Mapping gray matter development: implications for typical development and vulnerability to psychopathology. *Brain Cogn.* 2010;72:6-15.
11. Gould E, Reeves AJ, Graziano MS, et al. Neurogenesis in the neocortex of adult primates. *Science.* 1999;286(5439): 548-552.
12. Huttenlocher PR, Dabholkar AS. Regional differences in synaptogenesis in human cerebral cortex. *J Comp Neurol.* 1997;387(2):167-178.
13. Johnson JS, Newport EL. Critical period effects in second language learning: the influence of maturational

state on the acquisition of English as a second language. *Cognit Psychol.* 1989;21(1):60-99.

14. Merzenich MM, Nelson RJ, Stryker MP, et al. Somatosensory cortical map changes following digit amputation in adult monkeys. *J Comp Neurol.* 1984;224(4):591-605.
15. Mirescu C, Peters JD, Gould E. Early life experience alters response of adult neurogenesis to stress. *Nat Neurosci.* 2004;7(8):841-846.
16. Munte TF, Altenmuller E, Jancke L. The musician's brain as a model of neuroplasticity. *Nat Rev Neurosci.* 2002;3(6):473-478.
17. Nestler EJ, Hyman SE, Malenka RC. *Molecular Neuropharmacology. A Foundation for Clinical Neuroscience.* 2nd ed. New York, NY: McGraw-Hill; 2009.
18. Pantev C, Engelien A, Candia V, et al. Representational cortex in musicians. Plastic alterations in response to musical practice. *Ann N Y Acad Sci.* 2001;930:300-314.
19. Purves D, Augustine GJ, Fitzpatrick D, et al. *Neuroscience.* 5th ed. Sunderland, MA: Sinauer; 2011.
20. Silver J, Miller JH. Regeneration beyond the glial scar. *Nat Rev Neurosci.* 2004;5(2):146-156.
21. Takagi Y, Takahashi J, Saiki H, et al. Dopaminergic neurons generated from monkey embryonic stem cells function in a Parkinson primate model. *J Clin Invest.* 2005;115(1):102-109.
22. Taub E, Uswatte G. Constraint-induced movement therapy: bridging from the primate laboratory to the stroke rehabilitation laboratory. *J Rehabil Med.* 2003(41 suppl):34-40.
23. Wiesel TN. Postnatal development of the visual cortex and the influence of environment. *Nature.* 1982;299(5884):583-591.

CHAPTER 9

1. Bauer S, Kerr BJ, Patterson PH. The neuropoietic cytokine family in development, plasticity, disease and injury. *Nat Rev Neurosci.* 2007;8:221-232.
2. Clarke MC, Tanskanen A, Huttunen M, Whittaker JC, Cannon M. Evidence for an interaction between familial liability and exposure to infection in the causation of schizophrenia. *Am J Psychiatry.* 2009;166:1025-1030.
3. Coico R, Sunshine G. *Immunology: A Short Course.* 6th ed. Hoboken, NJ: Wiley-Blackwell; 2009.
4. Compston A, Coles A. Multiple sclerosis. *Lancet.* 2008;372:1502-1517.
5. Faulkner JR, Herrmann JE, Woo MJ, Tansey KE, Doan NB, Sofroniew MV. Reactive astrocytes protect tissue and preserve function after spinal cord injury. *J Neurosci.* 2004;24:2143-2155.
6. Glaser R, Kiecolt-Glazer JK. Stress-induced immune dysfunction: implications for health. *Nat Rev Immunol.* 2005;5:243-251.
7. Graeber MB, Streit WJ. Microglia: biology and pathology. *Acta Neuropathol.* 2005;119:89-105.
8. Hoofnagle JH, Seeff LB. Peginterferon and ribavirin for chronic hepatitis C. *N Engl J Med.* 2006;355:2444-2451.
9. Kadhim HJ, Duchateau J, Sebire G. Cytokines and brain injury: invited review. *J Intensive Care Med.* 2008;23:236-249.
10. LaFond RE, Lukehart SA. Biological basis for syphilis. *Clin Microbiol Rev.* 2006;19:29-49.
11. Lucas SM, Rothwell NJ, Gibson RM. The role of inflammation in CNS injury and disease. *Br J Pharmacol.* 2006;147:S232-S240.
12. Maes M, Yirmyia R, Noraberg J, et al. The inflammatory & neurodegenerative hypothesis of depression:

leads for future research and new drug developments in depression. *Metab Brain Dis.* 2009;24:27-53.
13. Martell BA, Orson FM, Poling J, et al. Cocaine vaccine for the treatment of cocaine dependence in methadone-maintained patients. *Arch Gen Psychiatry.* 2009;66:1116-1123.
14. McClure M, Wessely S. Chronic fatigue syndrome and human retrovirus XMRV. Three studies now refute the original study reporting the link. *BMJ.* 2010;340:489-490.
15. Miller AH, Maletic V, Raison CL. Inflammation and its discontents: the role of cytokines in the pathophysiology of major depression. *Biol Psychiatry.* 2009;65:732-741.
16. Owen N, Poulton T, Hay FC, Mohamed-Ali V, Steptoe A. Socioeconomic status, C-reactive protein, immune factors, and responses to acute mental stress. *Brain Behav Immun.* 2003;17:286-295.
17. Panagiotakos DB, Dimakopoulou K, Katsouyanni K, et al. Mediterranean diet and inflammatory response in myocardial infarction survivors. *Int J Epidemiol.* 2009;38:856-866.
18. Padgett DA, Marucha PT, Sheridan JF. Restraint stress slows cutaneous wound healing in mice. *Brain, Behav Immun.* 1998;12:64-73.
19. Potvin S, Stip E, Sepehry AA, Gendron A, Bah R, Kouassi E. Inflammatory cytokine alterations in schizophrenia: a systematic quantitative review. *Biol Psychiatry.* 2008;63:801-808.
20. Reichert WM. *Indwelling Neural Implants: Strategies for Contending with the In Vivo Environment.* Boca Raton, FL: CRC Press, Taylor & Francis Group; 2008.
21. Sanchez-Vellegas A, Delgado-Rodriquez M, Alonso A, et al. Association of the Mediterranean diet pattern with the incidence of depression. *Arch Gen Psychiatry.* 2009;66:1090-1098.
22. Silver J, Miller JH. Regeneration beyond the glial scar. *Nat Rev Neurosci.* 2004;5:146-156.
23. Sompayrac L. *How the Immune System Works.* 3rd ed. Malden, MA: Blackwell Publishing; 2008.
24. Sternberg EM. Neural regulation of innate immunity: a coordinated nonspecific host response to pathogens. *Nat Rev Immunol.* 2006;6:318-328.
25. Tyring S, Gottlieb A, Papp K, et al. Etanercept and clinical outcomes, fatigue, and depression in psoriasis: double-blind placebo-controlled randomised phase III trial. *Lancet.* 2006;367:29-35.
26. van Rossum CT, Shipley MJ, van de Mheen H, Grobbee DE, Marmot MG. Employment grade differences in cause specific mortality. A 25 year follow up of civil servants from the first Whitehall study. *J Epidemiol Community Health.* 2000;54:178-184.

CHAPTER 10

1. Breedlove SM, Watson NV, Rosenzweig MR. *Biological Psychology.* 6th ed. Sunderland, MA: Sinauer; 2010.
2. Chahine M, Chatelier A, Babich O, Grupp JJ. Voltage-gated sodium channels in neurological disorders. *CNS Neurol Disord Drug Targets.* 2008;7(2):144-158.
3. Datta A, Bansal V, Diaz J, et al. Gyri-precise head model of transcranial direct current stimulation: improved spatial focality using a ring electrode versus conventional rectangular pad. *Brain Stimul.* 2009;2:201-207.
4. Flöel A, Meinzer M, Kirstein R, et al. Short-term anomia training and electrical brain stimulation. *Stroke.* 2011;42:2065-2067.
5. Higgins ES, George MS. *Brain Stimulation Therapies for Clinicians.* Washington, DC: American Psychiatric Press; 2008.

6. Koch C. A theory of consciousness. *Sci Am Mind.* 2009;20(4):16-19.

7. Parent A. Giovanni Aldini: from animal electricity to human brain stimulation. *Can J Neurol Sci.* 2004;31(4):576-584.

8. Penfield W, Boldrey E. Somatic motor and sensory representation in the cerebral cortex of man as studied by electrical stimulation. *Brain.* 1938;60:389-443.

9. Penfield W. Engrams in the human brain. Mechanisms of memory. *Proc R Soc Med.* 1968;61(8):831-840.

10. Purves D, Augustine GJ, Fitzpatrick D, et al. *Neuroscience.* 5th ed. Sunderland, MA: Sinauer; 2011.

CHAPTER 11

1. Antonini A, Stryker MP. Rapid remodeling of axonal arbors in the visual cortex. *Science.* 1993;260(5115): 1819-1821.

2. Apkarian AV, Sosa Y, Sonty S, et al. Chronic back pain is associated with decreased prefrontal and thalamic gray matter density. *J Neurosci.* 2004;24(46):10410-10415.

3. Bear MF, Connors BW, Paradiso MA, eds. *Neuroscience: Exploring the Brain.* 3rd ed. Baltimore, MD: Lippincott Williams & Wilkins; 2007.

4. Beecher HK. Pain in men wounded in battle. *Ann Surg.* 1946;123(1):96-195.

5. Borckardt JJ, Weinstein M, Reeves ST, et al. Postoperative left prefrontal repetitive transcranial magnetic stimulation reduces patient-controlled analgesia use. *Anesthesiology.* 2006;105(3):557-562.

6. Boucher TJ, Okuse K, Bennett DL, et al. Potent analgesic effects of GDNF in neuropathic pain states. *Science.* 2000;290(5489):124-127.

7. Cho ZH, Chung SC, Jones JP, et al. New findings of the correlation between acupoints and corresponding brain cortices using functional MRI. *Proc Natl Acad Sci U S A.* 1998;95(5):2670-2673.

8. Coghill RC, McHaffie JG, Yen YF. Neural correlates of interindividual differences in the subjective experience of pain. *Proc Natl Acad Sci U S A.* 2003;100(14):8538-8542.

9. Coghill RC, Sang CN, Maisog JM, et al. Pain intensity processing within the human brain: a bilateral, distributed mechanism. *J Neurophysiol.* 1999;82(4):1934-1943.

10. Colloca L, Benedetti F. Placebos and painkillers: is mind as real as matter? *Nat Rev Neurosci.* 2005;6: 545-552.

11. Diatchenko L, Slade GD, Nackley AG, et al. Genetic basis for individual variations in pain perception and the development of a chronic pain condition. *Hum Mol Genet.* 2005;14(1):135-143.

12. Gwilym S, Filippini N, Douaud G, Carr AJ, Tracey I. Thalamic atrophy associated with painful osteoarthritis of the hip is reversed after arthroplasty. *Arthritis Rheum.* 2010;62:2930-2940.

13. Harden RN. Chronic neuropathic pain. Mechanisms, diagnosis, and treatment. *Neurologist.* 2005;11(2): 111-122.

14. Hocking B. Epidemiological aspects of "repetition strain injury" in Telecom Australia. *Med J Aust.* 1987;147(5):218-222.

15. Hohmann AG, Suplita RL, Bolton NM, et al. An endocannabinoid mechanism for stress-induced analgesia. *Nature.* 2005;435(7045):1108-1112.

16. Hooley JM, Delgado ML. Pain insensitivity in the relatives of schizophrenia patients. *Schizophr Res.* 2001;47(2-3):265-273.

17. Hunt SP, Mantyh PW. The molecular dynamics of pain control. *Nat Rev Neurosci.* 2001;2(2):83-91.

18. Jaffee JH, Strain EC. Opioid-related disorders. In: Sadock BJ, Sadock VA, eds. *Kaplan & Sadock's Comprehensive Textbook of Psychiatry.* 8th ed. Philadelphia, PA: Lippincott Williams & Wilkins; 2005:1265-1290.

19. Kandel ER, Schwartz JH, Jessell TM, eds. *Principles of Neural Science.* 4th ed. New York, NY: McGraw-Hill; 2000.

20. Mardy S, Miura Y, Endo F, et al. Congenital insensitivity to pain with anhidrosis (CIPA): effect of TRKA (NTRK1) missense mutations on autophosphorylation of the receptor tyrosine kinase for nerve growth factor. *Hum Mol Genet.* 2001;10(3):179-188.

21. McMahon SB, Cafferty WB, Marchand F, et al. Immune and glial cell factors as pain mediators and modulators. *Exp Neurol.* 2005;192(2):444-462.

22. Melzack R, Coderre TJ, Katz J, et al. Central neuroplasticity and pathological pain. *Ann N Y Acad Sci.* 2001;933:157-174.

23. Nagasako EM, Oaklander AL, Dworkin RH, et al. Congenital insensitivity to pain: an update. *Pain.* 2003;101(3):213-219.

24. Pariente J, White P, Frackowiak RS, et al. Expectancy and belief modulate the neuronal substrates of pain treated by acupuncture. *Neuroimage.* 2005;25(4):1161-1167.

25. Petrovic P, Kalso E, Petersson KM, et al. Placebo and opioid analgesia—imaging a shared neuronal network. *Science.* 2002;295(5560):1737-1740.

26. Premkumar L. Targeting TRPV1 as an alternative approach to narcotic analgesics to treat chronic pain conditions. *AAPS J.* 2010;12:361-370.

27. Price DD. Psychological and neural mechanisms of the affective dimension of pain. *Science.* 2000;288(5472): 1769-1772.

28. Purves D, Augustine GJ, Fitzpatrick D, et al. *Neuroscience.* 5th ed. Sunderland, MA: Sinauer; 2011.

29. Reynolds DV. Surgery in the rat during electrical analgesia induced by focal brain stimulation. *Science.* 1969;164(878):444-445.

30. Schrader H, Obelieniene D, Bovim G, et al. Natural evolution of late whiplash syndrome outside the medicolegal context. *Lancet.* 1996;347(9010):1207-1211.

31. Staiger TO, Gaster B, Sullivan MD, et al. Systematic review of antidepressants in the treatment of chronic low back pain. *Spine.* 2003;28(22):2540-2545.

32. Tajet-Foxell B, Rose FD. Pain and pain tolerance in professional ballet dancers. *Br J Sports Med.* 1995;29(1):31-34.

33. Wager TD, Rilling JK, Smith EE, et al. Placebo-induced changes in FMRI in the anticipation and experience of pain. *Science.* 2004;303(5661):1162-1167.

CHAPTER 12

1. Adinoff B. Neurobiologic processes in drug reward and addiction. *Harv Rev Psychiatry.* 2004;12(6): 305-320.

2. Adriani W, Spijker S, Deroche-Gamonet V, et al. Evidence for enhanced neurobehavioral vulnerability to nicotine during periadolescence in rats. *J Neurosci.* 2003;23(11):4712-4716.

3. Bassareo V, De Luca MA, Di Chiara G. Differential expression of motivational stimulus properties by dopamine in nucleus accumbens shell versus core and prefrontal cortex. *J Neurosci.* 2002;22(11):4709-4719.

4. Bolanos CA, Barrot M, Berton O, et al. Methylphenidate treatment during pre- and periadolescence alters behavioral responses to emotional stimuli at adulthood. *Biol Psychiatry.* 2003;54(12):1317-1329.

5. Buhusi CV, Meck WH. Differential effects of metham-phetamine and haloperidol on the control of an internal clock. *Behav Neurosci.* 2002;116(2):291-297.

6. Carlezon WA Jr, Mague SD, Andersen SL. Enduring behavioral effects of early exposure to methylphenidate in rats. *Biol Psychiatry.* 2003;54(12):1330-1337.

7. Ernst M, Nelson EE, Jazbec S, et al. Amygdala and nucleus accumbens in responses to receipt and omis-sion of gains in adults and adolescents. *Neuroimage.* 2005;25(4):1279-1291.

8. Fone KC, Nutt DJ. Stimulants: use and abuse in the treatment of attention deficit hyperactivity disorder. *Curr Opin Pharmacol.* 2005;5(1):87-93.

9. Garavan H, Pankiewicz J, Bloom A, et al. Cue-induced cocaine craving: neuroanatomical specificity for drug users and drug stimuli. *Am J Psychiatry.* 2000;157(11): 1789-1798.

10. Glass JM, Buu A, Adams KM, et al. Effects of alcohol-ism severity and smoking on executive neurocognitive function. *Addiction.* 2009;104(1):38-48.

11. Goldman D, Barr CS. Restoring the addicted brain. *N Engl J Med.* 2002;347(11):843-845.

12. Higgins ES. Do ADHS drugs take a toll on the brain? *Sci Am Mind.* 2009;20:38-43.

13. Kalivas PW, Volkow N, Seamans J. Unmanageable moti-vation in addiction: a pathology in prefrontal-accumbens glutamate transmission. *Neuron.* 2005;45(5):647-650.

14. Kolb B, Gorny G, Li Y, et al. Amphetamine or cocaine limits the ability of later experience to promote structural plasticity in the neocortex and nucleus accumbens. *Proc Natl Acad Sci U S A.* 2003;100(18):10523-10528.

15. Kringelback ML, Berridge KC. Toward a functional neuroanatomy of pleasure and happiness. *Trends Cogn Sci.* 2009;13:479-487.

16. Le AD, Harding S, Juzytsch W, et al. The role of cor-ticotrophin-releasing factor in stress-induced relapse to alcohol-seeking behavior in rats. *Psychopharmacology (Berl).* 2000;150(3):317-324.

17. Leknes S, Tracey I. A common neurobiology for pain and pleasure. *Nat Rev Neurosci* 2008;9:314-320.

18. Morgan D, Grant KA, Gage HD, et al. Social domi-nance in monkeys: dopamine D2 receptors and cocaine self-administration. *Nat Neurosci.* 2002;5(2):169-174.

19. Nestler EJ. Molecular basis of long-term plasticity underlying addiction. *Nat Rev Neurosci.* 2001;2(2): 119-128.

20. Nestler EJ, Hyman SE, Malenka RC. *Molecular Neuropharmacology. A Foundation for Clinical Neuroscience.* 2nd ed. New York, NY: McGraw-Hill; 2009.

21. Nestler EJ, Malenka RC. The addicted brain. *Sci Am.* 2004;290(3):78-85.

22. O'Connor MF, Wellisch DK, Stanton AL, Eisenberger NI, Irwin MR, Lieberman MD. Craving love? Enduring grief activates brain's reward center. *Neuroimage.* 2008;42:969-972.

23. Olds J. Pleasure centers in the brain. *Sci Am.* 1956;195: 105-112.

24. Pettit HO, Justice JB Jr. Effect of dose on cocaine self-administration behavior and dopamine levels in the nucleus accumbens. *Brain Res.* 1991;539(1):94-102.

25. Ricaurte GA, Mechan AO, Yuan J, et al. Amphetamine treatment similar to that used in the treatment of adult atten-tion-deficit/hyperactivity disorder damages dopaminergic nerve endings in the striatum of adult nonhuman primates. *J Pharmacol Exp Ther.* 2005;315(1):91-98.

26. Robbins TW, Everitt BJ. Drug addiction: bad habits add up. *Nature.* 1999;398(6728):567-570.

27. Robinson TE, Gorny G, Savage VR, et al. Widespread but regionally specific effects of experimenter- versus self-administered morphine on dendritic spines in the nucleus accumbens, hippocampus, and neocortex of adult rats. *Synapse.* 2002;46(4):271-279.

28. Robinson TE, Kolb B. Persistent structural modifica-tions in nucleus accumbens and prefrontal cortex neurons produced by previous experience with amphet-amine. *J Neurosci.* 1997;17(21):8491-8497.

29. Robinson TE, Kolb B. Structural plasticity associated with exposure to drugs of abuse. *Neuropharmacology.* 2004;47(suppl 1):33-46.

30. Rosenbloom M, Sullivan EV, Pfefferbaum A. Using magnetic resonance imaging and diffusion tensor imag-ing to assess brain damage in alcoholics. *Alcohol Res Health.* 2003;27(2):146-152.

31. Schultz W. Multiple reward signals in the brain. *Nat Rev Neurosci.* 2000;1(3):199-207.

32. See RE, Fuchs RA, Ledford CC, et al. Drug addic-tion, relapse, and the amygdala. *Ann N Y Acad Sci.* 2003;985:294-307.

33. Tremblay L, Schultz W. Relative reward preference in primate orbitofrontal cortex. *Nature.* 1999;398(6729): 704-708.

34. Volkow ND, Fowler JS. Addiction, a disease of compul-sion and drive: involvement of the orbitofrontal cortex. *Cereb Cortex.* 2000;10(3):318-325.

35. Volkow ND, Fowler JS, Wang GJ, et al. Role of dopa-mine in the therapeutic and reinforcing effects of meth-ylphenidate in humans: results from imaging studies. *Eur Neuropsychopharmacol.* 2002;12(6):557-566.

36. Volkow ND, Li TK. Drug addiction: the neurobiology of behaviour gone awry. *Nat Rev Neurosci.* 2004;5(12): 963-970.

37. Wilens TE, Faraone SV, Biederman J, et al. Does stimu-lant therapy of attention-deficit/hyperactivity disorder beget later substance abuse? A meta-analytic review of the literature. *Pediatrics.* 2003;111(1):179-185.

38. Wilson SJ, Sayette MA, Fiez JA. Prefrontal responses to drug cues: a neurocognitive analysis. *Nat Neurosci.* 2004;7(3):211-214.

CHAPTER 13

1. Arch JR. Central regulation of energy balance: inputs, outputs and leptin resistance. *Proc Nutr Soc.* 2005;64(1):39-46.

2. Ayyad C, Andersen T. Long-term efficacy of dietary treatment of obesity: a systematic review of studies published between 1931 and 1999. *Obes Rev.* 2000;1(2): 113-119.

3. Bear MF, Connors BW, Paradiso MA, eds. *Neuroscience: Exploring the Brain.* 3rd ed. Baltimore, MD: Lippincott Williams & Wilkins; 2006.

4. Berthoud HR. Mind versus metabolism in the control of food intake and energy balance. *Physiol Behav.* 2004;81(5):781-793.

5. Breedlove SM, Watson NV, Rosenzweig MR. *Biological Psychology.* 6th ed. Sunderland, MA: Sinauer; 2010.

6. Carlson NR. *Physiology of Behavior.* Boston, MA: Pearson Education Inc.; 2004.

7. Colman E. Anorectics on trial: a half century of federal regulation of prescription appetite suppressants. *Ann Intern Med.* 2005;143(5):380-385.

8. Cone RD. Anatomy and regulation of the central mela-nocortin system. *Nat Neurosci.* 2005;8(5):571-578.

9. Dallman MF, Pecoraro N, Akana SF, et al. Chronic stress and obesity: a new view of "comfort food". *Proc Natl Acad Sci U S A.* 2003;100(20):11696-11701.

10. Freeman MP. Nutrition and psychiatry. *Am J Psychiatry.* 2010:167;244-247.

11. Havel PJ. Peripheral signals conveying metabolic information to the brain: short-term and long-term regulation of food intake and energy homeostasis. *Exp Biol Med.* 2001;226(11):963-977.

12. Kaati G, Bygren LO, Pembrey M, Sjostrom M. Transgenerational response to nutrition, early life circumstances and longevity. *Eur J Hum Genet.* 2007; 15:784-790.

13. Kalm LM, Semba RD. They starved so that others be better fed: remembering Ancel Keys and the Minnesota experiment. *J Nutr.* 2005;135(6):1347-1352.

14. Keesey RE, Boyle PC. Effects of quinine adulteration upon body weight of LH-lesioned and intact male rats. *J Comp Physiol Psychol.* 1973;84(1):38-46.

15. Kroeze WK, Hufeisen SJ, Popadak BA, et al. H1-histamine receptor affinity predicts short-term weight gain for typical and atypical antipsychotic drugs. *Neuropsychopharmacology.* 2003;28(3):519-526.

16. Leibel RL, Rosenbaum M, Hirsch J. Changes in energy expenditure resulting from altered body weight. *N Engl J Med.* 1995;332(10):621-628.

17. Lorello C, Goldfield GS, Doucet E. Methylphenidate hydrochloride increases energy expenditure in health adults. *Obesity.* 2008:16;470-472.

18. Lowell BB, Spiegelman BM. Towards a molecular understanding of adaptive thermogenesis. *Nature.* 2000;404(6778):652-660.

19. Mineur YS, Abizaid A, Roa Y, et al. Nicotine decreases food intake through activation of POMC neurons. *Science.* 2011;332:1330-1332.

20. Ochner CN, Kwok Y, Conceicao E, et al. Selective reduction in neural responses to high calorie foods following gastric bypass surgery. *Ann Surg.* 2011:253;502-507.

21. Rapoport JL, Buchsbaum MS, Zahn TP, et al. Dextroamphetamine: cognitive and behavioral effects in normal prepubertal boys. *Science.* 1978;199(4328): 560-563.

22. Ravussin E, Valencia ME, Esparza J, et al. Effects of a traditional lifestyle on obesity in Pima Indians. *Diabetes Care.* 1994;17(9):1067-1074.

23. Schwartz MW, Woods SC, Porte D Jr, et al. Central nervous system control of food intake. *Nature.* 2000;404(6778):661-671.

24. Seeley RJ, Woods SC. Monitoring of stored and available fuel by the CNS: implications for obesity. *Nat Rev Neurosci.* 2003;4(11):901-909.

25. Strader AD, Woods SC. Gastrointestinal hormones and food intake. *Gastroenterology.* 2005;128(1):175-191.

26. Stunkard AJ, Sorensen TI, Hanis C, et al. An adoption study of human obesity. *N Engl J Med.* 1986;314(4): 193-198.

27. Vaisse C, Clement K, Durand E, et al. Melanocortin-4 receptor mutations are a frequent and heterogeneous cause of morbid obesity. *J Clin Invest.* 2000;106(2): 253-262.

28. Volkow ND, Wise RA. How can drug addiction help us understand obesity? *Nat Neurosci.* 2005;8(5):555-560.

CHAPTER 14

1. Bear MF, Connors BW, Paradiso MA. *Neuroscience: Exploring the Brain.* 3rd ed. Baltimore, MD: Lippincott Williams & Wilkins; 2007.

2. Birbaumer N, Veit R, Lotze M, et al. Deficient fear conditioning in psychopathy: a functional magnetic resonance imaging study. *Arch Gen Psychiatry.* 2005;62(7):799-805.

3. Blair RJ. Neurobiological basis of psychopathy. *Br J Psychiatry.* 2003;182:5-7.

4. Branchi I, Francia N, Alleva E. Epigenetic control of neurobehavioural plasticity: the role of neurotrophins. *Behav Pharmacol.* 2004;15(5-6):353-362.

5. Breedlove SM, Watson NV, Rosenzweig MR. *Biological Psychology.* 6th ed. Sunderland, MA: Sinauer; 2010.

6. Brower MC, Price BH. Neuropsychiatry of frontal lobe dysfunction in violent and criminal behaviour: a critical review. *J Neurol Neurosurg Psychiatry.* 2001;71:720-726.

7. Coccaro EF, Kavoussi RJ. Fluoxetine and impulsive aggressive behavior in personality-disordered subjects. *Arch Gen Psychiatry.* 1997;54:1081-1088.

8. Coccaro EF, Kavoussi RJ, Hauger RL, et al. Cerebrospinal fluid vasopressin levels: correlates with aggression and serotonin function in personality-disordered subjects. *Arch Gen Psychiatry.* 1998;55:708-714.

9. Damasio H, Grabowski T, Frank R, et al. The return of Phineas Gage: clues about the brain from the skull of a famous patient. *Science.* 1994;264:1102-1105.

10. Ehrenkranz J, Bliss E, Sheard MH. Plasma testosterone: correlation with aggressive behavior and social dominance in man. *Psychosom Med.* 1974;36:469-475.

11. Eisenegger C, Haushofer J, Fehr E. The role of testosterone in social interaction. *Trends Cogn Sci.* 2011:15;263-271.

12. Enserink M. Searching for the mark of Cain. *Science.* 2000;289:575-579.

13. van Erp AM, Miczek KA. Aggressive behavior, increased accumbal dopamine, and decreased cortical serotonin in rats. *J Neurosci.* 2000;20:9320-9325.

14. Fiore M, Amendola T, Triaca V, et al. Fighting in the aged male mouse increases the expression of TrkA and TrkB in the subventricular zone and in the hippocampus. *Behav Brain Res.* 2005;157(2):351-362.

15. Flynn JP. The neural basis of aggression in cats. In: Glass DC, ed. *Neurophysicology and Emotion.* New York, NY: Rockefeller University Press; 1967:40-60.

16. Gregg TR, Siegel A. Brain structures and neurotransmitters regulating aggression in cats: implications for human aggression. *Prog Neuropsychopharmacol Biol Psychiatry.* 2001;25:91-140.

17. Hare RD. *Without Conscience. The Disturbing World of the Psychopaths Among Us.* New York, NY: Guilford Press; 1999.

18. Higley JD, Mehlman PT, Higley SB, et al. Excessive mortality in young free-ranging male nonhuman primates with low cerebrospinal fluid 5-hydroxyindoleacetic acid concentrations. *Arch Gen Psychiatry.* 1996;53(6):537-543.

19. Kiehl KA, Smith AM, Hare RD, et al. Limbic abnormalities in affective processing by criminal psychopaths as revealed by functional magnetic resonance imaging. *Biol Psychiatry.* 2001;50:677-684.

20. Lee GP, Bechara A, Adolphs R, et al. Clinical and physiological effects of stereotaxic bilateral amygdalotomy for intractable aggression. *J Neuropsychiatry Clin Neurosci.* 1998;10(4):413-420.

21. Nelson RJ. *The Biology of Aggression.* New York, NY: Oxford University Press; 2006.

22. Ortiz J, Raine A. Heart rate level and antisocial behavior in children and adolescents: a meta-analysis. *J Am Acad Child Adolesc Psychiatry.* 2004;43(2):154-162.

23. de Quervain DJ, Fischbacher U, Treyer V, et al. The neural basis of altruistic punishment. *Science.* 2004;305(5688): 1254-1258.

24. Raine A. Annotation: the role of prefrontal deficits, low autonomic arousal, and early health factors in the

development of antisocial and aggressive behavior in children. *J Child Psychol Psychiatry*. 2002;43:417-434.

25. Raine A, Meloy JR, Bihrle S, et al. Reduced prefrontal and increased subcortical brain functioning assessed using positron emission tomography in predatory and affective murderers. *Behav Sci Law*. 1998;16(3): 319-332.

26. Sano K, Mayanagi Y. Posteromedial hypothalamotomy in the treatment of violent, aggressive behaviour. *Acta Neurochir Suppl (Wien)*. 1988;44:145-151.

27. Sheard MH, Marini JL, Bridges CI, et al. The effect of lithium on impulsive aggressive behavior in man. *Am J Psychiatry*. 1976;133:1409-1413.

28. Siegel A, Edinger H, Dotto M. Effects of electrical stimulation of the lateral aspect of the prefrontal cortex upon attack behavior in cats. *Brain Res*. 1975; 93:473-484.

29. Tricker R, Casaburi R, Storer TW, et al. The effects of supraphysiological doses of testosterone on angry behavior in healthy eugonadal men–a clinical research center study. *J Clin Endocrinol Metab*. 1996; 81:3754-3758.

30. Wagner GC, Beuving LJ, Hutchinson RR. The effects of gonadal hormone manipulations on aggressive target-biting in mice. *Aggress Behav*. 1980;6:1-7.

31. Yang Y, Raine A, Narr KL, et al. Localization of deformations within the amygdala in individual with psychopathy. *Arch Gen Psychiatry*. 2009;9:986-994.

CHAPTER 15

1. Bear MF, Connors BW, Paradiso MA, eds.*Neuroscience: Exploring the Brain*. 3rd ed. Baltimore, MD: Lippincott Williams & Wilkins; 2007.

2. Breedlove SM, Watson NV, Rosenzweig MR. *Biological Psychology*. 6th ed. Sunderland, MA: Sinauer; 2010.

3. Everson CA, Laatsch CD, Hogg N. Antioxidant defense responses to sleep loss and sleep recovery. *Am J Physiol Regul Integr Comp Physiol*. 2005;288(2): R374-R383.

4. Fosse R, Stickgold R, Hobson JA. Brain-mind states: reciprocal variation in thoughts and hallucinations. *Psychol Sci*. 2001;12(1):30-36.

5. Frank MG, Issa NP, Stryker MP. Sleep enhances plasticity in the developing visual cortex. *Neuron*. 2001; 30(1):275-287.

6. Guzman-Marin R, Suntsova N, Stewart DR, et al. Sleep deprivation reduces proliferation of cells in the dentate gyrus of the hippocampus in rats. *J Physiol*. 2003;549(pt 2):563-571.

7. Hobson JA. *Sleep*. New York, NY: Scientific American Library; 1989.

8. Hobson JA, Pace-Schott EF. The cognitive neuroscience of sleep: neuronal systems, consciousness and learning. *Nat Rev Neurosci*. 2002;3(9):679-693.

9. Horne JA. *Why We Sleep: The Functions of Sleep in Humans and Other Mammals*. Oxford: Oxford University Press; 1988.

10. Kryger MH, Roth T, Dement WC. *Principles and Practice of Sleep Medicine*. 4th ed. Philadelphia, PA: Elsevier Saunders; 2005.

11. Landrigan CP, Rothschild JM, Cronin JW, et al. Effect of reducing interns' work hours on serious medical errors in intensive care units. *N Engl J Med*. 2004;351(18):1838-1848.

12. Mahowald MW, Schenck CH. Insights from studying human sleep disorders. *Nature*. 2005;437(7063): 1279-1285.

13. Mansour HA, Monk TH, Nimgaonkar VL. Circadian genes and bipolar disorder. *Ann Med*. 2005;37(3): 196-205.

14. Meddis R. *The Sleep Instinct*. London: Routledge & Kegan Paul; 1977.

15. Mujhametov LM. Sleep in marine mammals. In: Borbely AA, ed. 1984.

16. Nofzinger EA, Buysse DJ, Germain A, et al. Functional neuroimaging evidence for hyperarousal in insomnia. *Am J Psychiatry*. 2004;161(11):2126-2128.

17. Ohayon MM, Carskadon MA, Guilleminault C, et al. Meta-analysis of quantitative sleep parameters from childhood to old age in healthy individuals: developing normative sleep values across the human lifespan. *Sleep*. 2004;27(7):1255-1273.

18. Pace-Schott EF, Hobson JA. The neurobiology of sleep: genetics, cellular physiology and subcortical networks. *Nat Rev Neurosci*. 2002;3(8):591-605.

19. Peigneux P, Laureys S, Fuchs S, et al. Are spatial memories strengthened in the human hippocampus during slow wave sleep? *Neuron*. 2004;44(3):535-545.

20. Purves D, Augustine GJ, Fitzpatrick D, et al. *Neuroscience*. 5th ed. Sunderland, MA: Sinauer; 2011.

21. Ralph MR, Lehman MN. Transplantation: a new tool in the analysis of the mammalian hypothalamic circadian pacemaker. *Trends Neurosci*. 1991;14(8):362-366.

22. Reiter RJ. The melatonin rhythm: both a clock and a calendar. *Experientia*. 1993;49(8):654-664.

23. Saper CB, Scammell TE, Lu J. Hypothalamic regulation of sleep and circadian rhythms. *Nature*. 2005;437(7063):1257-1263.

24. Siegel JM. Why we sleep. *Sci Am*. 2003;289(5): 92-97.

25. Siegel JM. Sleep viewed as a state of adaptive inactivity. *Nat Rev Neurosci*. 2009;10(10):747-753.

26. Sutherland GR, McNaughton B. Memory trace reactivation in hippocampal and neocortical neuronal ensembles. *Curr Opin Neurobiol*. 2000;10(2):180-186.

27. Taheri S, Lin L, Austin D, et al. Short sleep duration is associated with reduced leptin, elevated ghrelin, and increased body mass index. *PLoS Med*. 2004; 1(3):e62.

28. Van Dongen HP, Maislin G, Mullington JM, et al. The cumulative cost of additional wakefulness: dose-response effects on neurobehavioral functions and sleep physiology from chronic sleep restriction and total sleep deprivation. *Sleep*. 2003;26(2):117-126.

29. Walsh JK, Krystal AD, Amato DA, et al. Nightly treatment of primary insomnia with eszopiclone for six months: effects on sleep, quality of life, and work limitations. *Sleep*. 2007;30(8):959-968.

30. Wehr TA, Duncan WC Jr, Sher L, et al. A circadian signal of change of season in patients with seasonal affective disorder. *Arch Gen Psychiatry*. 2001;58(12): 1108-1114.

31. Wehr TA, Turner EH, Shimada JM, et al. Treatment of rapidly cycling bipolar patient by using extended bed rest and darkness to stabilize the timing and duration of sleep. *Biol Psychiatry*. 1998;43(11):822-828.

CHAPTER 16

1. Alexander GM, Hines M. Sex differences in response to children's toys in nonhuman primates (*Cercopithecus aethiops sabaeus*). *Evol Hum Behav*. 2002;23:467-479.

2. Allen LS, Hines M, Shryne JE, et al. Two sexually dimorphic cell groups in the human brain. *J Neurosci*. 1989;9(2):497-506.

3. Bear MF, Connors BW, Paradiso MA, eds. *Neuroscience: Exploring the Brain.* 3rd ed. Baltimore, MD: Lippincott Williams & Wilkins; 2007.

4. Ben Zion IZ, Tessler R, Cohen L, et al. Polymorphisms in the dopamine D4 receptor gene (DRD4) contribute to individual differences in human sexual behavior: desire, arousal and sexual function. *Molecular Psychiatry.* 2006;11(8):782-786.

5. Breedlove SM, Arnold AP. Hormonal control of a developing neuromuscular system. II. Sensitive periods for the androgen-induced masculinization of the rat spinal nucleus of the bulbocavernosus. *J Neurosci.* 1983;3(2):424-432.

6. Breedlove SM, Watson NV, Rosenzweig MR. *Biological Psychology.* 6th ed. Sunderland, MA: Sinauer; 2010.

7. Cohen LS, Altshuler LL, Harlow BL, et al. Relapse of major depression during pregnancy in women who maintain or discontinue antidepressant treatment. *JAMA.* 2006;295(5):499-507.

8. Colapinto J. *As Nature Made Him: The Boy Who was Raised As a Girl.* New York, NY: HarperCollins; 2000.

9. Conn J, Gillam L, Conway GS. Revealing the diagnosis of androgen insensitivity syndrome in adulthood. *Br Med J.* 2005;331(7517):628-630.

10. Dunn KM, Cherkas LF, Spector TD. Genetic influences on variation in female orgasmic function: a twin study. *Biol Lett.* 2005;1(3):260-263.

11. Hines M. Sex steroids and human behavior: prenatal androgen exposure and sex-typical play behavior in children. *Ann N Y Acad Sci.* 2003;1007:272-282.

12. Hines M, Ahmed SF, Hughes IA. Psychological outcomes and gender-related development in complete androgen insensitivity syndrome. *Arch Sex Behav.* 2003;32(2):93-101.

13. Jordan R, Hallam TJ, Molinoff P, Spana C. Developing treatments for female sexual dysfunction. *Clin Pharmacol Ther.* 2011;89(1):137-141.

14. Kinsley CH, Lambert KG. The maternal brain. *Sci Am.* 2006;294(1):72-79.

15. Laumann EO, Paik A, Rosen RC. Sexual dysfunction in the United States: prevalence and predictors. *JAMA.* 1999;281(6):537-544.

16. LeVay S. A difference in hypothalamic structure between heterosexual and homosexual men. *Science.* 1991;253(5023):1034-1037.

17. Nelson RJ. *An Introduction to Behavioral Endocrinology.* 3rd ed. Sunderland, MA: Sinauer; 2005.

18. Nottebohm F. The road we travelled: discovery, choreography, and significance of brain replaceable neurons. *Ann N Y Acad Sci.* 2004;1016:628-658.

19. Pfaus JG, Shadiack A, Van Soest T, et al. Selective facilitation of sexual solicitation in the female rat by a melanocortin receptor agonist. *Proc Natl Acad Sci U S A.* 2004;101(27):10201-10204.

20. Pope HG Jr, Cohane GH, Kanayama G, et al. Testosterone gel supplementation for men with refractory depression: a randomized, placebo-controlled trial. *Am J Psychiatry.* 2003;160(1):105-111.

21. Purves D, Augustine GJ, Fitzpatrick D, et al. *Neuroscience.* 5th ed. Sunderland, MA: Sinauer; 2011.

22. Rapp SR, Espeland MA, Shumaker SA, et al. Effect of estrogen plus progestin on global cognitive function in postmenopausal women: the Women's Health Initiative Memory Study: a randomized controlled trial. *JAMA.* 2003;289(20):2663-2672.

23. Reiner WG, Gearhart JP. Discordant sexual identity in some genetic males with cloacal exstrophy assigned to female sex at birth. *N Engl J Med.* 2004;350(4):333-341.

24. Roselli CE, Larkin K, Resko JA, et al. The volume of a sexually dimorphic nucleus in the ovine medial preoptic area/anterior hypothalamus varies with sexual partner preference. *Endocrinology.* 2004;145(2):478-483.

25. Rust J, Golombok S, Hines M, et al. The role of brothers and sisters in the gender development of preschool children. *J Exp Child Psychol.* 2000;77(4):292-303.

26. Savic I, Gracia-Falgueras A, Swaab DF. Sexual differentiation of the human brain in relation to gender identity and sexual orientation. *Prog Brain Res.* 2010;186:41-62.

27. Soares CN, Almeida OP, Joffe H, et al. Efficacy of estradiol for the treatment of depressive disorders in perimenopausal women: a double-blind, randomized, placebo-controlled trial. *Arch Gen Psychiatry.* 2001;58(6):529-534.

28. Schule C, Eser D, Baghai C, et al. Neuroactive steroids in affective disorders: target for novel antidepressant or anxiolytic drugs? *Neuroscience.* 2011;191:55-77.

29. Spitzer RL. Can some gay men and lesbians change their sexual orientation? 200 participants reporting a change from homosexual to heterosexual orientation. *Arch Sex Behav.* 2003;32(5):403-417; discussion 19-72.

30. Stahl SM. *Essential Psychopharmacology. Neuroscientific Basis of Practical Applications.* 2nd ed. New York, NY: Cambridge University Press; 2000.

31. Stein DG. Progesterone in the treatment of acute traumatic brain injury: a clinical perspective and update. *Neuroscience.* 2011;191:101-106.

32. Wallen K. Nature needs nurture: the interaction of hormonal and social influences on the development of behavioral sex differences in rhesus monkeys. *Horm Behav.* 1996;30(4):364-378.

33. Woolley CS, Weiland NG, McEwen BS, et al. Estradiol increases the sensitivity of hippocampal CA1 pyramidal cells to NMDA receptor-mediated synaptic input: correlation with dendritic spine density. *J Neurosci.* 1997;17(5):1848-1859.

34. Yang LY, Verhovshek T, Sengelaub DR. Brain-derived neurotrophic factor and androgen interact in the maintenance of dendritic morphology in a sexually dimorphic rat spinal nucleus. *Endocrinology.* 2004;145(1):161-168.

35. Zandi PP, Carlson MC, Plassman BL, et al. Hormone replacement therapy and incidence of Alzheimer disease in older women: The Cache County Study. *JAMA.* 2002;288(17):2123-2129.

36. Zucker KJ, Bradley SJ, Oliver G, et al. Psychosexual development of women with congenital adrenal hyperplasia. *Horm Behav.* 1996;30(4):300-318.

CHAPTER 17

1. Aron A, Fisher H, Mashek DJ, et al. Reward, motivation, and emotion systems associated with early-stage intense romantic love. *J Neurophysiol.* 2005;94(1):327-337.

2. Becker JB, Breedlove SM, Crews D, et al. *Behavioral Endocrinology.* 2nd ed. Cambridge, MA: MIT Press; 2002.

3. Bosch OJ, Meddle SL, Beiderbeck DI, et al. Brain oxytocin correlates with maternal aggression: link to anxiety. *J Neurosci.* 2005;25(29):6807-6815.

4. Breedlove SM, Watson NV, Rosenzweig MR. *Biological Psychology.* 6th ed. Sunderland, MA: Sinauer; 2010.

5. Bridges RS. Endocrine regulation of parental behavior in rodents. In: Krasnegor NA, Bridges RS, eds. *Mammalian Parenting: Biochemical, Neurobiological and Behavioral Determinants.* New York, NY: Oxford University Press; 1990.

6. Buchen L. In their nurture. *Nature.* 2010;467:146-148.

7. Carr L, Iacoboni M, Dubeau MC, et al. Neural mechanisms of empathy in humans: a relay from neural systems for imitation to limbic areas. *Proc Natl Acad Sci U S A*. 2003;100(9):5497-5502.
8. Dapretto M, Davies MS, Pfeifer JH, et al. Understanding emotions in others: mirror neuron dysfunction in children with autism spectrum disorders. *Nat Neurosci*. 2006;9(1):28-30.
9. Dawson G, Rogers S, Munson J, et al. Randomized, controlled trial of an intervention for toddlers with autism: the Early Start Denver Model. *Pediatrics*. 2010;125(1):e17-e23.
10. Emanuele E, Politi P, Bianchi M, et al. Raised plasma nerve growth factor levels associated with early-stage romantic love. *Psychoneuroendocrinology*. 2006;31:288-294.
11. Engh AL, Beehner JC, Bergman TJ, et al. Behavioral and hormonal responses to predation in female chacma baboons (*Papio hamadryas ursinus*). *Proc R Soc Lond B Biol Sci*. 2006;273(1578):707-712.
12. Felsenfeld G, Groudine M. Controlling the double helix. *Nature*. 2003;421(6921):448-453.
13. Francis D, Diorio J, Liu D, et al. Nongenomic transmission across generations of maternal behavior and stress responses in the rat. *Science*. 1999;286(5442):1155-1158.
14. Iacoboni M. Neural mechanisms of imitation. *Curr Opin Neurobiol*. 2005;15(6):632-637.
15. Klin A, Jones W, Schultz R, et al. Visual fixation patterns during viewing of naturalistic social situations as predictors of social competence in individuals with autism. *Arch Gen Psychiatry*. 2002;59(9):809-816.
16. Klin A, Jones W, Schultz R, et al. Defining and quantifying the social phenotype in autism. *Am J Psychiatry*. 2002;159(6):895-908.
17. Li M, Davidson P, Budin R, et al. Effects of typical and atypical antipsychotic drugs on maternal behavior in postpartum female rats. *Schizophr Res*. 2004;70(1):69-80.
18. Lim MM, Wang Z, Olazabal DE, et al. Enhanced partner preference in a promiscuous species by manipulating the expression of a single gene. *Nature*. 2004;429:754-757.
19. Liu D, Diorio J, Tannenbaum B, et al. Maternal care, hippocampal glucocorticoid receptors, and hypothalamic-pituitary-adrenal responses to stress. *Science*. 1997;277(5332):1659-1662.
20. McGowan PO, Sasaki A, D'Alessio AC, et al. Epigenetic regulation of the glucocorticoid receptor in human brain associates with childhood abuse. *Nat Neurosci*. 2009;12(3):342-348.
21. Mcgue M, Lykken DT. Genetic influence on risk of divorce. *Psychol Sci*. 1992;3(6):368-373.
22. Meyer-Lindenberg A, Domes G, Kirsch P, Heinrichs M. Oxytocin and vasopressin in the human brain: social neuropeptides for translational medicine. *Nat Rev Neurosci*. 2011;12:524-538.
23. Nelson RJ. *An Introduction to Behavioral Endocrinology*. 3rd ed. Sunderland, MA: Sinauer; 2005.
24. Numan M, Sheehan TP. Neuroanatomical circuitry for mammalian maternal behavior. *Ann N Y Acad Sci*. 1997;807:101-125.
25. Purves D, Augustine GJ, Fitzpatrick D, et al. *Neuroscience*. 5th ed. Sunderland, MA: Sinauer; 2011.
26. Redcay E, Courchesne E. When is the brain enlarged in autism? A meta-analysis of all brain size reports. *Biol Psychiatry*. 2005;58(1):1-9.
27. Rizzolatti G, Fogassi L, Gallese V. Neurophysiological mechanisms underlying the understanding and imitation of action. *Nat Rev Neurosci*. 2001;2(9):661-670.
28. Rosenblatt JS, Siegel HI, Mayer AD. Blood levels of progesterone, estradiol and prolactin in pregnant rats. *Adv Study Behav*. 1979;10:225-311.
29. Schultz RT, Anderson GM. The neurobiology of autism and the pervasive developmental disorders. In: Charney DS, Nestler EJ, eds. *Neurobiology of Mental Illness*. 2nd ed. Oxford: Oxford University Press; 2004: 954-967.
30. Taylor SE, Klein LC, Lewis BP, et al. Biobehavioral responses to stress in females: tend-and-befriend, not fight-or-flight. *Psychol Rev*. 2000;107(3):411-429.
31. Terkel J, Rosenblatt JS. Maternal behavior induced by maternal blood plasma injected into virgin rats. *J Comp Physiol Psychol*. 1968;65(3):479-482.
32. Walem H, Wastberg L, Henningsson S, et al. Genetic variation in the vasopressin receptor 1a gene (AVPR1A) associates with pair-bonding behavior in humans. *Proc Natl Acad Sci U S A*. 2008;105(37):14153-14156.
33. Weaver IC, Cervoni N, Champagne FA, et al. Epigenetic programming by maternal behavior. *Nat Neurosci*. 2004;7(8):847-854.
34. Werner E, Dawson G. Validation of the phenomenon of autistic regression using home videotapes. *Arch Gen Psychiatry*. 2005;62(8):889-895.
35. Wolff JJ, Gu H, Gerig G, et al. Differences in white matter fiber tract development present from 6 to 24 months in infants with autism. *Am J Psychiatry*. 2012; 169(6):589-600.
36. Young LJ, Wang Z. The neurobiology of pair bonding. *Nat Neurosci*. 2004;7(10):1048-1054.

CHAPTER 18

1. Barad M. Fear extinction in rodents: basic insight to clinical promise. *Curr Opin Neurobiol*. 2005;15(6): 710-715.
2. Bayley PJ, Gold JJ, Hopkins RO, et al. The neuroanatomy of remote memory. *Neuron*. 2005;46(5):799-810.
3. Bear MF, Connors BW, Paradiso MA, eds. *Neuroscience: Exploring the Brain*. 3rd ed. Baltimore, MD: Lippincott Williams & Wilkins; 2007.
4. Breedlove SM, Watson NV, Rosenzweig MR. *Biological Psychology*. 6th ed. Sunderland, MA: Sinauer; 2010.
5. Corkin S. What's new with the amnesic patient H.M.? *Nat Rev Neurosci*. 2002;3(2):153-160.
6. Frankland PW, Bontempi B. The organization of recent and remote memories. *Nat Rev Neurosci*. 2005;6(2): 119-130.
7. Genoux D, Haditsch U, Knobloch M, et al. Protein phosphatase 1 is a molecular constraint on learning and memory. *Nature*. 2002;418(6901):970-975.
8. Guan JS, Haggarty SJ, Giacometti, et al. HDAC2 negatively regulates memory formation and synaptic plasticity. *Nature*. 2009;459(7243):55-60.
9. Hebb DO. *The Organization of Behavior*. New York, NY: Wiley; 1949.
10. Hofmann SG, Smits JAJ, Asnaani A, et al. Cognitive enhancers for anxiety disorders. *Pharmacol Biochem Behav*. 2011;99:275-284.
11. Kandel ER, Schwartz JH, Jessell TM, eds. *Principles of Neural Science*. 4th ed. New York, NY: McGraw-Hill; 2000.
12. Kirn J, O'Loughlin B, Kasparian S, et al. Cell death and neuronal recruitment in the high vocal center of adult male canaries are temporally related to changes in song. *Proc Natl Acad Sci U S A*. 1994;91(17):7844-7848.
13. Lamprecht R, LeDoux J. Structural plasticity and memory. *Nat Rev Neurosci*. 2004;5(1):45-54.

14. Leuner B, Falduto J, Shors TJ. Associative memory formation increases the observation of dendritic spines in the hippocampus. *J Neurosci*. 2003;23(2):659-665.
15. Leuner B, Mendolia-Loffredo S, Kozorovitskiy Y, et al. Learning enhances the survival of new neurons beyond the time when the hippocampus is required for memory. *J Neurosci*. 2004;24(34):7477-7481.
16. Luria AR. *The Mind of a Mnemonist*. New York, NY: Basic Books; 1968.
17. Maviel T, Durkin TP, Menzaghi F, et al. Sites of neocortical reorganization critical for remote spatial memory. *Science*. 2004;305(5680):96-99.
18. Meiri N, Rosenblum K. Lateral ventricle injection of the protein synthesis inhibitor anisomycin impairs long-term memory in a spatial memory task. *Brain Res*. 1998;789(1):48-55.
19. Mikaelsson MA, Miller CA. The path to epigenetic treatment of memory disorders. *Neurobiol Learn Mem*. 2011;96:13-18.
20. Nader K, Schafe GE, Le Doux JE. Fear memories require protein synthesis in the amygdala for reconsolidation after retrieval. *Nature*. 2000;406(6797):722-726.
21. Nobler MS, Sackeim HA. Neurobiological correlates of the cognitive side effects of electroconvulsive therapy. *J ECT*. 2008;24(1):40-45.
22. Purves D, Augustine GJ, Fitzpatrick D, et al. *Neuroscience*. 5th ed. Sunderland, MA: Sinauer; 2011.
23. Ressler KJ, Rothbaum BO, Tannenbaum L, et al. Cognitive enhancers as adjuncts to psychotherapy: use of D-cycloserine in phobic individuals to facilitate extinction of fear. *Arch Gen Psychiatry*. 2004;61(11):1136-1144.
24. Sackeim HA, Prudic J, Ruller R, et al. The cognitive effects of electroconvulsive therapy in community settings. *Neuropsychopharmacology*. 2007;32:244-454.
25. Santini E, Ge H, Ren K, et al. Consolidation of fear extinction requires protein synthesis in the medial prefrontal cortex. *J Neurosci*. 2004;24(25):5704-5710.
26. Van Hoesen GW. The parahippocampal gyrus: new observations regarding its cortical connections in the monkey. *Trends Neurosci*. 1982;5:345-350.

CHAPTER 19

1. Andreasen NC. *The Creating Brain: The Neuroscience of Genius*. New York, NY: Dana Press; 2005.
2. Beckett C, Maughan B, Rutter M, et al. Do the effects of early severe deprivation on cognition persist into early adolescence? Findings from the English and Romanian adoptees study. *Child Dev*. 2006;77(3):696-711.
3. Breslau N, Lucia VC, Alvarado GF. Intelligence and other predisposing factors in exposure to trauma and posttraumatic stress disorder. *Arch Gen Psychiatry*. 2006; 63(11):1238-1245.
4. Carlsson I, Wendt PE, Risberg J. On the neurobiology of creativity. Differences in frontal activity between high and low creative subjects. *Neuropsychologia*. 2000;38(6):873-885.
5. Carson SH, Peterson JB, Higgins DM. Decreased latent inhibition is associated with increased creative achievement in high-functioning individuals. *J Pers Soc Psychol*. 2003;85(3):499-506.
6. Cooper NJ, Keage H, Hermens D, et al. The dose-dependent effect of methylphenidate on performance, cognition and psychophysiology. *J Integr Neurosci*. 2005;4(1):123-144.
7. Dierssen M, Ramakers GJA. Dendritic pathology in mental retardation: from molecular genetics to neurobiology. *Genes Brain Behav*. 2006;5(suppl 2):48-60.

8. Dietrich A, Kanso R. A review of EEG, ERP, and neuroimaging studies of creativity and insight. *Psychol Bull*. 2010;136(5):822-848.
9. Glascher J, Rudrauf D, Colom R, et al. Distributed neural system for general intelligence revealed by lesion mapping. *Proc Natl Acad Sci U S A*. 2010;107(10): 4705-4709.
10. Gottfredson LS. The general intelligence factor. *Sci Am Presents: Exploring Intell*. 1998;9(4):24-29.
11. Gray JR, Thompson PM. Neurobiology of intelligence: science and ethics. *Nat Rev Neurosci*. 2004;5(6):471-482.
12. Harris JC. Chauvet Cave: the panel of horses. *Arch Gen Psychiatry*. 2011;68(9):869-870.
13. Jamison KR. Manic-depressive illness and creativity. *Sci Am*. 1995;272(2):62-67.
14. MacCabe JH, Lambe MP, Cnattingius S, et al. Excellent school performance at age 16 and risk of adult bipolar disorder: national cohort study. *Br J Psychiatry*. 2010;196:109-115.
15. Maher B. Poll results: look who's doping. *Nature*. 2008;452:674-675.
16. McDaniel MA. Big-brained people are smarter: a meta-analysis of the relationship between *in vivo* brain volume and intelligence. *Intelligence*. 2005; 33(4):337-346.
17. Mell JC, Howard SM, Miller BL. Art and the brain: the influence of frontotemporal dementia on an accomplished artist. *Neurology*. 2003;60(10):1707-1710.
18. Nottebohm F. The road we travelled: discovery, choreography, and significance of brain replaceable neurons. *Ann N Y Acad Sci*. 2004;1016:628-658.
19. Plomin R, DeFries JC. The genetics of cognitive abilities and disabilities. *Sci Am*. 1998;278(5):62-69.
20. Purpura DP. Dendritic spine "dysgenesis" and mental retardation. *Science*. 1974;186(4169):1126-1128.
21. Roth G, Dicke U. Evolution of the brain and intelligence. *Trends Cogn Sci*. 2005;9(5):250-257.
22. Schoenemann PT, Sheehan MJ, Glotzer LD. Prefrontal white matter volume is disproportionately larger in humans than in other primates. *Nat Neurosci*. 2005; 8(2):242-252.
23. Shaw P, Greenstein D, Lerch J, et al. Intellectual ability and cortical development in children and adolescents. *Nature*. 2006;440(7084):676-679.
24. Shaywitz SE, Shaywitz BA. Dyslexia (specific reading disability). *Biol Psychiatry*. 2005;57(11):1301-1309.
25. Simonton DK. Are genius and madness related? Contemporary answers to an ancient question. *Psychiatr Times*. 2005;22(7):21-23.
26. Smith ME, Farah MJ. Are prescription stimulants "Smart Pills"? The epidemiology and cognitive neuroscience of prescription stimulant use by normal healthy individuals. *Psychol Bull*. 2011;137(5):717-741.
27. Stix G. Turbocharging the brain. *Sci Am*. 2009;301(4): 46-55.

CHAPTER 20

1. Banaschewski T, Becker K, Scherag S, Franke B, Coghill D. Molecular genetics of attention-deficit/hyperactivity disorder: an overview. *Eur Child Adolesc Psychiatry*. 2010;19:237-257.
2. Bear MF, Connors BW, Paradiso MA, eds. *Neuroscience: Exploring the Brain*. 3rd ed. Baltimore, MD: Lippincott Williams & Wilkins; 2007.
3. Ben-Pazi H, Shalev RS, Gross-Tsur V, et al. Age and medication effects on rhythmic response in ADHD: possible oscillatory mechanisms? *Neuropsychologia*. 2006;44:412-416.

4. Bobb AJ, Castellanos FX, Addington AM, et al. Molecular genetic studies of ADHD: 1991 to 2004. *Am J Med Genet B Neuropsychiatr Genet*. 2005;132(1):109-125.

5. Cardinal RN, Pennicott DR, Sugathapala CL, et al. Impulsive choice induced in rats by lesions of the nucleus accumbens core. *Science*. 2001;292(5526):2499-2501.

6. Cardinal RN, Winstanley CA, Robbins TW, et al. Limbic corticostriatal systems and delayed reinforcement. *Ann N Y Acad Sci*. 2004;1021:33-50.

7. Castellanos FX, Lee PP, Sharp W, et al. Developmental trajectories of brain volume abnormalities in children and adolescents with attention-deficit/hyperactivity disorder. *JAMA*. 2002;288(14):1740-1748.

8. Castellanos FX, Tannock R. Neuroscience of attention-deficit/hyperactivity disorder: the search for endophenotypes. *Nat Rev Neurosci*. 2002;3(8):617-628.

9. Castner SA, Williams GV, Goldman-Rakic PS. Reversal of antipsychotic-induced working memory deficits by short-term dopamine D1 receptor stimulation. *Science*. 2000;287(5460):2020-2022.

10. Faraone SV, Biederman J, Mick E. The age-dependent decline of attention deficit hyperactivity disorder: a meta-analysis of follow-up studies. *Psychol Med*. 2006; 36(2):159-165.

11. Franke B, Meale BM, Faraone SV. Genome-wide association studies in ADHD. *Human Genetics*. 2009;126: 13-50.

12. Fuster JM. Unit activity in prefrontal cortex during delayed-response performance: neuronal correlates of transient memory. *J Neurophysiol*. 1973;36(1):61-78.

13. Greenberg LM, Crosby RD. A summary of developmental normative data on the T.O.V.A. ages 4 to 80+. Unpublished manuscript available through The TOVA company; 1992.

14. Landhuis CE, Poulton R, Welch D, Hancox RJ. Does childhood television viewing lead to attention problems in adolescence? Results from a prospective longitudinal study. *Pediatrics*. 2007;120:532-537.

15. Larisch R, Sitte W, Antke C, et al. Striatal dopamine transporter density in drug naive patients with attention-deficit/hyperactivity disorder. *Nucl Med Commun*. 2006;27(3):267-270.

16. Levesque J, Beauregard M, Mensour B. Effect of neurofeedback training on the neural substrates of selective attention in children with attention-deficit/hyperactivity disorder: a functional magnetic resonance imaging study. *Neurosci Lett*. 2006;394(3):216-221.

17. Lillard AS, Peterson J. The immediate impact of different types of television on young children's executive function. *Pediatrics*. 2011;128:644-649.

18. McEvoy SP, Stevenson MR, McCartt AT, et al. Role of mobile phones in motor vehicle crashes resulting in hospital attendance: a case-crossover study. *BMJ*. 2005;331(7514):428.

19. Mozley PD, Acton PD, Barraclough ED, et al. Effects of age on dopamine transporters in healthy humans. *J Nucl Med*. 1999;40(11):1812-1817.

20. Nakao T, Radua J, Rubia K, Mataix-Cols D. Gray matter volume abnormalities in ADHD: voxel-based meta-analysis exploring the effects of age and stimulant medication. *Am J Psychiatry*. 2011;168(11):1154-1163.

21. Nutt DJ, King LA, Phillips LD. Drug harm in the UK: a multicriteria decision analysis. *Lancet*. 2010;376:1558-1565.

22. Phillips AG, Ahn S, Floresco SB. Magnitude of dopamine release in medial prefrontal cortex predicts accuracy of memory on a delayed response task. *J Neurosci*. 2004;24(2):547-553.

23. Purves D, Augustine GJ, Fitzpatrick D, et al. *Neuroscience*. 5th ed. Sunderland, MA: Sinauer; 2011.

24. Shaw P, Lerch J, Greenstein D, et al. Longitudinal mapping of cortical thickness and clinical outcome in children and adolescents with attention-deficit/hyperactivity disorder. *Arch Gen Psychiatry*. 2006;63(5):540-549.

25. Tamm L, Menon V, Reiss AL. Parietal attentional system aberrations during target detection in adolescents with attention deficit hyperactivity disorder: event-related fMRI evidence. *Am J Psychiatry*. 2006;163(6):1033-1043.

26. Toplak ME, Dockstader C, Tannock R. Temporal information processing in ADHD: findings to date and new methods. *J Neurosci Methods*. 2006;151(1):15-29.

27. Volkow ND, Wang GJ, Fowler JS, et al. Evidence that methylphenidate enhances the saliency of a mathematical task by increasing dopamine in the human brain. *Am J Psychiatry*. 2004;161(7):1173-1180.

28. Volkow ND, Wang GJ, Fowler JS, et al. Imaging the effects of methylphenidate on brain dopamine: new model on its therapeutic actions for attention-deficit/hyperactivity disorder. *Biol Psychiatry*. 2005;57(11): 1410-1415.

CHAPTER 21

1. Autry A, Adachi M, Nosyreva E, et al. NMDA receptor blockade at rest triggers rapid behavioural antidepressant responses. *Nature*. 2011;475:91-95.

2. Berton O, McClung CA, Dileone RJ, et al. Essential role of BDNF in the mesolimbic dopamine pathway in social defeat stress. *Science*. 2006;311(5762): 864-868.

3. Berton O, Nestler EJ. New approaches to antidepressant drug discovery: beyond monoamines. *Nat Rev Neurosci*. 2006;7(2):137-151.

4. Caspi A, Sugden K, Moffitt TE, et al. Influence of life stress on depression: moderation by a polymorphism in the 5-HTT gene. *Science*. 2003;301:386-389.

5. Deuschle M, Schweiger U, Weber B, et al. Diurnal activity and pulsatility of the hypothalamus-pituitary-adrenal system in male depressed patients and healthy controls. *J Clin Endocrinol Metab*. 1997;82(1):234-238.

6. Drevets WC. Neuroimaging and neuropathological studies of depression: implications for the cognitive-emotional features of mood disorders. *Curr Opin Neurobiol*. 2001;11(2):240-249.

7. Duman RS. The neurochemistry of depressive disorders: preclinical studies. In: Charney DS, Nestler EJ, eds. *Neurobiology of Mental Illness*. 2nd ed. New York, NY: Oxford University Press; 2004:421-439.

8. Dwivedi Y, Rizavi HS, Conley RR, et al. Altered gene expression of brain-derived neurotrophic factor and receptor tyrosine kinase B in postmortem brain of suicide subjects. *Arch Gen Psychiatry*. 2003;60(8): 804-815.

9. Haldane M, Frangou S. New insights help define the pathophysiology of bipolar affective disorder: neuroimaging and neuropathology findings. *Prog Neuropsychopharmacol Biol Psychiatry*. 2004;28(6):943-960.

10. Haldane M, Frangou S. Functional neuroimaging studies in mood disorders. *Acta Neuropsychiatr*. 2006;18:88-99.

11. Hamilton JP, Etkin A, Furman DJ, et al. Functional neuroimaging of major depressive disorder: a meta-analysis and new integration of baseline activation and neural response data. *Am J Psychiatry*. 2012;169:693-703.

12. Holsboer F. Stress, hypercortisolism and corticosteroid receptors in depression: implications for therapy. *J Affect Disord*. 2001;62(1-2):77-91.

13. Koss S, George MS. Functional magnetic resonance imaging investigations in mood disorders. In: Soares JC, ed. *Brain Imaging in Affective Disorders.* New York, NY: Marcel Dekker Inc; 2003.

14. Mamounas LA, Blue ME, Siuciak JA, et al. Brain-derived neurotrophic factor promotes the survival and sprouting of serotonergic axons in rat brain. *J Neurosci.* 1995;15(12):7929-7939.

15. Manji HK, Quiroz JA, Sporn J, et al. Enhancing neuronal plasticity and cellular resilience to develop novel, improved therapeutics for difficult-to-treat depression. *Biol Psychiatry.* 2003;53(8):707-742.

16. McQuade R, Young AH. Future therapeutic targets in mood disorders: the glucocorticoid receptor. *Br J Psychiatry.* 2000;177:390-395.

17. Moore GJ, Bebchuk JM, Wilds IB, et al. Lithium-induced increase in human brain grey matter. *Lancet.* 2000;356(9237):1241-1242.

18. Nobler MS, Oquendo MA, Kegeles LS, et al. Decreased regional brain metabolism after ECT. *Am J Psychiatry.* 2001;158(2):305-308.

19. Rajkowska G, Miguel-Hidalgo JJ, Wei J, et al. Morphometric evidence for neuronal and glial prefrontal cell pathology in major depression. *Biol Psychiatry.* 1999;45(9):1085-1098.

20. Risch N, Herrell R, Lehner T, et al. Interaction between the serotonin transporter gene (5-HTTLPR), stressful life events, and risk of depression. *JAMA.* 2009;301(23):2462-2471.

21. Santarelli L, Saxe M, Gross C, et al. Requirement of hippocampal neurogenesis for the behavioral effects of antidepressants. *Science.* 2003;301(5634):805-809.

22. Tsankova NM, Berton O, Renthal W, et al. Sustained hippocampal chromatin regulation in a mouse model of depression and antidepressant action. *Nat Neurosci.* 2006;9(4):519-525.

23. Videbech P, Ravnkilde B. Hippocampal volume and depression: a meta-analysis of MRI studies. *Am J Psychiatry.* 2004;161(11):1957-1966.

24. Wolkowitz OM, Wolf J, Shelly W, et al. Serum BDNF levels before treatment predict SSRI response in depression. *Prog Neuropsychopharmacol Biol Psychiatry.* 2011;35:1623-1630.

25. Wong ML, Licinio J. Research and treatment approaches to depression. *Nat Rev Neurosci.* 2001;2(5):343-351.

26. Zobel AW, Nickel T, Sonntag A, et al. Cortisol response in the combined dexamethasone/CRH test as predictor of relapse in patients with remitted depression. A prospective study. *J Psychiatr Res.* 2001;35(2):83-94.

CHAPTER 22

1. Abi-Dargham A, Krystal JH, Anjilvel S, et al. Alterations of benzodiazepine receptors in type II alcoholic subjects measured with SPECT and [123I]iomazenil. *Am J Psychiatry.* 1998;155(11):1550-1555.

2. Barlow DH, Gorman JM, Shear MK, et al. Cognitive-behavioral therapy, imipramine, or their combination for panic disorder: a randomized controlled trial. *JAMA.* 2000;283(19):2529-2536.

3. Baxter LR Jr, Schwartz JM, Bergman KS, et al. Caudate glucose metabolic rate changes with both drug and behavior therapy for obsessive-compulsive disorder. *Arch Gen Psychiatry.* 1992;49(9):681-689.

4. Berton O, McClung CA, Dileone RJ, et al. Essential role of BDNF in the mesolimbic dopamine pathway in social defeat stress. *Science.* 2006;311(5762):864-868.

5. Breedlove SM, Watson NV, Rosenzweig MR. *Biological Psychology.* 6th ed. Sunderland, MA: Sinauer; 2010.

6. Calder AJ, Lawrence AD, Young AW. Neuropsychology of fear and loathing. *Nat Rev Neurosci.* 2001;2(5):352-363.

7. Charney DS. Neuroanatomical circuits modulating fear and anxiety behaviors. *Acta Psychiatr Scand Suppl.* 2003(417):38-50.

8. Furmark T, Tillfors M, Marteinsdottir I, et al. Common changes in cerebral blood flow in patients with social phobia treated with citalopram or cognitive-behavioral therapy. *Arch Gen Psychiatry.* 2002;59(5):425-433.

9. Gilbertson MW, Shenton ME, Ciszewski A, et al. Smaller hippocampal volume predicts pathologic vulnerability to psychological trauma. *Nat Neurosci.* 2002;5(11):1242-1247.

10. Gross C, Hen R. The developmental origins of anxiety. *Nat Rev Neurosci.* 2004;5(7):545-552.

11. Kirschbaum C, Prussner JC, Stone AA, et al. Persistent high cortisol responses to repeated psychological stress in a subpopulation of healthy men. *Psychosom Med.* 1995;57(5):468-474.

12. Kushner MG, Abrams K, Borchardt C. The relationship between anxiety disorders and alcohol use disorders: a review of major perspectives and findings. *Clin Psychol Rev.* 2000;20(2):149-171.

13. LeDoux JE. Emotion, memory and the brain. *Sci Am.* 1994;270(6):50-57.

14. LeDoux JE. *The Synaptic Self: How Our Brains Become Who We Are.* New York, NY: Viking; 2002.

15. Likhtik E, Pelletier JG, Paz R, et al. Prefrontal control of the amygdala. *J Neurosci.* 2005;25(32):7429-7437.

16. Lorberbaum JP, Kose S, Johnson MR, et al. Neural correlates of speech anticipatory anxiety in generalized social phobia. *Neuroreport.* 2004;15(18):2701-2705.

17. Mahan AL, Ressler KJ. Fear conditioning, synaptic plasticity and the amygdala: implications for post-traumatic stress disorder. *Trends Neurosci.* 2012;35(1):24-35.

18. Maren S, Ferrario CR, Corcoran KA, et al. Protein synthesis in the amygdala, but not the auditory thalamus, is required for consolidation of Pavlovian fear conditioning in rats. *Eur J Neurosci.* 2003;18(11):3080-3088.

19. Mashour GA, Walker EE, Martuza RL. Psychosurgery: past, present, and future. *Brain Res Brain Res Rev.* 2005;48(3):409-419.

20. Montgomery SM, Ehlin A, Sacker A. Breast feeding and resilience against psychosocial stress. *Arch Dis Child.* 2006;91(12):990-994.

21. Otto MW, Smits JAJ, Reese HE. Combined psychotherapy and pharmacotherapy for mood and anxiety disorders in adults: review and analysis. *Clin Psychol: Sci Pract.* 2005;12(1):72-86.

22. Purves D, Augustine GJ, Fitzpatrick D, et al. *Neuroscience.* 5th ed. Sunderland, MA: Sinauer; 2011.

23. Richter EO, Davis KD, Hamani C, et al. Cingulotomy for psychiatric disease: microelectrode guidance, a callosal reference system for documenting lesion location, and clinical results. *Neurosurgery.* 2004;54(3):622-628; discussion 8-30.

24. Shin LM, Wright CI, Cannistraro PA, et al. A functional magnetic resonance imaging study of amygdala and medial prefrontal cortex responses to overtly presented fearful faces in posttraumatic stress disorder. *Arch Gen Psychiatry.* 2005;62(3):273-281.

25. Stein DJ. Obsessive-compulsive disorder. *Lancet.* 2002;360(9330):397-405.

26. Ursin H, Baade E, Levine S. *Psychobiology of Stress: A Study of Coping Men.* New York, NY: Academic Press; 1978.
27. Vyas A, Pillai AG, Chattarji S. Recovery after chronic stress fails to reverse amygdaloid neuronal hypertrophy and enhanced anxiety-like behavior. *Neuroscience.* 2004;128(4):667-673.
28. Willyard C. Remembered for forgetting. *Nat Med.* 2012;18:482-484.
29. Yen CP, Kung SS, Su YF, et al. Stereotactic bilateral anterior cingulotomy for intractable pain. *J Clin Neurosci.* 2005;12(8):886-890.

CHAPTER 23

1. Abdolmaleky HM, Cheng KH, Russo A, et al. Hypermethylation of the reelin (RELN) promoter in the brain of schizophrenic patients: a preliminary report. *Am J Med Genet B Neuropsychiatr Genet.* 2005; 134(1):60-66.
2. Adityanjee, Aderibigbe YA, Theodoridis D, et al. Dementia praecox to schizophrenia: the first 100 years. *Psychiatry Clin Neurosci.* 1999;53(4):437-448.
3. Akbarian S, Kim JJ, Potkin SG, et al. Gene expression for glutamic acid decarboxylase is reduced without loss of neurons in prefrontal cortex of schizophrenics. *Arch Gen Psychiatry.* 1995;52(4):258-266.
4. Baumeister AA, Francis JL. Historical development of the dopamine hypothesis of schizophrenia. *J Hist Neurosci.* 2002;11(3):265-277.
5. Black DN, Taber KH, Hurley RA. Metachromatic leukodystrophy: a model for the study of psychosis. *J Neuropsychiatry Clin Neurosci.* 2003;15(3):289-293.
6. Davis KL, Stewart DG, Friedman JI, et al. White matter changes in schizophrenia: evidence for myelin-related dysfunction. *Arch Gen Psychiatry.* 2003;60(5):443-456.
7. Dierks T, Linden DE, Jandl M, et al. Activation of Heschls gyrus during auditory hallucinations. *Neuron.* 1999;22(3):615-621.
8. Evans K, McGrath J, Milns R. Searching for schizophrenia in ancient Greek and Roman literature: a systematic review. *Acta Psychiatr Scand.* 2003;107(5):323-330.
9. Glantz LA, Gilmore JH, Lieberman JA, et al. Apoptotic mechanisms and the synaptic pathology of schizophrenia. *Schizophr Res.* 2006;81(1):47-63.
10. Glantz LA, Lewis DA. Decreased dendritic spine density on prefrontal cortical pyramidal neurons in schizophrenia. *Arch Gen Psychiatry.* 2000;57(1):65-73.
11. Gogtay N, Sporn A, Rapoport J. Structural brain MRI studies in childhood-onset schizophrenia and childhood atypical psychosis. In: Lawrie S, Johnstone E, Weinberger D, eds. *Schizophrenia: From Neuroimaging to Neuroscience.* New York, NY: Oxford University Press; 2004.
12. Hakak Y, Walker JR, Li C, et al. Genome-wide expression analysis reveals dysregulation of myelination-related genes in chronic schizophrenia. *Proc Natl Acad Sci U S A.* 2001;98(8):4746-4751.
13. Ho, BC, Andreasen NC, Ziebell S, et al. Long-term antipsychotic treatment and brain volumes. *Arch Gen Psychiatry.* 2011;68(2):128-137.
14. Hof PR, Haroutunian V, Friedrich VL Jr, et al. Loss and altered spatial distribution of oligodendrocytes in the superior frontal gyrus in schizophrenia. *Biol Psychiatry.* 2003;53(12):1075-1085.
15. Howes OD, Kapur S. The dopamine hypothesis of schizophrenia: version III—the final common pathway. *Schizophr Bull.* 2009;35(3):549-562.

16. Hubl D, Koenig T, Strik W, et al. Pathways that make voices: white matter changes in auditory hallucinations. *Arch Gen Psychiatry.* 2004;61(7):658-668.
17. Hulshoff Pol HE, Schnack HG, Bertens MG, et al. Volume changes in gray matter in patients with schizophrenia. *Am J Psychiatry.* 2002;159(2):244-250.
18. Kong A, Frigge ML, Masson G, et al. Rate of *de novo* mutations and the importance of father's age to disease risk. *Nature.* 2012;488:471-475.
19. Lawrie S, Johnstone E, Weinberger D. *Schizophrenia: From Neuroimaging to Neuroscience.* New York, NY: Oxford University Press; 2004.
20. Lewis DA, Hashimoto T, Volk DW. Cortical inhibitory neurons and schizophrenia. *Nat Rev Neurosci.* 2005; 6(4):312-324.
21. Lewis DA, Lieberman JA. Catching up on schizophrenia: natural history and neurobiology. *Neuron.* 2000; 28(2):325-334.
22. Liberman RP, Musgrave JG, Langlois J. Taunton State Hospital, Massachusetts. *Am J Psychiatry.* 2003; 160(12):2098.
23. McClellan JM, Susser E, King MC. Maternal famine, de novo mutations, and schizophrenia. *JAMA.* 2006; 296(5):582-584.
24. Pedersen CB, Mortensen PB. Urbanization and traffic related exposures as risk factors for schizophrenia. *BMC Psychiatry.* 2006;6:2.
25. Selemon LD. Increased cortical neuronal density in schizophrenia. *Am J Psychiatry.* 2004;161(9): 1564.
26. Selemon LD, Goldman-Rakic PS. The reduced neuropil hypothesis: a circuit based model of schizophrenia. *Biol Psychiatry.* 1999;45(1):17-25.
27. Sporn AL, Greenstein DK, Gogtay N, et al. Progressive brain volume loss during adolescence in childhood-onset schizophrenia. *Am J Psychiatry.* 2003;160(12): 2181-2189.
28. Suddath RL, Christison GW, Torrey EF, et al. Anatomical abnormalities in the brains of monozygotic twins discordant for schizophrenia. *N Engl J Med.* 1990;322(12): 789-794.
29. Tamminga C, Hashimoto T, Volk DW, et al. GABA neurons in the human prefrontal cortex. *Am J Psychiatry.* 2004;161(10):1764.
30. Tienari P, Wynne LC, Sorri A, et al. Genotype-environment interaction in schizophrenia-spectrum disorder. Long-term follow-up study of Finnish adoptees. *Br J Psychiatry Suppl.* 2004;184:216-222.
31. Torrey EF, Miller J. *The Invisible Plague: The Rise of Mental Illness from 1750 to the Present.* New Brunswick, NJ: Rutgers University Press; 2001.
32. Walker E, Kestler L, Bollini A, et al. Schizophrenia: etiology and course. *Annu Rev Psychol.* 2004;55: 401-430.
33. Weinberger DR, Berman KF, Zec RF. Physiologic dysfunction of dorsolateral prefrontal cortex in schizophrenia. I. Regional cerebral blood flow evidence. *Arch Gen Psychiatry.* 1986;43(2):114-124.

CHAPTER 24

1. Baas PW, Qiang L. Neuronal microtubules: when the MAP is the roadblock. *Trends Cell Biol.* 2005;15(4): 183-187.
2. Bennett DA, Schneider JA, Wilson RS, et al. Education modifies the association of amyloid but not tangles with cognitive function. *Neurology.* 2005;65(6):953-955.
3. Blennow K, de Leon MJ, Zetterberg H. Alzheimer's disease. *Lancet.* 2006;368(9533):387-403.

4. Braak H, Braak E. Frequency of stages of Alzheimer-related lesions in different age categories. *Neurobiol Aging*. 1997;18(4):351-357.

5. Erickson EI, Voss MW, Prakash RS, et al. Exercise training increases size of hippocampus and improves memory *PNAS*; 2011;108:3017-3022.

6. Finger S. *Origins of Neuroscience: A History of Explorations into Brain Functions*. Oxford: Oxford University Press; 1994.

7. Fox NC, Schott JM. Imaging cerebral atrophy: normal ageing to Alzheimer's disease. *Lancet*. 2004;363(9406): 392-394.

8. Fuso A, Seminara L, Cavallaro RA, et al. S-adenosylmethionine/homocysteine cycle alterations modify DNA methylation status with consequent deregulation of PS1 and BACE and beta-amyloid production. *Mol Cell Neurosci*. 2005;28(1):195-204.

9. Hayflick L. The future of ageing. *Nature*. 2000;408(6809): 267-269.

10. Herholz K, Salmon E, Perani D, et al. Discrimination between Alzheimer dementia and controls by automated analysis of multicenter FDG PET. *Neuroimage*. 2002; 17(1):302-316.

11. Kandel ER, Schwartz JH, Jessell TM, eds. *Principles of Neural Science*. 4th ed. New York, NY: McGraw-Hill; 2000.

12. Lemere CA, Maier M, Jiang L, et al. Amyloid-beta immunotherapy for the prevention and treatment of Alzheimer disease: lessons from mice, monkeys, and humans. *Rejuvenation Res*. 2006;9(1):77-84.

13. Mattson MP. Pathways towards and away from Alzheimer's disease. *Nature*. 2004;430(7000):631-639.

14. Mattson MP, Magnus T. Ageing and neuronal vulnerability. *Nat Rev Neurosci*. 2006;7(4):278-294.

15. Morgan D, Diamond DM, Gottschall PE, et al. A beta peptide vaccination prevents memory loss in an animal model of Alzheimer's disease. *Nature*. 2000;408(6815) 982-985.

16. Mortimer JA. Brain reserve and the clinical expression of Alzheimer's disease. *Geriatrics*. 1997;52 (suppl 2):S50-S53.

17. Qin W, Chachich M, Lane M, et al. Calorie restriction attenuates Alzheimer's disease type brain amyloidosis in squirrel monkeys (*Saimiri sciureus*). *J Alzheimers Dis*. 2006;10:417-422.

18. Ridley RM, Baker HF, Windle CP, et al. Very long term studies of the seeding of beta-amyloidosis in primates. *J Neural Transm*. 2006;113:1243-1251.

19. Schenk D, Hagen M, Seubert P. Current progress in beta-amyloid immunotherapy. *Curr Opin Immunol*. 2004;16(5):599-606.

20. Snowdon DA, Kemper SJ, Mortimer JA, et al. Linguistic ability in early life and cognitive function and Alzheimer's disease in late life. Findings from the Nun Study. *JAMA*. 1996;275(7):528-532.

21. Tuszynski MH, Thal L, Pay M, et al. A phase 1 clinical trial of nerve growth factor gene therapy for Alzheimer disease. *Nat Med*. 2005;11(5):551-555.

22. Wang J, Ho L, Zhao Z, et al. Moderate consumption of Carernet Sauvignon attenuates AB neuropathology in a mouse model of Alzheimer's disease. *FASEB J*. 2006;20:2313-2320.

23. Winblad B, Andreasen N, Minthon L, et al. Safety, tolerability, and antibody response of active Aβ immunotherapy with CAD106 in patients with Alzheimer's disease: randomized, double-blind, placebo-controlled, first-in-human study. *Lancet Neurol*. 2012;11: 597-604.

24. Wolfe MS. Shutting down Alzheimer's. *Sci Am*. 2006;294(5):72-79.

25. Yang L, Rieves D, Ganley C. Brain amyloid imaging—FDA approval of florbetapir F18 injection. *N Engl J Med*. 2012;367(10):885-887.

Answers to End-of-Chapter Questions

CHAPTER 1

Part 1
1. L
2. E
3. B
4. D
5. F
6. C
7. J
8. A
9. H
10. G
11. K
12. I

Part 2
13. P
14. N
15. O
16. M
17. Q

CHAPTER 2
1. b
2. c
3. a
4. c
5. d
6. a
7. b
8. d

CHAPTER 3
1. c
2. a
3. b
4. d
5. a
6. b
7. d
8. a

CHAPTER 4
1. c
2. b
3. d
4. a
5. d
6. c
7. a
8. d

CHAPTER 5
1. c
2. b
3. c
4. a
5. d
6. b
7. d
8. d

CHAPTER 6
1. d
2. c
3. a
4. b
5. c
6. d
7. b

CHAPTER 7
1. c
2. d
3. a
4. c
5. b
6. b
7. a

CHAPTER 8
1. d
2. a
3. b
4. c
5. c
6. a
7. d
8. b

CHAPTER 9
1. d
2. c
3. d
4. a
5. c
6. b

CHAPTER 10
1. e
2. c
3. a
4. g
5. h
6. b
7. d
8. f

CHAPTER 11
1. c
2. b
3. a
4. d
5. c
6. d
7. b
8. a

CHAPTER 12
1. c
2. a
3. d
4. b
5. a
6. c
7. d
8. a
9. b

CHAPTER 13
1. d
2. b
3. a
4. c
5. b
6. a
7. d
8. c

CHAPTER 14
1. a
2. c
3. b
4. d
5. c
6. d
7. a
8. b

CHAPTER 15
1. a
2. b
3. d
4. a
5. c
6. c
7. d
8. c

CHAPTER 16
1. d
2. a
3. c

4. b
5. d
6. c
7. a
8. b

CHAPTER 17
1. c
2. d
3. b
4. a
5. b
6. a
7. d
8. c

CHAPTER 18
1. b
2. a
3. d
4. c
5. a
6. d
7. c
8. b

CHAPTER 19
1. a
2. c
3. d
4. b
5. b
6. c

CHAPTER 20
1. d
2. c
3. b
4. a
5. c
6. b
7. 1. C
   2. B
   3. D
   4. A

CHAPTER 21
1. b
2. a
3. c
4. d
5. a
6. b
7. c
8. d

CHAPTER 22
1. b
2. c
3. d
4. a
5. a
6. d
7. b
8. c

CHAPTER 23
1. d
2. b
3. a
4. c
5. d
6. a
7. c
8. 1. E
   2. D
   3. B
   4. F
   5. A
   6. C

CHAPTER 24
1. d
2. c
3. a
4. c
5. d
6. b

Index

Note: Locators followed by 'f' and 't' refer to figures and tables respectively.